# THE HAIR AND SCALP

And whan the alopecya is remo=
ued: whiche thynge is knowen by the
good colour of the skynne, ye shal ap=
ply suche thynges as haue nature to
engendre heere, as is thys lynimente
folowyng .R. of the iuyce of smalage.
ʒ.ii. of the iuyce of fenell, and parcelie.
.añ.ʒ.i. of ÿ iuice of enula campana.ʒ.
vi. the iuice of apium tisus, ʒ.ii. of oile
of eldern, and terebentyne .añia.ʒ.r. of
shyppe pytche, greke pytche, and ly=
quide pitche. aña.ʒ.b. of dyaquilõ gũ=
med, mugwort, sothernwoode some=
what stamped, of rosemary, of may=
denheere fyne stamped. aña . the .iii.
parte of an handfull, of odoryferous
wyne, halfe a cyathe, of vynegre. ʒ.ii.
Let them seethe all togyther, tyll the
wyne, iuyce, and vynegre be cõsumed,
than strayne them , and adde to the
straynyng, of newe odoryferous wax
as moche as shall suffyce, of saffrã.ʒ.
ʃ. of pyeos.ʒ.i.ʃ.make it after the ma
ner of a cerote. Thys lynymente is of
good operatyon , to engendre heeres
in the heed, and in the chynne.

Before ye apply this lynimente, ye
muste rubbe the place wyth a courfe
clothe . Note that when alopecya and
albaras ben olde, the cure is in a ma=
ner impossyble. Thus we ende thys
present Chapter.

# THE HAIR AND SCALP

## A CLINICAL STUDY
### (WITH A CHAPTER ON HIRSUTIES)

BY

## AGNES SAVILL, M.A., M.D.(GLASG.), F.R.C.P.I.

CONSULTING PHYSICIAN TO FITZROY SQUARE SKIN HOSPITAL;
FORMERLY HONORARY DERMATOLOGIST TO THE ROYAL
SURREY COUNTY HOSPITAL, GUILDFORD, SURREY;
PHYSICIAN TO ST. JOHN'S HOSPITAL FOR SKIN DISEASES,
LEICESTER SQUARE; TO THE SKIN DEPARTMENT, SOUTH LONDON
HOSPITAL FOR WOMEN; AND CHIEF (DURING THE 1914–18
WAR) OF THE ELECTROTHERAPEUTIC DEPARTMENT,
SCOTTISH WOMEN'S HOSPITAL, ROYAUMONT,
FRANCE

FOURTH EDITION

LONDON
EDWARD ARNOLD & CO.

*Printed in Great Britain by*
*Butler & Tanner Ltd., Frome and London*

# FOREWORD

It is only fitting that " The Hair and Scalp " and the diseases thereof should be written by a woman because women, much more than men, are concerned with the preservation and appearance of their hair ; also, they are concerned regarding hirsuties. A fundamental and scientific background is first given by Doctor Savill in chapters on the physiology of the hair, and one on its molecular structure and elastic properties, by Doctor Astbury. Doctor Savill scientifically describes in simple English the normal care of the hair and beneficial or harmful effects of such treatment as permanent waving, singeing, bleaching, and dyeing of the hair. Excellent concise descriptions are given of the multiple dermatoses affecting the scalp and hair, either primarily or secondarily, and emphasis is placed on their relation to internal diseases. Only a person of Doctor Savill's wide experience as a practitioner, gynæcologist, dermatologist, and editor for years of *Savill's Clinical Medicine* could bring all these important findings together in a single, small volume. She has incorporated into the book all that is of value from older treatises on the hair, including the extensive observations of Sabouraud, under whom she studied. She has correlated these data with the newest observations, many of which are her own.

I am thoroughly familiar with the second edition of this book which I regard as one of the best on the subject. It has been my privilege to have had an extensive correspondence with Doctor Savill during the past two years in regard to possible publication of a third edition of this work in the United States. Exigencies of the war, however, have prevented my seeing the proof. I am sure this third edition will continue to be a distinguished and outstanding contribution.

HAMILTON MONTGOMERY, M.D.

ROCHESTER, MINNESOTA.

▼

# PREFACE TO THE FOURTH EDITION

Owing to the war some time has passed since the reprint of the third edition, and therefore few pages have escaped alteration for this fourth edition ; some sections have been omitted, many rewritten. Amongst new additions are : grouped and compound hairs, cases of sudden blanching and of exfoliative dermatitis, meningioma, the influence of the vitamins and the endocrine glands on the condition of the hair, a section on the cold permanent wave, reports of grey, lustreless states of the hair and of lanugo hypertrichosis in famine-stricken districts. Thorough revision was necessary for ringworm, sarcoidosis, trichomycosis nodosa, folliculitis decalvans, pseudo-pelade, and the composition of spirit lotions. The last two diseases have long been confused and wrongly described, owing to their rarity and consequent difficulty in diagnosis. The cold permanent wave, first introduced by Professor Speakman of Leeds University, popularized in America during the war years and now revived in Britain, has aroused much interest and controversy concerning its advantages, its drawbacks, even its dangers for certain individuals. I have been fortunate in that Dr. Hamilton Montgomery has despatched to me every article which he found on that subject in the medical journals and the popular press of America. I am most grateful to him for that assistance and also for many suggestions and important information regarding nævo-carcinoma and other malignant conditions ; to my every question he gave patient consideration and sent full replies, with references to articles in American journals and the Proceedings of the Mayo Clinic which otherwise would have escaped my notice.

Ringworm has become so complicated that I asked Dr. Arthur Rook to rewrite the chapter ; while retaining some of the paragraphs on treatment, he has been responsible for the alterations in the revision of ringworm, and has succeeded in making a clear summary of the modern classification of the fungi, and has compiled useful tables which aid diagnosis and the choice of treatment suitable for the many types of infection. I am glad to thank him also for many suggestions throughout the book concerning rare diseases and modern methods of treatment. Other colleagues to whom I am indebted are Dr. H. W. Barber, who has been most kind in answering questions on endocrinology, a subject which specially interests him, and has allowed me to reproduce his Table from *Modern Trends in Dermatology*, a summary of the stages of pityriasis which were first enunciated so clearly by Sabouraud. Dr. Benjamin Sieve sent a concise report of 800 cases of canities treated with para-aminobenzoic acid, combined with elimination of sepsis and careful adjustment of the endocrine balance required for the individual patient ; his original articles display a persistence of investigation and treatment which deserved the success obtained. I have also to thank Dr. Clara Warren for her summary of the method of staining hairs and fungi which she employs in her clinic ; Dr. A. C. Roxburgh, who has lent me the illustration of pseudo-pelade from his popular book, *Common Diseases of the Skin* ; Dr. Martin Scott, for two original photographs from his collection, " Grouped and Compound Hairs and Trichotillomania," and for his offer of micro-photographs which I was obliged, reluctantly, to refuse, because their addition would have demanded a new chapter and have altered the character of a book which has a clinical approach. Professor Astbury revised his chapter on the Molecular and Elastic properties of the Hair which has always been a popular and most valuable contribution to this volume. I should also like to take this opportunity to thank Dr. H. J. Wallace and his team of dermatologists who have always given me so warm a welcome on my visits to the Guildford clinic which I directed during the second World War.

As one of the older generation I have watched the rise, decline and fall of many new remedies and hope that my younger colleagues will forgive my guarded references to those which at present ride on the crest of the wave ; time alone can determine their value. Specialism is tending to replace the wisdom of the general practitioner whose approach to the patient is that of one who knows the whole man—his family, his habits, his heredity and his environment. Soporific drugging is too much relied upon to relieve the mental tension of this age of unrest, but it cannot in the long run perform the healing work of Nature which the wise physicians of ancient Greece well understood was obtained by sunlight, fresh air, training in correct methods of relaxation and of exercise, and above all, by the cultivation of a quiet and detached attitude of the spirit.

AGNES SAVILL.

# PREFACE TO THE FIRST EDITION

All forms of illness, however slight, should fall within the sphere of the physician. The public, however, have for so long associated the idea of medicine with serious disease that they hesitate to consult a medical practitioner for maladies connected with the scalp and the hair. Women in particular believe that those regions of the human body belong to the domain of cosmetics. Even in the case of obvious disease of the scalp the advice of the dermatologist is often not requested until the patient has tried several of the preparations described in the glowing advertisements which adorn the popular magazines. This attitude of the layman has some justification ; few busy practitioners show much sympathy with the young woman who complains of scanty or lustreless hair.

The common diseases of the scalp and hair, apparently so simple, provide some of the most puzzling problems in medicine. Although volumes have been written on the subject of the ordinary baldness of men, on dandruff and on oiliness of the scalp, these conditions are still attributed to divergent causes by opposing schools of dermatology. In these days of an overburdened curriculum, few have time for such study. In his daily round, the practitioner deals with serious, acute and fatal illness ; in comparison with such emergencies, it is only natural that he should regard the maladies of the scalp as of comparatively little importance. But to the average sufferer they seem far from trivial ; to women they may indeed colour all life with tragedy.

Sabouraud's illuminating and eloquent volumes, *Maladies du Cuir Chevelu*, fascinated me on their first appearance. Before 1914 I had collected notes of a large number of cases which confirmed his work. During the eventful years which followed, these records were laid aside and forgotten. When, once again, I felt the attraction of the subject, new methods of hairdressing had come about. To write on the hair, and exclude consideration of the " permanent wave," seemed to me an evasion of responsibility. At last I was fortunate enough to secure the help of Dr. W. T. Astbury ; he has written a chapter with the first authoritative account of the molecular structure of the hair in a medical book.

When dealing with the care of the hair and the common disorders of the scalp, I found that it was impossible to avoid discussion of disease ; even when the history of so apparently simple a condition as dandruff

ix

is followed up the province of disease is encroached upon. It was necessary to differentiate so many diseases that it became difficult to decide which to omit ; thus the manuscript grew. Finally, in order to simplify diagnosis and to render the book more useful to the student and busy practitioner, I decided to arrange the material on the lines of Savill's Clinical Medicine. The chief symptom complained of by the patient is investigated and is followed by a list of its possible causes. The disease is fully described in the chapter which deals with its characteristic symptom, and the other possible causes are passed in review and briefly differentiated. To assist ready reference, several forms of type are employed. Thick black type denotes the complete description of a disease; capitals imply that it is being dealt with briefly, as one of several diseases sharing the symptom which is not its chief feature. Space is devoted to the simple disorders rather than the rare diseases ; the latter are summarized as concisely as possible, and are usually in small type. I am conscious that any work written on these lines for the first time must be full of defects and omissions ; I shall be most grateful to those who write to me to point them out.

I gladly take this opportunity of thanking those colleagues who have generously helped me by discussing the rare diseases and by lending photographs : Dr. H. G. Adamson, Dr. H. W. Barber, Dr. Louis Forman, Dr. J. M. H. MacLeod, Dr. R. Sabouraud, Dr. J. H. Sequeira, and the late Dr. Goodwin Tomkinson.

AGNES SAVILL.

DEVONSHIRE PLACE, W.1.

# CONTENTS

xi

# THE HAIR AND SCALP

## CHAPTER I

## STRUCTURE AND PHYSIOLOGY OF THE HAIR

The hair structure—Sebaceous glands—Sweat glands—Blood, nerve and muscle supply—Hairfall—Microscopical appearance of hair—Colour of the hair—Number of the hairs—Rate of growth—Physical properties—Medico-legal points.

**Hair Structure.** The intricate details of the structure of the hair can be studied in anatomical text-books. A brief summary of the formation and development of the hair is given here, because this knowledge is necessary in order to understand the principles governing the care and treatment of the scalp and hair in health and disease.

Each hair emerges from a follicle or indentation in the skin. The follicle is like a long narrow pocket; the skin is folded in as if a tiny finger had pushed the epidermis down into the dermis and the underlying subcutaneous tissue. The bottom of this depression is penetrated by an upward growing finger of connective tissue, which is called the papilla. From this papilla the hair develops. The hair, as it grows from the top and sides of the papilla, has the appearance of being folded over it like an inverted bowl. The papilla forms the *root of the hair* ; that part of the hair root which surrounds the top and sides, and turns in below at the neck of the papilla, is known as the *hair bulb*. The hair grows upward to the mouth of the follicle, and when it passes beyond the surface of the skin it becomes the *hair shaft*, which terminates in a *point*, at a variable distance, according to the length of the hair. The *cross-section* of a human hair may be circular, flat, oval, triangular or kidney-shaped. The straight hair is the round hair ; curly hair is oval or flattened. A soft hair is round or oval ; whereas a thick, wiry hair, such as that of the beard, moustache or pubis, may show on a cross-section a triangular or kidney outline. Illustrations of all these types of hair are given in Glaister's book, *Examination of Hairs and Wool*, which is elsewhere quoted in these pages.

The *papilla* is the small projection upwards of the tissue which lies below the skin or epidermis, and pushes up into the bottom of the follicle. It is shaped somewhat like a teat, having a rounded top, sloping curved sides and a narrower neck. In the papilla are capillaries conveying a blood supply, arterial and venous. From the top of the papilla grow the cells which form the medulla of the hair ; from the sides of the papilla grow the cells which become the cortex of the hair; from tl neck of the papilla grow the cells of the hair cuticle and of the interna root sheath.

One can picture the *follicle* if one imagines the epidermis as pushe( into the subcutaneous tissue, and at the bottom of this canal, piercec by circulatory vessels and probably nerves, which supply the upgrowing papilla. At the level of the upper third of the narrow follicle, the duct of the sebaceous gland opens into it. From this point the arrangement of the epidermal cells is altered, and there is formed the external root sheath. The external root sheath starts at the level of the sebaceous gland with several layers of cells of the prickle cell variety; at the bottom of the follicle these have diminished to one layer. The internal root sheath starts at the neck of the papilla and its cells grow upward to the neck of the follicle. The three layers of cells composing the internal root sheath are often referred to, and have been given distinctive names. There is the outer layer of Henlé, the middle layer of Huxley, and the inner layer, or cuticle of the follicle, which interlocks with the cuticle of the hair. The cells of the follicle cuticle grow pointing inward and downward. As these cells interlock with those of the hair cuticle, rough pulling out of a hair often brings away this sheath attached to it. Thus, in brief, the external root sheath is continuous with the epidermis, whilst the internal root sheath grows upward from the papilla.

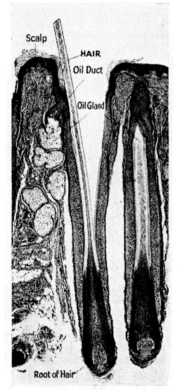

Scalp
HAIR
Oil Duct
Oil Gland
Root of Hair

Fig. 1.—Vertical section of a human scalp. Mag. × 25. (Section and Microphotograph by F. J. Pittock.)

The **hair shaft.** The hair itself has three parts: the central part or medulla, the middle part or cortex, and the outer part or cuticle.

The *medulla* starts from the top of the papilla; it becomes narrower above the level of the papilla. The medulla cells contain keratohyalin and sometimes granules of pigment. These cells have fine projections like those of the prickle cells of the epidermis. At a high level in the follicle the cells of the medulla shrink and leave air spaces between them ; they lie like flattened plates stacked in rows. At the free, distal end or tip of the hair the medulla may be absent, or its cells are fewer in number and have large spaces between them. Sometimes the medulla does not extend along the entire length of the hair ; it may appear to be interrupted at intervals throughout the shaft. A vacant space or a

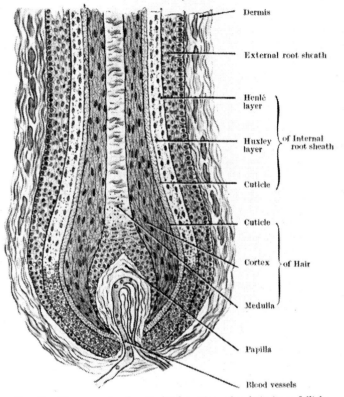

Dermis

External root sheath

Henlé layer

Huxley layer } of Internal root sheath

Cuticle

Cuticle

Cortex } of Hair

Medulla

Papilla

Blood vessels

FIG. 2.—Diagram of a longitudinal section of a hair in a follicle.
(*After MacLeod.*)

solid core may take its place. The size of the medulla varies ; thin hairs may have a large medulla and some apparently normal hairs may have no trace of a medulla or only a narrow one. Pincus states that strong hairs have a good medulla, but he found many hairs in which the medulla was absent. Some believe that the size of the medulla depends upon the age of the hair. I have seen thick hairs with a thin medulla and with no medulla ; and thin dark and also thin white fallen hairs, with a marked medulla (see pp. 13 and 14). Downy or lanugo hairs have no medulla. When a hair is about to fall, a space forms between the bulb of the hair and the medulla. Considerable study is being given to the factors which influence the medulla in the wool of sheep. Many observers record a definite correlation between the diameter of the hair shaft and the size of the medulla ; the more vigorous the hair growth of the sheep, the greater the medulla.[1]

The *cortex* forms the chief part of the hair. It consists of long, spindle-shaped cells longitudinally arranged and firmly adherent to each other. Minute air spaces are believed to lie in and between some of the

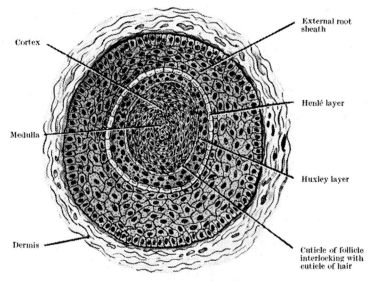

Cortex

Medulla

Dermis

External root sheath

Henlé layer

Huxley layer

Cuticle of follicle interlocking with cuticle of hair

FIG. 3.—Diagram of cross-section of a hair and follicle. (*After MacLeod.*)

cells of the cortex. The pigment which gives a hair its colour lies, diffused and in granules, in the cells of the cortex. The cortex springs from the columnar cells which grow from the sides of the papilla. As they pass upward in the follicle these cells assume first an oval, then a spindle shape ; the nuclei disappear and the cells undergo keratinization, so that the free hair shaft is so cornified that when there is no pigment, it appears translucent. Keratin is a firm substance which can resist strong mineral acid (up to 50 per cent.) for a considerable time, but is readily acted upon by alkalis. It contains sulphur, which is present

[1] References to recent research on this subject are given in " Growth Changes in Wool Fibres," by K. M. RUDALL. *J. Textile Inst.*, 1935, **26**, T.358.

in the form of cystine, an amino-acid. The keratin of the hair contains a higher proportion of cystine than does any other protein.[1] The cortex forms the body of the hair, and surrounds the central medulla. The cortex, in its turn, is surrounded by the protecting cuticle layer.

The *cuticle* starts from the upper portion of the neck of the papilla. The cells there are soft, polygonal or round in shape. As they pass up over the bulb of the hair these cells become flattened and horny. The nuclei of the cells disappear, and the horny, flat cells begin to lie along the hair surface like the tiles or slates of a house, five fitting into the length of one. The free ends of these overlapping, sloping, flat cells of the hair cuticle point upward and outward, and interlock with the cells of the cuticle of the follicle, which are arranged in the opposite direction, with the free ends pointing downward and inward. If a hair is rubbed lengthways between the finger and thumb, the shaft travels towards its root, because of the ratchet action of the projecting free edge of the cuticle cells pointing along to the tip. The horny cells which form the hair cuticle are translucent, and they contain no pigment.

Occasionally more than one hair is contained in one follicle. Twin hairs may spring from the papilla at the bottom of the follicle. These may join about the middle of the follicle, owing to a merging of the cuticle cells, and may separate again higher up. Under the title " compound hairs " Loewenthal[2] described that condition where two or more

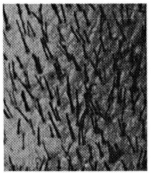

Fig. 4.—Compound and Grouped Hairs.

(*Photograph kindly lent by Dr. Martin Scott.*)

hairs spring from their individual papillæ, grow up in the one follicle, and emerge as separate hairs. New and old hairs may thus develop side by side. Sections were cut to investigate this little recognized condition.

There are three main **types of hair.** (1) Long, soft hair is found on the scalp, beard, the axilla and the pubis. These hairs grow in groups of two, four, and rarely, five. This is seen especially with the hairs of the scalp. In these groups the hairs may be of different ages and therefore of different lengths. The follicles of the long soft hairs lie obliquely, thus causing the hairs to lie in a sloping direction along the surface of

---

[1] The sulphur content of the hair in various races of mankind and in animals is discussed at length in *Arch. Derm. and Syph. Ap.*, 1933, **27**, 584.

[2] *J. Invest. Derm.*, 1947, **8**, 262.

the skin. The medulla is more often absent in the hair of women. (2) The second type of hair is the stiff, short and coarser hair which is found in the eyelashes, eyebrows, and within the orifices of the nose and the external meatus of the ear ; they have no arrector pili muscle. In some situations the follicles of these hairs lie almost at right angles to the skin surface ; such hairs stand out from the skin. (3) The third type of hair is the downy lanugo hair which is present over almost the whole smooth skin of the body ; no hairs are found on the palms, soles, lip margins, nipples, umbilicus, near the anus and uro-genital orifices, the tips and the third phalanges of the fingers and toes. These lanugo hairs have no medulla and many have no colour. The arrector pili muscle is usually absent and the sebaceous gland is often comparatively large.

**The Sebaceous Gland.** The oil which lubricates the hairs is supplied by the sebaceous gland. Two, three, or even six glands may supply each follicle. The size of the gland bears no relation to the size of the hair which it lubricates. With strong hairs the sebaceous glands may be quite small ; with insignificant hairs the sebaceous glands may be large. The gland is surrounded by a network of capillary blood vessels which anastomose with these in the cutis ; the lymphatics also are numerous, around both the follicle and the sebaceous gland. Sympathetic nerves are in control. Excitation of the cervical ganglion in animals has led to hyper-secretion, and it has been noted that the same excess of secretion may occur in chronic cases showing the Parkinson syndrome—e.g., in encephalitis lethargica and senile paralysis agitans. Some sebaceous glands open on to the skin surface without any connection with a hair. The sebaceous gland is lobulated, of the racemose variety of gland, resembling a bunch of grapes. The inner layer of cells which lines the gland undergoes a fatty change. Fine granules of fat appear within the cells and gradually become more numerous, the nucleus of each cell disappears, the fat granules increase until the cells burst and throw out the fat into the duct of the gland. The pressure of accumulating fat granules pushes the sebum up to the skin surface. With the warmth of the body the sebum, naturally of a butter-like consistence, becomes oily and suitable for its function of lubrication. The shiny, greasy appearance of some skins is due to excess of this sebaceous oil. The glands empty their content into the follicle at the level of its upper third. It is said that the amount of sebum excreted daily on the scalp is as much as that over the whole body. The oil gives the hair its lustre, and protects the hair from both too dry and too moist an atmosphere ; it lies on the surface of the cuticle and is also drawn by capillary attraction into its substance.

The sebaceous gland excretion amounts daily to 1 or 2 gm. ; it is less in cold weather and in children.    Analysis of the secretion shows fats (olein, palmitin and stearin), and fatty acids (oleic, palmitic and stearic), inorganic salts, cholesterol, epithelial debris and water.   With cholesterol there is always associated a small proportion of ergosterol. The importance of this compound lies in the fact that, when exposed to ultra-violet light, it is converted to vitamin D.   The secretion is influenced by diet.   It is especially affected by carbohydrates, easily fermenting, and by fats of the readily absorbed type.   In some individuals a noticeable increase of the activity of the sebaceous gland occurs when the general health is impaired.   The sebaceous glands are also much influenced by the condition of the endocrine glands.   They become very active at puberty, and during the later months of pregnancy ; they are less active after middle age, and in old age their deficiency leads to dryness of the skin.   This activity is stimulated by androgen secretion and hence increased in some women after the menopause.   They become hypertrophied in certain cases of hyperpituitarism, whilst in pituitary deficiency their secretion appears to be diminshed.

A. Policard and Y. Tritchkovitch [1] confirm the observations of previous workers, showing that sebum is not a product of fatty degeneration of the cell, but rather of fat secretion.   They conducted experiments in order to discover whether the cells of the sebaceous glands not only elaborated fat from fatty acids in the blood, but also whether they could take up directly fatty particles from the blood.   Scarlet red dye was given with food ; this dye is soluble only in fat.   In normal glands, as in thin subjects, no deep colouring within the gland was seen.   In normal glands, the cells manufacture a fat of a special composition.   In other cases, those of overfed, obese animals, the glands were deeply coloured throughout, and the colour extended to the basal membrane, close to the capillaries.   Thus it appeared that the cells were capable of fixing directly the fats circulating in the blood, especially after digestion.   This action of the sebaceous glands in overfed animals explains the fact that the secretion in such cases has been found to contain fats which present the same chemical characters as those in the diet.   Hence it is proved that the diet influences the character of the sebaceous secretion.   On a carbohydrate diet Kuznitsky [2] found that more fat was excreted than on a fatty diet.   It is known too that chemical substances, such as bromide and iodine, can be eliminated in the sebaceous secretion.

The amount and composition of sebum on the scalp of three individuals of different type was investigated by Butcher and Parnell.[3]   The cholesterol and the fat content was measured ; the cholesterol was highest in the case with most desquamation of the scalp.

[1] Sur le mode de fonctionnement des glandes sébacées.   A. POLICARD and Y. TRITCHKOVITCH, Lyon Méd., 1922, 131, 981.
[2] KUZNITSKY, Arch. f. Dermat. u. Syph., 1913, 114, 691.
[3] J. Invest. Derm., 1947, 9, 67.

**Sweat glands** open on the surface of the scalp. The sweat glands lie deeper than the sebaceous glands, being situated in the dermis. Water is their chief excretion. The small percentage of solids contained in the sweat consists chiefly of sodium chloride ; the other organic salts are the same as those of the blood, but in weaker proportions. Of the inorganic constituents may be mentioned creatinin, urea, uric acid, ethereal sulphates of indol and skatol, and albumin. Perspiration of the scalp may be profuse in hot weather, especially in the tropics, and the sufferer frequently mistakes it for an excess of oiliness.

**Blood Supply of the Scalp.** The blood supply of the scalp resembles that of the skin elsewhere in the body. It originates in the subcutaneous tissue and passes upward. Arteries and veins are present between the fat lobules. In the corium two vascular plexuses are found : one is deep-seated, near the subcutaneous tissue ; the other is superficial, in the sub-papillary layer. The **blood supply of the hair** comes from both of those sources. There is a network of arterial capillaries in the connective tissue surrounding the follicle, and nourishing its substance. The upper part of the hair follicle is supplied chiefly by the superficial plexus of vessels. The vessels from the deeper plexus run from below into the hair papilla ; and some of these supply also the lower part of the hair follicle. Hence the hair papilla is not influenced by defects of the superficial plexus (the sub-papillary circulation). Deficient nourishment to the papilla, arriving from the deeper plexus, would lead to decreased growth of the cells of the papilla and of the lower part of the follicle.

**Nerve Supply.** A complex network of nerves surrounds the hair follicle, just below the level of the sebaceous gland ; fine filaments traverse the wall of the follicle and pass to the root sheath. It is now believed that nerves also enter the hair papilla.

The hair has a **muscle supply,** the arrector pili. This muscle runs in an oblique or slanting direction from the papillary layer of the dermis to the connective tissue outside the follicle, to which it is attached at the level just below the entrance of the sebaceous gland. The action of this muscle is the erection of the hair. The soft, downy, lanugo hairs have no arrector pili muscles, but have often unusually large sebaceous glands. Indeed, the sebaceous gland may be so large that the tiny hair is in comparison a mere appendage to the gland. The follicle lies obliquely to the surface of the skin ; when the muscle contracts, it draws the follicle into a direction at a right angle to the skin surface, and hence causes the hair to stand up from its normal direction of lying along the skin. This action of the hair muscle is dramatically evident on the backs of angry cats and dogs. In man it is frequently seen when the skin is cold ; the arrector pili muscles then draw up the hair follicles and cause the appearance popularly known as " goose skin." Sometimes a similar action occurs under the stress of emotions of fear and anger. The terrible experiences endured in war lead to a hyper-activity of the thyroid and the adrenal glands which can continue for months when memories haunt by day and by night in dreams. This leads to exaggeration of the pilomotor reflex. Sir Arthur Hurst described how goose-skin and erection of the hairs can be elicited in these cases by gently stroking the skin of the chest. In a normal person no reaction would be thus obtained. Some men showed the extraordinary phenomenon of having their hair on end for several months after their return from France, whence they had escaped by Dunkirk. The hair of the head literally stood up like the bristles of a hedgehog.[1]

**Hairfall.** When a hair has attained to the natural limit of its age, it falls out and its place is taken by a young new hair. On the scalp the natural life limit of a hair has been estimated at eighteen months, two, four and six years. When the hair becomes old, an air space forms between the medulla and the top of the papilla, and the cuticle at

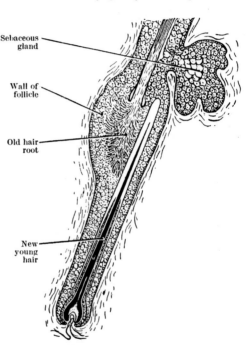

Fig. 5.—Shows old hair root attached to side of follicle, the " bed hair " ; also freshly formed new hair below. (*After Unna.*)

this level disappears for some time before the hair falls. When the life of the hair has reached its span, its bulb loosens and separates from the papilla. In animals, at certain times of the year a periodical shedding of the hair takes place. In man, periods of profuse hairfall, in health, are not marked ; there is continuous growth, fall and replacement of the hair. When the hair has loosened from the papilla it rises in the follicle, remaining for a time attached to the prickle cell layer at the

[1] " Medical Diseases of War." 4th edition, 1944. Edward Arnold and Co., London.

level of the middle of the follicle.   The papilla atrophies and the follicle
falls in over it.   The detached hair bulb passes upwards and appears to
grow from the edge of the follicle (see Fig. 5).   At this stage it is known
as the " bed hair " ;  it has no root sheath, cuticle or medulla, and its
pigment lies in stripes or heaps (see Fig. 6).   When the " bed hair "
reaches the level of the sebaceous gland it is pushed out by the pressure
from below of the new hair, and the fall is also hastened by traction from
above, caused by daily brushing and combing, or by washing or friction.
The new hair begins to appear at the bottom of the follicle about the
time when its predecessor has risen to the level of the middle of the
follicle.   Cells push down, from the old shrunken root sheath, to the
bottom of the follicle.   The old papilla revives and the new hair begins
to grow from it.   Others maintain [1] that the old papilla dies, and that
a fresh one is formed for each new hair.   The new hair rises and passes
out of the mouth of the follicle, sometimes together with the old hair,
but more frequently pushing it out in front of it.   The new hair then
lives its span, provided no interference with its blood supply from below,
or injury from above, occurs to shorten its life.   Then, in its turn, it
loosens from the papilla, passes upwards, becomes a " bed hair " in the
follicle and is pushed out by the new hair forming below it.

Disease can bring about profuse hairfall.   This is dealt with in the
sections on hairfall (p. 84).   When a hair has fallen out, the new one
begins to grow and is seen in the scalp in about six to ten weeks.   When
a hair has been pulled out, its successor appears much more rapidly.

A consideration of the above brief description of the anatomy and
development of the hair shows that the chief nourishment of the hair
depends on the state of the papilla, and that anything which interferes
with or alters the blood supply of the hair papilla is at once reflected
in the condition of the hair.   The papilla obtains its blood supply, as
mentioned above, from the deep circulatory plexus under the skin, and
the middle of the follicle has its arterial supply from the more superficial
plexus, known as the sub-papillary circulation.   A great deal has been
written on the formation of fresh hairs and their connection with the two
sources of blood supply to the follicle and the hair papilla.   The reader
who is interested in this subject should consult the work of Professor Unna.

Certain foods appear to influence the hair.   Experiments with animals
showed that a loss of fur occurred when they were given a diet poor in
quantity or quality of protein.[2]   Therefore it was thought that hair

[1] See an interesting illustrated article by ARNOLDO VENEZIANI, Giorn. Ital. d. Mal.
Ven. e. d. Pelle, 1901, **36**, 582.

[2] G. A. HARTWELL, *Biochem. Journ.*, 1925, **19**, 75 ; and H. D. LIGHTBODY and
H. B. LEWIS: *J. Biol. Chem.*, 1929, **82**, 663.

growth would be stimulated by supplying to the diet preparations rich in sulphur and cystine. Very conflicting, however, are the reports of this form of therapy on human beings. The influence of diet is discussed later, where the treatment of hairfall and of canities is considered.

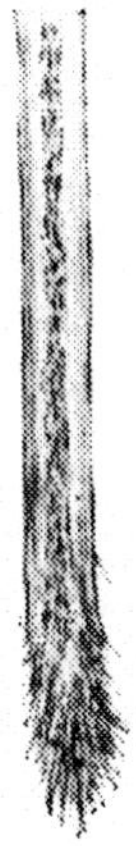

**Microscopical Appearance of the Hair.** When we desire to examine a hair under the microscope, the hair should be very gently pulled out in the direction of the axis of the follicle. The selected hair should be free from extraneous grease. To remove oil or grease the hair can be shaken up with ether in a tube or allowed to rest in ether on the slide. The hair is laid on the microscope slide, and a cover glass placed gently over it. A few drops of distilled water or of chemically pure glycerine are placed on the slide by the edge of the cover glass and are drawn in, by capillary attraction, beneath the cover glass. The hair can then be examined, first with the low-power, then with the high-power lens. Glaister states that for microscopic examination in medicolegal work the structure of the cells and pigment is seen to best advantage after the hair has lain for twenty-four hours in Canada balsam.

FIG. 6.—Hair pulled when about to fall out. Note branched condition of root of a " bed hair." × 50.

For a close study of the structure of the cells of the hair, the oil immersion lens is necessary. In cases of suspected fungus infection, the low- or a medium-power lens is sufficient. The hair is examined after soaking for ten minutes in liquor potassæ or 30 per cent. caustic potash ; spores and mycelium then show up clearly. There are several good methods for staining the hair (see Ringworm, p. 200).

Under the microscope the appearance of the hair root varies according to whether it is a falling hair, or a hair which has been pulled out. If it is a hair about to fall, the end presents a rounded cone, branched like a broom, and the cuticle, root sheath and medulla are absent (see Fig. 7). A *complete*

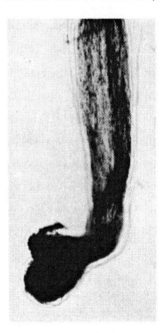

FIG. 7.—From dark-haired woman of thirty. Shows indented bulb of a pulled, young hair, with sheath attached. Microphotograph Mag. × 120.

hair shows a bulb-shaped end, hollowed out if it is a young hair, where it has fitted on to the papilla ; the medulla, cortex and cuticle are visible ; a hair in this condition is seen when a young hair is tugged or pulled out (see Fig. 7).   Or the hair root may have the appearance of the hair which has fallen out between these two periods—the rounded end may be narrow or may have a prolongation like a tap-root or a tail, which is the lower part of the shrunken follicle, attached to the hair root (see Figs. 8a and b).   If a

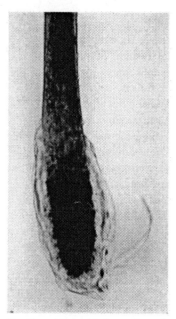

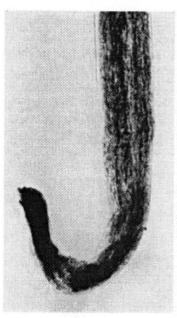

FIG. 8a.—Adjacent hair root from the same subject.  It had passed the stage of having an indented bulb over the papilla.  Note attached and torn inner root sheath, owing to hair having been pulled out roughly.   Microphotograph Mag. × 120.

FIG. 8b.—Adjacent hair from the same subject.  A hair which has been pulled out at a late stage. The bulb has no indentation ; the root is narrow and shows the shrunken part of lower follicle attached to it.   Microphotograph Mag. × 120.

hair has been forcibly *pulled* out, there is also seen, normally attached to it, part of the internal root sheath, which is broken off and frayed above.

When focussing the lens upon a hair, it should be remembered that a hair is not a flat, but a round object, and therefore one must alter the focus in order to observe the middle and the edge of the hair shaft. Focussing upon the edge of the hair reveals the overlapping free ends of the cuticle cells, looking like a saw.   Focussing upon the middle of the hair shows the cuticle cells like dark lines arranged as tiles on a roof.

This network shows up particularly well when the hair has soaked in glycerine during several hours. Focussing in order to observe the hair at a deeper level brings into view the cortex. The long spindle cells which compose the cortex resemble muscle fibres ; when one follows the hair shaft down to the root, these cortex cells become more visible. In the cortex lies the colouring matter of the hair. Down the centre of the hair, the medulla lies like a dark streak. Sometimes it forms a long, continuous line, like the leaden core of a pencil, but more often it is discontinuous, showing thick spindle-shaped nodes with narrow lines of junction (see Fig. 9). In dark hair the medulla is usually dark, but it may be almost invisible, being the same shade as the fluid pigment of the cortex ; in a photograph it might be missed, but careful regulation of the focus of the microscope reveals it to the examining eye. In white hair, the medulla may show as a pale streak with delicate light and shade, like a white cloud with glistening and grey points ; on the other hand, it may be quite dark (see Fig. 9). The dark appearance of the medulla is sometimes due to pigment content, but often to the presence of air, which looks dark by transmitted light. For a study of the structure of the cells of the medulla, it is recommended to let the hair lie in glycerine or oil for a time so that the air can be dispelled from the cavities between the cells. This subject is dealt with again in the chapter on Grey Hair.

Pohl Pincus examined hairs under polarized light and found that he could distinguish from the colouring of the root and adjacent shaft whether the hair had fallen in health or disease. Where the fall had been caused by disease (acute or chronic infections), or emotional states (such as prolonged grief or mental depression), the normal process of cornification was interfered with, and the colours under polarized light underwent modifications characteristic of these conditions.[1]

In view of the recent work carried out on animal hairs, these observations of Pincus may be regarded as of only historical value. When a structure is examined by polarized light the effects observed vary both with the nature of the substance and its thickness ; the colour depends largely upon the thickness of the hair.

FIG. 9.—Two white hairs, both alike to the eye. Unaltered in appearance after prolonged soaking in oil. Note dark medulla in one, and apparent absence of any medulla in adjoining hair.

[1] " Polarisirte Licht als Erkennungs-Mittel für die Erregungs-Zustande der Nerves der Kopfhaut," J. POHL PINCUS, Berlin, 1886.

The **colour of the hair** depends chiefly on the shade and the amount of pigment in the cortex. Air spaces, when present in the outer part of the cortex, affect the colour of the hair ; when viewed by transmitted light these air spaces appear dark, and by direct light as bright points. The importance of air spaces is borne out by research in the case of Ringed hair, described on page 34. The air globules may be small and round, or long and oval, or of irregular shape, and are said to be distinguished from pigment granules by the fact that on regulation of the focus of the microscope, they appear to glisten. In my experience, air cavities which can cause difficulty in diagnosis from pigment granules in the cortex are exceedingly rare. I believe that their existence in the cortex has been exaggerated ; but that their influence on the apparent colour of the medulla is of great importance. In normal hair, the colouring of the cortex occurs in the form of pigment granules, which lie in heaps and in scattered grains, and also in the form of a paler colouring matter diffused in the substance of the cortex cells. Most books describe this diffused colour as " fluid pigment."

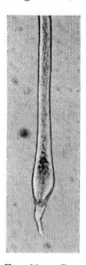

Fig. 10. — Grey hair, naturally fallen. Shows pigment above hair bulb, and a few pigment granules in cortex. Lower part of follicle is attached, a frequent appearance in a fallen old hair. Microphotograph Mag. × 50.

The pigment in the hair is believed to be produced in the cells of the hair bulb ; as these grow upward the pigment continues to be formed in the cells of the cortex. Cells containing pigment are seen on the papilla and higher up on the hair bulb. Even in grey hairs showing no pigment granules along the shaft, and in entirely white hairs, I have seen dark streaks and granules of pigment on the hair bulb (see Figs. 10 and 11). Light hair is said to have no granules, only diffuse colouring in the cortex ; but in red gold hairs I have often seen delicate granules of pigment. I have found that when no pigment at all is visible, the hair appears white ; when there are a few dark granules, or a trace of diffused pigment, the hair appears grey. Even when the hair has a thick dark medulla, the absence of all colour in the cortex makes it seem to the eye a white hair. Such a hair is shown in Fig. 9. See Chapter II, where the subject is discussed more fully.

The question of the origin of pigment is a highly involved physiological and chemical problem. The pigment in the hair belongs to the melanin type. Research on the origin of the pigment in the skin has led to the abandonment of the theory that its source lies in the dermis. Meirowsky [1] has reviewed the work of the past hundred years on the problem of pigment formation. In 1917, Bruno Bloch found that by treating frozen sections of freshly excised skin with a colourless chemical substance, 3·4 dihydroxyphenylalanine (shortened to " dopa "), melanin was produced in the basal layer of the epidermis and the corresponding cells of the hair follicles. He concluded that these cells contain a ferment, dopa-oxydase, which activates the oxidation of the dopa to melanin. Bloch made many tests, and found that dopa was the most effective chemical ; it is closely allied to adrenalin. The dopa reaction is negative in vitiligo, scar tissue, albinos and in the bulbs of white hairs ; it is increased in conditions where hyperpigmentation is usual, as after exposure to X-ray and ultraviolet ray. Although it is agreed that melanin is formed in the epidermis, there is no certainty regarding the origin of the dendritic cells in which it is found. It is suggested that they are modified epithelial cells which produce pigment and also constitute a special system evolving from the undifferentiated epidermis just as the Langerhans cells develop from the pancreas. Under the influence of irradiation, pigment forms in most of the Malpighian cells and in the basal cells of the epidermis. Apparently the nucleus of the cell undergoes a transformation into pigment. Adrenalin and its oxidation products seem to be the precursors of melanin. The origin of pigment in the dermis is not known. Melanin formation is discussed by Fitzpatrick and H. Montgomery.[2]

Sorby [3] dissolved out the pigment from hairs, and found that golden hair contained a mixture of red and yellow pigment ; dark-red hair had red and black ; sandy brown had mixed red, black and yellow pigments ; dark brown was formed by black pigment ; black hair was due to the presence of a great amount of black pigment and white hair was conspicuous by the absence of all pigment. Danforth states that all shades of red hair have diffuse pigment ; brown to black have granules, and glossy black hair has both diffuse and granular pigment. Arnow [4] has shown that human red hair is an oxidation product of melanin. It is probable that the various shades of hair are due to different stages in the oxidation of the same pigment base.

The **number of hairs** on the scalp has been calculated to be about

[1] MEIROWSKY, Brit. Journ. Dermat., 1940, 52, 205.
[2] FITZPATRICK, MONTGOMERY et al., Science, 1950, 112, 223 ; see also LERNER and FITZPATRICK, Physiol. Rev., 1950, 30, 91.
[3] SORBY, " Colouring Matter found in the Human Hair," J. Anthrop. Inst., 1878, 8, 1.
[4] ARNOW, Biochem. J., 1938, 32, 1281.

1000 to the square inch; hence about 120,000 hairs clothe the adult head. I believe that Erasmus Wilson [1] was one of the first to make these calculations; he quotes Withof as having made similar measurements. The finer the hairs, the more numerous. Stelwagon found that blond hair averages 140,000; red hair, 90,000; brown hair, 109,000; black hair, 108,000.

As regards the **diameter** of the hair, Wilson measured the diameter of 2000 hairs taken from thirty-eight individuals, and states that flaxen hair is the finest, black hair the coarsest. In the Anglo-Saxon race the finest hairs varied from $\frac{1}{1500}$ to $\frac{1}{500}$ inch, the coarsest from $\frac{1}{400}$ to $\frac{1}{140}$ inch in diameter. The hair of the head in women was on the average slightly thicker than that of men: it varied from $\frac{1}{500}$ to $\frac{1}{250}$ inch, whereas in men the variation was from $\frac{1}{525}$ to $\frac{1}{300}$ inch. The hair of a child is finer than that of an adult. Observations were also made on hairs from the heads of three South American Indians and a New Zealand chief; these gave measures ranging from $\frac{1}{1000}$ to $\frac{1}{200}$ inch. A hair is not necessarily of uniform diameter; especially in grey and in white hair, the diameter of the cortex often varies throughout the length of the hair. In some cases this condition is so marked that to the finger the hair conveys a sensation of being beaded; I have seen the same condition in the hairs on a woman's chin. Usually, the medulla is clearly visible in the thickened portions, and is sometimes absent in the narrow regions. The hair is coarse in some cases of hyperpituitarism and microcytic anæmia; in Addisonian anæmia the hair is fine.

Dr. U. Matsuura gives details of a laborious investigation [2] into the alterations of the thickness of the hair in health and disease. With micrometer measurements of the cross section of hair roots and shafts, he was able to detect that disease caused variations in the hair width. He could estimate the duration of an illness, whether it was slight or severe, and also whether the hair had come from a patient who had recently died. He drew up charts of the altered thickness of the hairs in several maladies and found that these provided evidence of the condition of the patient which corresponded with the charts of the temperature and the body weight. The thicker the hair, the greater its reduction during ill health. In serious illness, with marked thinning of the hair, the medulla became broken up; this feature developed a few days later than the thinning of the hair shaft. Previously Pincus had observed that the medulla was narrowed and broken up after prolonged and severe emotional disturbance.

The painstaking work of Dr. Matsuura has been long overlooked. It is of interest that research on the wool of sheep has proved the existence of

---

[1] ERASMUS WILSON, " Healthy Skin," 6th edition, London, 1859.
[2] U. MATSUURA, *Archiv. f. Derm. u. Syph.*, 1902, **62**, 273.

a similar relationship. Alteration in the thickness of the wool fibres is a well-known phenomenon in sheep. When a sheep is " off-colour " the fact is reflected in its wool. Ill-health and starvation bring about a sudden thinning which is recognised by all who deal with sheep.

The **rate of growth** of the hair is of practical interest. When the hair has been cut short, for æsthetic reasons, we are often asked how long a period of time must elapse before the hair can again become long ? So long ago as 1882, Pincus of Berlin published a small book of careful clinical observations on the hair in health and disease, with notes of elaborate investigations into the subject of the duration of the life and the rate of growth of the hairs of the head. He noticed that every hair has its own special duration of life and its own characteristic length. Not every hair on the scalp attains the average length peculiar to the scalp ; along the margin of the scalp there are always found a number of short hairs. In a normal scalp, i.e. one which is unaffected by any local or general disease, the average life of a hair is from two to six years. The rate of growth of a hair varies with its age. When the hair reaches the level of the skin it grows very rapidly, from 2 to 5 milli-metres every ten days, or about $\frac{3}{4}$ inch per month. When the hair is older, 10 to 14 inches in length, it grows more slowly, at about half its previous rate. When the hair is older still, the rate of growth is so slow that any addition to its length is only visible in six weeks. Other observers have stated that the rate of hair growth is greatest in young women, between the ages of sixteen and twenty-four, when a growth of 7 inches in a year has been seen. As a rule, after sixty-five no long hair makes further growth. During illness and during pregnancy the hair grows very slowly. After severe illness the hair sometimes grows very quickly during convalescence. So much for the scientific pro-nouncements ; it is a commonplace observation that in a family some members require their hair cut twice as frequently as others of about the same age and in the same state of health.

The hair appears to grow faster in summer ; between March and July it is said to make more headway than between August and February. Every follicle has its individual cycle ; even adjacent follicles may show different rates of growth. Those with long and strong hairs are more continuously active than those with short hairs. The rate of growth is affected by the general health, the condition of the endocrine system and by nutrition. Much work remains to be done on these influences, and also upon the effect of the nervous system, especially emotions of anxiety and fear.

**Life Span of a Hair.** Even in health, a certain number of hairs fall out every day. The proportion of short and long hairs varies in health and disease. Pincus introduced a simple method for deciding whether the proportion of short to long hairs in the daily loss remained normal. When the hair is worn uncut, the fallen hairs can be collected morning and evening for three successive days, and divided into two bundles, hairs over and hairs under 6 inches long. Pincus found it a good working rule that in health the short hairs did not exceed in number one-quarter of the total loss. When the proportion of the short hairs was higher than a quarter of the total fall, disease was present. When the hair is worn cut, as in men, even the long hairs do not measure 6 inches ; the longest hairs are usually 4½ inches. Therefore, when the hair is worn cut, it is necessary to note which hairs have blunt or cut ends, and which have uncut or pointed ends. If these are separated, and counted, the proportion of the pointed hairs to the cut hairs should not be higher than a quarter or a fifth of the total loss. Disease is present if the pointed hairs number a third or more of the total daily loss.

Influence of **Cutting** and **Shaving**. Recent research tends to confirm the observations of Pincus (p. 47). Without referring to these, Bulliard [1] describes his independent experiments which proved that cutting does not stimulate hair growth. Hair grows rapidly at first and reaches a stage when it grows slowly. Thus a hair which is cut during the first period is seen growing very fast ; if it has been cut during its later, i.e. its slower stage, it grows very little. Hence the ragged appearance soon assumed by cut hair ; for those cut in their young stage grow quickly and pass by the hairs which have been cut at the later period of their life span. Frequent cutting and shaving did not hasten growth.

Raymond Seymour [2] investigated the factors which modify the rate and abundance of hair growth. As the rate of growth was found to vary in different individuals, the experiments were made with hairs from the same subject ; as it also varies with the position of the hair— lip, chin and scalp—a careful study, continued over two and three years, was made of the effect of shaving upon the rate of growth. He concluded (1) that in some manner undetermined the actual cutting of the hair appears to stimulate the growth of facial hair in man ; (2) the rate of growth is most rapid immediately subsequent to the cutting, and decreases as the time of cutting becomes more remote ; (3) no direct relationship with temperature or season was proved. The apparent contradiction

[1] H. BULLIARD, *Ann. Derm. et Syph.*, June, 1923, 6^me, Sér. **4**, 386.
[2] R. J. SEYMOUR, *Amer. Journ. Physiol.*, 1926, **78**, 281.

of these findings with those of Bulliard is explained by the fact that the cuttings took place within short periods of time, 12 to 48 hours, and the rate of growth was therefore measured, not in days or weeks, but in hours. Seymour's experiments confirmed the fact that the hair growth is most rapid at the level of the skin. Danforth quotes the experiments of many workers on the results of cutting and shaving, and concludes that there is no proof that they accelerate the rate of the hair growth.

Mildred Trotter [1] made experiments with grease, shaving and sunlight, in order to discover whether the popular belief in the hair-stimulating properties of these agents has any basis in fact. She found that the use of petrolatum for eight months had no effect on the rate of growth ; nor had shaving. Actinic rays hastened the growth of hair in the growing period, but had no effect on its later development. However, many young women are convinced that the hairs on their legs and arms grow noticeably faster during the summer bathing season than during the winter.

Whitaker [2] reasoned that if, as Danforth maintained, the hair on the chest, breast, abdomen and limbs of men is a sex characteristic, the local application of testosterone should stimulate the growth of the hair on these regions. For five months he rubbed in daily on one side a simple preparation of alcohol, on the other a measured amount of male hormone. The subjects did not know on which side the control experiment was being made ; the testosterone was applied in alcohol so that the same sensation was felt. The men were between 30 and 40 years of age. The experiment succeeded ; the hair growth on the hormone region was stimulated. On the other hand, Danforth [3] obtained no result from similar experiments on the hairs on the backs of the fingers, although such hairs are a sex characteristic.

Miss D. H. Strangeways [4] conducted a study on the conditions affecting hair growth in the guinea-pig. It was found that the general health of the animal influenced the hair growth. During the last weeks of pregnancy the number and the length of fibres growing in a marked region of the body became progressively less, and the rate of growth was slower than in the normal animal. The period of gestation in the guinea-pig is about nine weeks ; during the last four or five weeks little hair growth took place, and normal growth was not resumed till ten weeks after parturition. The amount of hair growing in a definite area was not constant, and the variation was

[1] *Arch. Derm. and Syph.*, 1923, **7**, 93.
[2] *University Hospital Bulletin, Ann Arbor, Michigan*, 1942, **8**, June.
[3] DANFORTH, *Physiol. Rev.*, 1939, **19**, 94.
[4] *J. Agricult. Sc.*, 1933, **23**, 369, 379.

due chiefly to alteration in the number of active follicles on that part. Apparently some follicles cease to produce hair for a time—" resting follicles." In young and in older animals an equal weight of hair was produced in a given time. Yet in the older animal the individual hairs were longer and thicker, but there were fewer of them ; i.e. a certain number of follicles ceased to produce hair for a time. When several animals were placed in a cold room the hair growth was reduced for two to three weeks, then returned to normal. Increased production of hair occurred in the late spring and autumn after the moulting season, but the time of onset and the duration varied greatly in different animals.

Experiments with re-growth after shaving confirmed on the whole the findings of Pincus, Trotter and Bulliard. After many experiments the following conclusion was formed : " It seems probable that shaving may in some way cause an increase in the number of follicles which are active on an area, but not an increase in the rate of growth in length of the fibres."

Danforth discusses the problem of the active and the resting stages of the hair follicles. When animals moult at definite seasons the follicles remain quiescent for a time ; when the hairs resume growth they rapidly attain maturity and are then stationary for several months. Thus the resting stage of the follicle is longer than the active period. In man, individual hairs have been observed on the tragus and the eyebrows ; in some cases the hairs took about two months to reach maturity, then remained three months without growth. On the face and scalp the follicles appear to be continuously active ; when one hair falls out it is at once replaced by fresh growth. Mildred Trotter also found that resting cycles differed in certain follicles during pregnancy.[1]

H. E. Schmidt [2] observed that hair growth was apparently stimulated by light. Hairs developed on the exposed arms of nurses carrying out Finsen light work. He found that this effect was not due to any specific effect of light rays, but to increased vascularity and better nutrition of the follicles. He experimented with two guinea-pigs placed in separate boxes exposed to sunlight. Although one box had red glass, which prevented the passage of the actinic rays, the hair growth was greater in this than in the neighbouring box. This result justified the conclusion that warmth was more conducive than light to hair growth.

The average **length** of uncut hair is 22 to 28 inches. Longer hair is sometimes seen in women, but it is rare to find even long hair exceed 36 inches. Some writers have stated that they have seen hair 7 and 9 feet long ; there are frequent allusions to such cases in romantic poems and tales. I have seen one woman with hair so long that it reached a foot below the waist, and many with hair just beyond the waist level.

HAIR WHORLS. The hair lies along certain natural lines to which the names " hair streams " or " whorls " have been applied. Everyone knows

---

[1] *Surg. Gyn. and Obstet.*, 1935, **60**, 1092.
[2] *Arch. f. Derm. u. Syph.*, 1902, **62**, 329.

that when they brush their hair, it tends to part and to lie flat along one direction rather than another.   Thus it runs forward from the vertex to the brow ; at the vertex there is a junction, from which the natural partings of the hair turn along several directions.   Such appear to be relics of the animal state ; the rain would fall off the body along certain suitable hair lines. Those whom this subject interests will find it is fully studied in anatomical books and in Erasmus Wilson's *Healthy Skin*.

BAYONET HAIRS.   Pincus describes this form of hair shaft as occurring chiefly when baldness is beginning.   There is a bayonet-shaped part of the shaft near the hair point, so that the hair bends sharply at the area of narrow cross-section.

**Physical Properties.**   The hair is elastic ; it stretches when pulled. It is by virtue of this property that it does not break under the strain entailed by the daily pulling which it endures when brushed and combed, pinned and curled.   Less pain is felt when a growing hair is pulled out than when the hair has reached the limit of its length.   Under exceptionally vigorous toilet operations the hair may be stretched sufficiently to break it, as, for example, when a long hair is tugged hard near a tangled knot or dragged tightly round a curling-pin.   The hair absorbs water from the atmosphere and, in doing so, becomes lengthened and more round.   When the atmosphere is damp and the hair absorbs moisture, naturally curly hair becomes more curly, and straight hair, which has been artificially curled by heat or by curling-pins, becomes straight again.

Leftwich [1] carried out a series of simple clinical experiments in order to find out (1) how far hair could be stretched without being broken, (2) whether after being stretched, the elastic property of a hair enabled it to be restored to its original length and (3) whether and how far its elasticity and strength were affected by some of the toilet preparations in common use.   For these tests he selected healthy people and hairs which appeared to be of similar strength.   He measured the strength of a hair by pulling it firmly and evenly over both sides of a Salter's letter balance, and noted the weight registered at the instant the hair broke.   By this method of testing its resistance to a steady pull, he found that an average hair broke at 7 oz.   I made a large number of similar tests and found individual variations, not only in the hairs of different people, but even in hairs from adjacent parts of the scalp, and in different parts of the same long hair.   When trying to verify some of Leftwich's experiments, I encountered another obstacle, one which did not exist in his day—the " permanent wave."   The modern methods of waving and curling the hair demand study of the property

[1] R. W. LEFTWICH, *Preservation of the Hair*, Bristol, 1901.

of elasticity possessed by the human hair. The question of the elasticity of the hair is dealt with by Mr. Astbury in a special section (see Chapter IV). I destroyed the notes of over fifty of my simple clinical experiments when I found how profound a study of elasticity had been made by modern science.

Leftwich tested the effect of curling-tongs. After one curling a 7-oz. hair broke at 6 to 6½ oz. In another case, the strength of several hairs, after being curled daily for a week, remained unaltered. Hair which had been stretched, so as to curl on pins or paper, broke more easily. The weak point in these experiments is that the degree of heat used with the tongs was not estimated, and hence Leftwich's advocacy of curling-tongs cannot be accepted (see also pp. 56 and 73).

So far as clinical and everyday care of the hair is concerned, Leftwich's experiments showed that the degree of elasticity is affected by water, steam and other fluids employed in lotions. Leftwich found that hair which did not normally break till it carried a 7-oz. weight, broke at 6½ oz. after immersion in rectified spirit ; at 4½ to 5 oz. in a solution of soft soap (1 part in 8 of water) ; at 5¼ oz. in cold tap water, and less when soap was added. Soda and borax also reduced the resisting power of the hair. I could not confirm these figures.

I tested the weight-supporting strength of several long, fine grey hairs, by laying a hair on a Salter's letter balance, and pulling steadily downwards on each side. This natural hair broke at 6 oz. One hair, apparently similar in thickness, which had lain in almond oil three-quarters of an hour, broke at 5 oz. Three hairs which had lain in glycerine three-quarters of an hour broke just under 6 oz. ; another broke at 4 oz. A long white hair was cut into two parts. One part broke at 5 oz. ; the other part, after immersion one and a half hours in almond oil, broke at less than 5 oz. Another white hair cut from the scalp close to the first was divided into two and placed in almond oil for an hour ; then one part broke at 5¾ oz., the other part broke at 2 oz. A long, permanently waved, dark hair was divided into three ; one part was placed in almond oil, one in water, the other in glycerine. After an hour's immersion the strength was tested on a Salter's letter balance ; all broke at 4 instead of the normal 7 oz.

With both permanently waved and natural hairs these experiments were therefore found to yield contradictory results. One could only deduce that, as a general rule, permanently waved hair broke more readily than natural hair ; this was true even when it had lain immersed in oil for an hour. After immersion in water or glycerine the results obtained, even with hairs from the same scalp, were so varied that no rule could be formulated regarding their effect upon the strength of the hair.

Tests were next made with the hair of two healthy children who lived in the country, and had never used any local applications to the scalp. A lock of hair was cut off close to the scalp, and three days later, the same tests were carried out, in each case on four hairs.

*Margaret æt. two and a half.* Measured with Salter's letter balance, the hair broke at 5 oz. Three hairs were placed for forty minutes in water, in glycerine and in almond oil. The breaking-point after the immersion in

| Water | was 6 oz. |
| Glycerine | ,, 5½ oz. |
| Oil | ,, not quite 5 oz. |

*Kathleen æt. twelve.* Tested with Salter's balance the natural hair broke at 5½ oz.
After forty minutes' immersion in

| Water | the hair broke at 4½ oz. |
| Glycerine | ,, ,, ,, ,, 6½ oz. |
| Oil | ,, ,, ,, ,, just under 8 oz. |

These tests therefore were contradictory. In the case of the younger child oil did not make the hair less readily broken ; in the older child one could have deduced that oil greatly increased the strength of the hair. But that hair may have been a naturally stronger or thicker hair.

It is apparent that much more stringent precautions would be required in order to determine what is the effect upon the hair of the various toilet preparations in common use. The only point of agreement between my experiments and those of Leftwich is that the average doubled natural hair can sustain a weight of 7 oz. before it breaks.

For the examination of hairs for **medico-legal** purposes, Smith and Glaister advise, first, thorough cleansing. Place the hair in a test-tube containing equal parts of ether and rectified spirit ; shake the fluid several times, at intervals of a few minutes, for a quarter of an hour. After drying the hair in filter paper, clean the hair with benzol or oil of turpentine ; dry and mount it in fresh Canada balsam and let it stand for twenty-four to forty-eight hours before examination. The structure of the hair is by this method made more clear. The cuticle cells are made more distinct by employing a weak solution of potash. Many dyes can be distinguished by means of chemical tests. A dyed hair lacks lustre and is more brittle. Under the microscope details of the cells of a dyed hair are seen as through a mist ; the colour is more a uniform tinting than the streaks and heaps of the normal pigmentation of the hair.

The medico-legal subject can receive only brief reference here. In medico-legal work the examination of hairs may play an important part in tracking down the criminal or exculpating the innocent person. It may be necessary to decide whether hairs found on clothes, in or near a wound, or on some object such as a car or missile, are identical with those of the suspected individual. This may be a simple matter if the hairs have a characteristic colour, or degree of coarseness or fineness, or if they are dyed. On the other hand, this decision may be very difficult. Sometimes I have plucked several adjacent hairs from a scalp, and have found thick, thin, well-pigmented hairs and almost colourless hairs, hairs with thick medulla and hairs with scarcely any, or no visible medulla. The part of the body from which the hairs have come can be recognized, as a rule without difficulty, by one who is accustomed to such investigation. Usually it is easy to tell that a hair has fallen out naturally, when its span of life was over ; in such a case the root is narrow, the outer edge of its end split so that it resembles a broom, and the medulla, cuticle and sheath are usually absent (see Fig. 6). When a hair has been forcibly pulled out, the internal root sheath is attached to it and is broken. When the root is that of a young hair, it shows a bulb with the characteristic indentation which fitted over the papilla [1] (see Fig. 7). At later stages the root is narrower and rounded (Fig. 8a) or has a tap-like root (Figs. 8b and 10). The condition of the hair shaft may reveal that it has been cut, singed, or injured in such a way that its connection with some suspected weapon is rendered impossible, probable or certain. Again, when hairs are found in or near a wound, or on clothing or other objects, the microscope reveals whether such hairs are of human or animal origin. The microscopic appearance also enables the expert to distinguish from what type of animal the hair has come. Medico-legal questions have arisen in connection with hair which has been burnt ; above a certain temperature it is impossible to tell whether a burnt hair is of human or animal origin.[2] The effect of singeing is described, with illustrations, on page 50 et seq. To obtain a cross-section of a hair a special and delicate technique is required ; but it can yield invaluable and definite evidence to the skilled examiner. The comparative size of the medulla and cortex, and the arrangement of their cells differs in the various animals and in man. Medico-legal books must be consulted for details of the appearance [3] of the hair of various animals.

Questions are frequently asked about the arsenic contents of the hair. This subject is of importance when there is any question of

---

[1] Great care must be taken in preparing and mounting these specimens. Fig. 7 showed a perfect young hair bulb with surrounding sheath ; three days later it had twisted round in the Canada balsam. Too much balsam had been used ; hence the hair had not remained flat. It is surprising how seldom one sees this indented hair root ; the roots of most pulled, and all naturally fallen hairs, show the later stages, i.e. after the bulb has separated from the top of the papilla and begun to rise up within the follicle.

[2] PIÉDELIÈVRE and DÉROBERT, Ann. méd. légale, 1934, 14, 748, and MÉLISSINOS and DÉROBERT, Ann. méd. légale, 1934, 14, 899.

[3] SMITH and GLAISTER, " Recent Advances in Forensic Medicine," London, 1931, and J. GLAISTER, " Examination of Hairs and Wool," Cairo, 1931.

poisoning by arsenic. Keratin tissues, and therefore the hair, can contain more arsenic, weight for weight, than other tissues of the body. Arsenic can be found in the hair when no trace of the metal is in the organs of the body. This finding does not tell whether the arsenic has been absorbed during life, or whether it has soaked into the hair from some contamination in the vicinity. When hair is placed in a solution of arsenic, as time passes it absorbs arsenic in increasing amounts, up to seven times the strength of that in the solution by which it is surrounded. When more arsenic is found in the proximal than in the distal parts of the hair, although it is highly probable that the drug has been absorbed from the body fluids, this holds true only if there has been no contamination from without. Arsenic which has been absorbed from an external source can be removed in part by soaking the hair in distilled water for a long time. When the arsenic in the hair has been absorbed from the body during life, it cannot be removed by prolonged soaking,[1] a fact which obviously may prove of medico-legal value.

[1] SYDNEY SMITH and E. HENDRY, *Brit. Med. J.*, 1934, ii, 675.

# CHAPTER II

## CANITIES: GREY HAIR

Definition—Sudden blanching—Rapid blanching—Microscopical appearance of grey and white hair—Yellow tinge—Prematurely grey hair—The Albino—Leucotrichia —Ringed hair—Aetiology of canities—Treatment of canities—Altered colour of hair.

Grey and white hair are conditions so common that they should require no definition. Yet confusion exists, even in medical writings, as to what, precisely, constitutes "grey hair." What is frequently described as a head of grey hair turns out on closer examination to be a liberal sprinkling of white hairs amongst more numerous dark-brown or black hairs. True grey hair is comparatively rare; it is hair which contains a mixture of shades in its texture, usually brown or black fading into paler hues and white. A grey hair resembles shot silk; on moving it round, one sees that it glistens more than does an ordinary dark hair, and no sharp demarcation of the dark and the pale portions can be distinguished. This type of hair reflects or takes on the colours of the walls, furnishings or other surrounding lighter or darker objects. This phenomenon of several shades mingled in one, and influenced by adjacent colours, is well known to artists. Thus, in a dark oak-panelled room, a head of grey hair may look as if it glowed with a rich yellow brown. This chameleon property accounts for the pathetic fallacy which leads many a woman in the late forties to believe that her hair still retains its youthful dark colour. In bright sunlight this delusion is shattered.

In normal people the grey hair of middle age precedes the development of the snow-white hair of old age. Often the change of colour is associated either with a thickening or a thinning of the shaft of the hair. A few white hairs may be seen about the age of thirty-five, but in most people greyness appears during the forties. Although few have no grey or white hairs by their fiftieth year, it is not uncommon to see the change postponed until the middle fifties or even later. The alteration of colour over the entire scalp develops very gradually. Often the increasing number of grey hairs is arrested or at least there seems to be no further advance over a number of years; but as a general rule greyness is slowly but surely progressive. When grey hairs begin to appear in the twenties or early thirties the condition is described as *premature greyness* (p. 33). Occasionally, grey hairs appear before the age of twenty and the whole head may be white at forty.

26

Greyness of the hair starts, as a rule, on the temples, and gradually extends to the vertex ; the hair on the occiput is the last to lose colour. In the case of men the beard is often the first to whiten. The hair on the body (axilla and pubis) is usually the last to turn grey, and may even retain colour to the end of life. Sometimes the hair regains some or all of its former colour when the greyness has been due to disease of the scalp or to general ill-health, and both conditions have been cured. The hair may regain its colour after middle age, or in old age, but this is rare. V. C. Isdell [1] records the case of his own father, Dr. James Isdell of Dublin. At sixty-two, the hair of his head and beard were completely grey. Twenty-two years later, when he died, at the age of eighty-three, all the hair of his head had returned to its original dark colour, except for a few grey hairs on each temple. The beard had been shaved off for some years.

Normally, the greyness of a hair starts at its root. Exceptional cases are met with in which the greyness is seen at the root and the tip, whilst the middle of the hair shaft retains its colour ; in other rare cases the free end of the hair shaft is grey. Some observers claim that hairs on the head turn grey first at the tip, because they frequently find hairs which are dark near the scalp and grey farther along the shaft. The probable explanation is that these are grey hairs which are becoming rejuvenated from the root. After alopecia areata, the white hairs which return have been observed to become dark from root to tip.[2] Sabouraud made the same observation ; the entirely white hair becomes coloured, slowly taking on the shade of the hair on other parts of the head. It is said that brunettes become grey sooner than blondes, but this may be due to the fact that the greyness is more noticeable with dark than with fair hair.

**Sudden blanching** of the hair has been reported by so many competent observers that the existence of the phenomenon is probable. Charcot [3] wrote in criticism of Kaposi, who had denied the possibility of rapid blanching of the hair. Scientific exactitude, Charcot declared, had nothing in common with the prejudice which led certain types of mind to regard with disfavour all observations which presented any unusual character ; scepticism was no less blameworthy than naïve credulity. Kaposi expressed disbelief in sudden whitening of the hair because he considered it impossible for pigment granules suddenly to disappear or air spaces suddenly to develop, under the influence of emotion, in the hairs of the scalp. Most dermatologists quote historical

[1] *Med. Times*, 1884, ii, 680.      [2] *Brit. Journ. Dermat.*, 1912, **24**, 427.
[3] *Gazette Hébdomadaire de Méd.*, 1861, **8**, 445.

cases of sudden whitening of the hair as if they were legends. Among historical examples always cited are those of Marie Antoinette and Sir Thomas More, whose hair turned grey during the night preceding their execution. Henry of Navarre showed white hairs in the moustache a few hours after hearing that the edict of Nemours had been conceded. Erasmus Wilson quotes a number of reports of which particulars were given to him by reliable witnesses, but says that he had no belief in the sudden conversion of dark hair to snowy whiteness until a case came under his notice. Pincus likewise writes about several subjects in which the blanching occurred after sudden grief. Xavier, in *La Chronique Medicale* of April, 1934, cites many cases. Lee McCarthy [1] adds his testimony to the belief that sudden blanching may occur, even in a night. In subjects with a hereditary tendency to early greyness this may be precipitated by illness, especially severe nervous shock.

A man aged fifty-two, whose truthfulness I cannot doubt, told me that at the age of thirty-six his hair turned grey in a single night. His history was that he was motor-cycling in a thick fog on a dark night. Towards midnight he fell into a canal and spent a long time trying to reach the bank. Exhausted, he collapsed. When he regained consciousness he was told by the police that he had been picked up insensible at 6 a.m. His hair had turned grey that night. R. McNeill Love reported a case of sudden blanching.[2] In reply to my letter asking for particulars he answered: " The patient to whom I referred was a male aged sixty-five who was nearly blown up by V bombs twice in one night. I saw him the following day and did not recognize him at first. Nor did his friends."

Sometimes the blanching of the hair takes place with abnormal rapidity. One of my patients, an intelligent observer, aged 65, said that her golden brown hair had developed its present shade of marked greyness within a week of the tragic death of her only son 20 years previously. His doctor had remarked on the change at the funeral. Sir Arthur Hurst quoted two instances of rapid greying after terrifying experiences ; one was a boy of seventeen. Jackson [3] knew a case whose hair and beard changed from black to white and back again three times in thirty years : the change from black to white was rapid ; the return to colour took five years. The hair has become white during attacks of mental insanity, remained so for a few days or hours, then restored its natural colour. Dr. Claye Shaw [4] wrote that it was not uncommon to

[1] LEE McCARTHY, " Diseases of the Hair," 1940.
[2] *Brit. Med. Journ.*, 1947, ii, 160.
[3] G. T. JACKSON and C. W. McMURTRY, Treatise on "Diseases of the Hair," London, 1913.
[4] *St. Bart's Hospital Rep.*, 1884, **20**, 169.

see symmetrical white bands or tracts of hair develop during insanity and the usual colour restored during convalescence. Brown-Séquard [1] described how the hairs of the beard can change colour very rapidly. He pulled out the few white hairs he had, so that he could observe how soon a black hair became white. He had not long to wait. Where only black hairs had been seen, and a few hairs which showed white only close to the root, he saw, two days later, five hairs, white along their entire length. Subsequent similar observations, carried out over five weeks in bright summer morning light, showed that black hairs could change rapidly to white, sometimes even during less than one night. Unfortunately, he made no microscopic examination and he does not mention the length of the hairs.

Carefully noted details of a remarkable case of rapid alteration in colour of the hair are described by Raymond.[2] The patient was a French woman, thirty-eight years of age, with black hair. After she had suffered a period of great grief, she had been told of severe financial loss. The bad news arrived when she was menstruating, and the flow was at once checked. She became very ill and complained of acute neuralgia. After the patient had endured two days of excruciating pain in the head and shoulders, on January 30, 1882, at 2 a.m. the hair was still its normal deep-black colour. On January 31, at 7 a.m., much of the hair had turned white. Some of the original dark colour remained at the sides and back of the scalp ; the hair on the upper part of the head was red, and the shorter hairs were white. No alteration of colour had taken place on the hairs on the body. The severe neuralgic pains continued, and on February 1 practically all the hair of the head had changed colour. By February 2, most of the hair which had turned red on January 31 had become white. Then the hair began to fall out. The pain diminished. In fifteen days hardly any hairs were left on the head except a few on the sides and the occiput. On March 3 her remaining hairs on the sides and the occipital region were of mixed colours—white, red and black. A fortnight later, she was almost bald. The eyebrows and the eyelashes had remained black throughout.

Darier reported the case of a man of fifty, whose hair had become white and thin in two months ; under treatment with thyroid an abundant dark re-growth took place, and the pigment of the white hairs became restored. In this connection may be recalled the undoubted fact of repigmentation of the white hairs which usually follow alopecia areata. The colour returns too rapidly to be accounted for by a re-growth of fresh dark hair.

[1] *Arch. de Physiol.*, 1869, **2**, 442.    [2] *Révue de méd.*, 1882, **2**, 770.

*Ringed hair* must be mentioned here, because it is a form of grey hair, in which the hair shows alternate bands of grey or white and of dark hair. It is discussed on page 34.

*Microscopical appearance.* Grey hair and white hair are natural as age advances. Practically universal as the condition is, there is still uncertainty as to its cause. In the charming language of his time, some fifty years ago, Pincus wrote : " The blanching of the hair is preceded by a number of changes of the whole body brought on by age. The greyness is then in accordance with nature, and harmonizes with the general course of human existence." After patient study, Pincus arrived at the conclusion that white hair had no pigment, and grey hair had a deficiency of pigment. In certain forms of grey hairs he found pigment, but owing to the presence of air between the outer cells of the cortex the rays of light were reflected and thus a white appearance was given to the hair. In cases of ordinary canities due to age, he found there was a decrease in the amount of pigment in the middle layer cells of the papilla, but some still remained in the external layers ; the mixture of pigmented and non-pigmented regions caused the grey colour. As time passed, pigment formation ceased and hence the hair became white. Metchnikoff believed that the pigment was lost owing to the activity of certain wandering cells which absorbed it, removing the pigment granules from the hair to the dermis.

I have examined several hundred GREY HAIRS, and find that (1) at the root of the hairs which have fallen naturally or been pulled out, there is usually a quantity of pigment (see Figs. 10 and 11) ; (2) the cortex may have a few grains of pigment, but more often it has no pigment granules at all ; (3) there is often a pale yellow diffuse pigment throughout the cortex ; and (4) the medulla may be dark, may have the same pale yellowish colour as in the cortex, or may show no colour at all.

WHITE HAIRS are said to look white because they contain air spaces which thicken the hair shaft and render it opaque to reflected light. I have examined a large number of white hairs from the scalp of (1) a healthy man of seventy-four ; (2) a young girl of twenty, who had a lock of white hair on a dark head ; (3) a woman of forty-five, with a similar white lock ; (4) a woman of forty-eight ; (5) a woman under sixty ; and (6) an old lady of eighty. The following were the observations made :

(1) The man's white hair showed a little pigment at the hair roots (see Fig. 11), no medulla, and a colourless and airless cortex. In this case the hair in youth had been a vivid chestnut shade.

(2) Two adjacent hairs of the girl's white tress showed no pigment at the roots, a colourless cortex, and a dark medulla. Even after prolonged

soaking in oil the medulla in one hair remained dark.  To the eye, this particular hair closely resembled the adjoining hair in which the medulla, after several hours in oil, had become colourless.

(3) In the white lock of the woman of forty-five, most of the white hairs (microscopically examined) were colourless, but some showed a little pale diffused brown colour in portions of the cortex.  One coarse, hard, white hair, with a trace of brown at some parts of the shaft when regarded with the naked eye, showed under the microscope, in the portion white to the eye, long black blotches ; so I removed it from the Canada balsam, cleaned it with xylol and left it to soak in oil for some hours.  When it was again examined, the black blotches had gone ; in their place were seen long narrow splits in the cortex, and the hair appeared brown, with both diffused and granular pigment.  As I have seen only one other white hair behave in this manner, I believe that the theory of air spaces in the cortex reflecting the light can account for comparatively few cases of white hair.  Compare Ringed Hair (p. 34) in this connection. Five other hairs examined from the same white tress were found to have no pigment at the roots, a colourless cortex, and no medulla for over an inch up.  The distal ends of two hair shafts had a thick medulla which was dark in some hairs and pale in others.  A few of the finer hairs showed a pale yellow diffused colour along both cortex and medulla ; to the eye these hairs appeared grey rather than white.

(4) The woman of forty-eight had thick, wavy black hair, streaked with white. The white hairs showed a broad colourless cortex, and thick dark medulla, and except in a few hairs, no pigment at the roots. After soaking in oil all night, the thick dark medulla remained unaltered in ap-

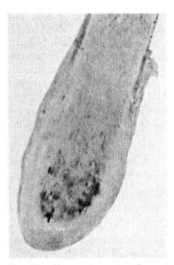

FIG. 11.—Shows pigment at the root of a pulled thick white hair.  Note attached and broken internal root sheath.    Microphotograph Mag. × 120.

pearance.  If all white hairs resembled those of this lady, they would provide evidence in favour of the theory that in age there is formed a large medulla, which gives an opaque white appearance to the shaft.  However, I have known this woman for many years ; her dark hair has always been of a hard wiry quality.  This is the type of thick, hard hair which has given rise to the impression that a thick medulla is the cause of the snow-white shade of a vigorous old age.

(5) The woman under sixty had all her life had very fine hairs ; as she aged, this quality did not alter.  In the white hairs the roots showed no pigment, and the cortex was colourless.  The medulla was very variable, sometimes dark, sometimes pale, often absent, sometimes narrow in the thick hairs and wide in the thin hairs.  Soaking in oil and glycerine, and boiling in water made no alteration in appearance.

(6) The old lady of eighty had had dark hair in youth and had become grey in the early thirties. Her hair used to be of a clearer white than the majority of her hairs at the age of eighty-two, when a considerable number had the yellow tinge to which so many elderly women object. Under the microscope the yellow-tinged hairs showed throughout the cortex a very pale yellow diffused colour, no medulla, no pigment granules, and no trace of pigment at the hair roots. Several of the pure white hairs showed (a) a thick dark medulla, not altered by prolonged soaking in glycerine or in oil, and (b) a very thick cortex, entirely colourless, without granules or any sign of air spaces. Thus the thick white hairs in this lady resembled those of Case 4.

When examining white hairs in Canada balsam one occasionally sees black portions which might be mistaken by a novice for splashes of pigment. Curiously enough, they sometimes occur in the shaft just above the scalp level. The grey-black colour, the absence of granules, the curiously angular outline, are distinctive points in favour of air spaces rather than pigment; and the diagnosis is confirmed when, after the hair has been immersed in oil, these dark blotches are no longer visible. Such hairs, however, remain white. The air spaces had developed because the hair was brittle; their disappearance, with the oil soaking into their cavities, did not remove a screen of air which hid pigment, as in the case of the woman with a lock of white hair (Case 3).

After I had made the above observations I was fortunate enough to read the summary of a research by R. M. Strong[1] on the subject of white hair. His work led him to disagree with the widely accepted theory that hair looks white because of air spaces in the cortex. He states: " Hair and feathers are white for the same reason that powdered ice or glass and other transparent substances in a fine state of division appear white. . . . White in hair and feather structures is due to failure or absence of pigment formation in the follicle before cornification takes place. I know of no critical evidence that either hair or feather structure can become white in any other way."

I was glad to find this summary of a thorough study of white hair, because it provided a convincing explanation of the appearance (so frequently seen when grey and white hairs are observed under the low- and then the high-power lens) of minute, bright spots adjoining the nuclei of the cells of the cortex and recurring at regular intervals along the shaft. These do not disappear on boiling the hair; nor on leaving it to soak in oil or glycerine; they are visible in hairs which have lain in Canada balsam for thirty years; hence I could not believe that they were air spaces. They had rather the appearance of light reflected from glass, as if the cell structure at these sites was very hard, as indeed it is.

[1] R. M. STRONG, "The Causes of Whiteness in Hair and Feathers," *Science*, 1921, N.S. 54, 356.

In dark hair they are probably also present, but are concealed by the thick granules of pigment.

As regards the **yellow tinge** which is so often seen along part of the shaft of grey and white hair, many hairdressers tell their women clients that this is due to " rheumatism," " acidity " or " uric acid." When hairs with a yellow tinge are examined under the microscope, no pigment granules are found. The whole cortex shows a beautiful golden yellow shade, resembling the glow of amber. It is like the yellow diffused pigment often seen in normal grey hairs (see p. 30), except that the shade is more pronounced. This points to pigment extending up from the root, not to deposition of colouring matter from without. Sometimes a yellow colour is caused by the dye coming off the cotton covering of the metal curlers used on damp hair at night. As these curlers are sometimes made of lead, it is probable that these act as a slow dye when their covering is not sufficiently protective. A white-haired man over sixty was suspected of using a dye ; the golden colour was eventually traced to the use of a lotion containing liq. carbonis detergens. Whilst his hair was dark and turning grey in his fifties this colour had not been noticed. Excess of cholesterol was found in the blood of another man. In other cases the colour is due to hair washes which contain lead or other dyes concealed under the innocent title of the bottle label ; see the chapter on hair dyes. Again, simple lotions containing carbolic acid, naphthol or soda, and the tragacanth and other gummy preparations used for stiffening the hair, may in some cases colour the hair shaft. Resorcin in hair lotions is a well-known cause of a yellow colour developing on grey or white hair. In the case of the old lady of eighty (described above), of the above external causes the only one possible was the lotion of weak phenol in glycerine and water which had kept her scalp clean and her hair thick for twenty years.

When the hair is beginning to turn grey, the greyness becomes rapidly much more noticeable if the patient uses lotions containing ammonia or other alkalis, or too high a percentage of spirit. On the other hand, applications of oil delay for a considerable time the appearance of greyness.

**Prematurely grey hair** often runs in families. When the hair begins to turn grey before, or soon after the age of twenty, in healthy people with a healthy scalp there can usually be elicited a history of early greyness in the family. There is no foundation for the popular belief that early greyness is due to a rheumatic diathesis.

The **Albino** shows defective production of pigment on both the body and the head. The hair may be white or have a red or yellow tinge. The pigmentary deficiency is a recessive hereditary feature ; the albino may have normal parents and children.[1]

In **Leucotrichia** or **Poliosis** there is a congenital deficiency or absence of pigment in a localized area.  Sometimes only one lock of hair is grey.  The condition is a dominant hereditary trait ; therefore it appears in several successive generations.

**Ringed Hair** is so rare that many dermatologists have never seen a case.  By reflected light there are seen alternating bands of light and dark hair, of varying width, from 0·2 to 0·6 mm.  A few, many or all of the hairs of the scalp may be affected ; the ringed appearance may not occur along the whole length of the shaft.  The diameter of the hair-shaft is not altered as in monilethrix and trichorrhexis nodosa ; this normal size of the shaft distinguishes Ringed hair from the other conditions with which it has so often been confused.  As a rule the malady begins at birth and it has occurred in several members of a family.

Pincus found pigment was present in the white parts of the hair, but the colour was rendered invisible to the eye because the outer layers of the cortex were loosened, so that air cavities developed between the cells.  These air cavities prevented the light from reaching the more deeply situated coloured region of the hair shaft, but reflected it, so that the hair gave the appearance of being white.  Lee Cady and Mildred Trotter published an important study of Ringed hair [2] confirming what Pincus described.  The portions of the hair which to the eye appeared white were found to be dark by transmitted light, because they were opaque.  The medulla in some of those parts showed expansion.  In other hairs were seen large blotches of darkness, and after the hair had been soaked in 5 per cent. sodium hydroxide, these disappeared, showing that the dark patches had been air cavities, probably containing carbon dioxide.  When the dark patches had been thus dispelled, the ringed appearance of the hair had also vanished.  This treatment had no effect upon normal hairs.  After many tests they concluded that Ringed hair was caused by the presence of gas-filled spaces in the medulla and also in the cortex, which rendered the outer cortical cells opaque and concealed the pigment from the eye.  They concluded that a similar cause may often be in operation in the case of normal white hair.

*Ætiology.*  A certain number of grey hairs often develop in patients who have some form of chronic toxæmia.  Diseases of the intestinal canal in particular have in many cases hastened the onset of canities.  For three years I watched the gradual appearance of grey hairs in a woman over thirty ; within eight months after the removal of her appendix colour was restored to her complexion and to most of her hair.  By the following year, however, she had again many grey hairs.  In two of my patients who had *B. coli* infection (one a woman over forty-five) the hair was much less grey six months after cure in one case, and within

---

[1] COCKAYNE, " Inherited Abnormalities of the Skin and its Appendages," London, 1933, H. Milford.

[2] *Archiv. Derm. and Syph.*, 1922, **6**, 301.

two months in the other. I had details of the case of a middle-aged man whose thick, dark hair turned grey within six months, during which he suffered from progressive malaise and fatigue ; his ill-health was soon afterwards found to be due to malignant disease of the alimentary canal.

Hot climates, malaria, anæmia and tuberculosis have all been credited with causing premature greyness ; on the other hand, such conditions are not usually associated with early greyness. Greyness may accompany both forms of dysfunction of the *thyroid* gland, hyper- and hypothyroidism. With Graves' disease canities, vitiligo and alopecia areata, sometimes even all three together, have been associated. In myxoedema greyness often accompanies the hairfall which is so characteristic in that disease. Premature greyness has been associated with *hypopituitary disorders*, as in Simmonds' disease. Premature greyness has also been attributed · to excessive study, prolonged mental work, anxiety, worry and other causes of lowered vitality ; in some cases the removal of the cause has been accompanied by a return of colour to the hair.

I have observed that unhealthy *local conditions of the scalp* are sometimes accompanied by grey hair. Thus, for example, sparse grey hairs are often seen scattered over the vertex and temples in quite young people whose scalps are affected with pityriasis sicca or with true seborrhœa. In many of these cases there exists also alimentary toxæmia and low vitality. I have seen the natural colour of the hair restored in the younger patients after the local cause had been cured and the general health improved. The *nervous system* can certainly influence the onset of canities, but the method of its action is still obscure. Neuralgia of the fifth nerve has been associated with white hair on the region supplied by the nerve. After hemiplegia canities has been noticed on the paralysed side. Dental trouble has been associated with white hair over the region of the beard supplied by the same nerve. Many of the hairs which remain on *skin which has atrophied*, after over-exposure to X-ray or radium, are white, and never regain colour. Hairs returning on a long-standing alopecia areata patch are usually white at first, and soon become coloured.

Laboratory experiments [1] conducted in different parts of the world point to the importance of *vitamin B deficiency* as a cause of greying of the hair. The vitamin B complex has many constituents ; apparently grey hair is due to the absence of the unknown factor which is at present described as the " filtrate factor " ; this contains both an anti-greying and a growth component. The greying in experiments on rats was preceded by altered texture of the hair ; it became brittle and dry. The

---

[1] A. MORGAN *et al.*, *J. Nutrition*, 1938, **15**, 27, and 1940, **19**, 233.
G. LUNDE and H. KRINGSTED, *J. Nutrition*, 1940, **19**, 321.

depigmentation began in the follicle. Damage was found in the adrenal glands, thyroid, skin and testes of the rats. Cure was sometimes obtained, but slowly, with adrenal gland injections and thyroid ; the real cure came with the administration of vitamin B, especially in the form which exists in certain brands of brewers' yeast, in liver and in rice bran filtrate.

In a series of 800 patients, of both sexes, varying in age from sixteen to seventy-four, Benjamin F. Sieve investigated the effects of para-aminobenzoic acid on achromotrichia.[1] Eighty-two per cent. showed definite response, with darkening and improvement in lustre and texture of the hair. Para-aminobenzoic acid was administered in 100 mg. tablets containing a specially purified grade of the aromatic amine. Best results were obtained by giving 100 mg. three or four times daily, in divided doses, with meals and at bedtime. In achromotrichia, oral was as successful as parenteral medication. It was essential to give the entire vitamin B complex in conjunction with $p$-aminobenzoic acid. The patients took a potent elixir of the vitamin B complex, 5 cc. twice daily, with breakfast and dinner. Darkening of the hair was observed in the majority after six weeks' treatment ; a few showed no change for ten to fifteen weeks ; almost complete darkening required from twelve to eighteen months. When medication was stopped, pigmentation began to recede in four to ten weeks. One tablet twice daily was an adequate maintenance dose. $P$-aminobenzoic acid was ineffective in the presence of a septic focus or endocrine imbalance ; these had to be corrected. The effects produced by $p$-aminobenzoic acid are believed at present to be due to its action on the intestinal flora. Recently Sieve added hydrolysed protein in the form of amino-acids, and the lipoids of whole liver with the vitamin B complex ; these factors enhanced the action of $p$-aminobenzoic acid. He concluded that when endocrine dyscrasia has been corrected, infection eradicated, and substitution vitamin therapy given, a physiological balance is established, and the best results are obtained. $P$-aminobenzoic acid did not act on the hair alone ; it aided brittle finger-nails, certain types of dry skin, and apigmented and hyperpigmented areas of the skin and mucous membranes. The primary reaction to the drug was in most cases a feeling of well-being, increased appetite and bowel activity. At any time when sulphonamide therapy is being taken $p$-aminobenzoic acid must be stopped.

Reports have been published of children and infants with greying, dry, brittle, " staring " hair, and hairfall from temples and vertex. These sufferers

---

[1] BENJAMIN F. SIEVE, *Science*, 1941, **94**, 257 ; and *Med. World*, 1943, **62**, 251 ; *Amer. J. Dig. Dis.*, 1946, **13**, 80 ; 1947, **14**, 16.

were chiefly non-Europeans in tropical America and South Africa ; some have been seen also in parts of Europe where the diet was deficient. In America the dietetic deficiency was not severe enough to cause the other changes noted in South Africa and tropical America—œdema, oral and gastro-intestinal symptoms, such as diarrhœa and steatorrhœa, with enlarged liver, and depigmentation of the skin of the body. A provisional diagnosis was made of pellagra, but feeding with vitamins, especially vitamin B, gave no relief. Indeed, such therapy in subjects with enlarged liver appeared in some victims to aggravate their condition. Hog's stomach, 10 G. daily, brought about dramatic improvement : the œdema disappeared in about a week or 10 days, and the other symptoms soon also were cured. Liver therapy did good, but was not so rapid or dramatic as with hog's stomach.[1] Illustrations of the microscopical changes in the hairs and the livers are given by Chavarria.[2]

Much has been written about the rôle played by the different components of the B complex on grey hair. Rats and chickens fed on a diet low in B complex,[3] but supplemented with synthetic forms of thiamine, riboflavin, nicotinic acid and pyridoxin, showed signs of deficiency, with skin changes. No such signs of deficiency developed when yeast and liver were eaten ; therefore it was deduced that the natural food contains additional members of the B complex. In the so-called filtrate factor of the B complex, panto-thenic acid is present, but the experimenters could not find that the anti-grey hair constituent resided in that acid. Other workers [4] considered that their experimenters on a certain strain of rats pointed to the pantothenic acid as the active cause of the prevention of grey hair. Apparently inositol and p-aminobenzoic acid are both growth factors for yeast or bacteria ; the latter can inhibit the development of bacteria. Nutrition was adequately main-tained on six B factors : thiamine, riboflavin, pyridoxin, choline, niacin and calcium pantothenate. The addition of inositol precipitated a syndrome prevented by p-aminobenzoic acid ; and the addition of p-aminobenzoic acid precipitated a syndrome prevented by inositol. Normal nutrition was main-tained with eight B complex components : the above mentioned six plus inositol and p-aminobenzoic acid. Biotin, another part of the Vitamin B complex, promotes the growth of yeast and many micro-organisms ; its deficiency leads to dermatitis in rats fed on a diet rich in eggwhite. In man a similar dermatitis has been cured by large doses of biotin. It is now obtain-able in synthetic form.[5]

Recently Vitamin $B_{12}$ has been isolated ; its deficiency apparently is pro-ductive of Addisonian anæmia. A distinguished physician told me that after having for nearly a year taken tablets of vitamin B whole complex his grey

[1] GILLMAN, T., and GILLMAN, J., Arch. Int. Med., 1945, 76, 63, and J.A.M.A., 1945, 129, 12.
[2] Chavarria et al., J.A.M.A., 1946, 132, 570.
[3] SULLIVAN, MAURICE and NICHOLLS, Arch. Derm. and Syph., 1942, 45, 917.
[4] MARTIN, Amer. J. Physiol., 1942, 136, 124.
[5] Other references to this complicated subject are : Rosenberg, Chemistry and Physiology of the Vitamins ; Arch. Derm. and Syph. 1941, 43, 230 ; J.A.M.A., 1942, 118, 1199 ; Lancet, 1944, i, 826. A good summary of the constituents of the vitamin B complex is given by H. M. Sinclair, The Practitioner, 1949, 162, 235.

hair had become markedly darker. Another medical man, a victim to asthma all his life, had been obliged to take daily adrenalin medication ; although his family history was one of early baldness he retained thick dark hair after the age of sixty. He knew three other asthmatic friends with exactly similar experience. This led him to question : does adrenalin affect the growth and the pigmentation of the hair ? H. W. Barber tells me that he has noticed that allergic patients with the asthma-prurigo complex often retain colour in their hair.

Many explanations of sudden and rapid blanching of the hair have been advanced. Some maintain that the altered circulation allows loosening of the cells and thus air enters the spaces between the cells of the cortex, that these reflect the light and cause the hair to appear white, although there may still be pigment present. This may be true in a few cases, just as was found in the apparent white portions of Ringed hair (see above) and in Case 3 which I describe on page 30. Jackson stated that the change of colour is due to air bubbles in the cortex rendering the cortex opaque, and so hiding the pigment. He added : " This is proved by placing one of the affected hairs in hot water, ether or turpentine, when the air bubbles will be driven out and the hair will resume its natural colour." [1]  However, in his description of sudden as distinguished from unduly rapid blanching of the hair, he, like other dermatologists, does not quote cases which have come under his personal observation.

It seems a reasonable theory that with sudden and profound emotion there may occur constriction of the vessels supplying the hair papillæ, and that when these cells are deprived of their normal nutriment their function of pigment formation must be in abeyance. Dr. William Brown frequently noticed that the hair of shell shock patients became definitely more grey within two weeks after the shattering crisis, too short a time for the growth of new grey hairs. See also Sir Arthur Hurst's observations (p. 28).

With *prolonged* depressing emotion the changes in the circulation resemble those produced by disease and by age ; the slow decrease of pigment formation and alteration of the cortex cells in such conditions is readily understood. A more scientific explanation has been provided by the observation that Simmonds' disease (often associated with greyness) may follow sudden shock. It is probable that this effect is due to interference with the hypothalamic pituitary relationship. The hair has for too long been regarded as a dead object from the time it reaches the level of the skin. May not the medulla be a channel along which the hair shaft can receive nourishment and pigment ? Its structure, with its

---

[1] I have boiled many ordinary grey and white hairs in water and never found any restoration of colour gained by thus driving out air.

loose cells and definite cavities, lends itself to this function. In the event of sudden deprivation of circulation in the papilla, the medulla may absorb the fluid pigment from the cortex and may convey no further supply from below ; this would account for rapid greying of the appearance of the hair. Future research will determine whether this occurs more rapidly in hairs which have a medulla than in those which have none. Other arguments against the hypothesis of the hair being regarded as a dead object are : (1) Cut and singed hair ends behave as if they still had life (pages 47 to 52) ; (2) repigmentation of white hair has been watched in alopecia areata and similar cases ; and (3) the appearance and diameter of the hair varies with health and with constitutional disease (p. 16).

**Treatment of Canities.** Most cases do not consult the physician until they are beyond the stage when treatment can benefit the colour of the hair. Where obvious disease of the scalp is present, with correct local treatment the greyness can be arrested and in young people the colour of the hair as a whole is restored temporarily, if not permanently. When white hairs begin to appear in the twenties, treatment seems at first to be effective ; but I have been impressed by the fact that in several of these young patients, whom I had the opportunity of observing after a few years' interval, the greyness had soon returned. The general health must be attended to in every case. I attribute great importance to the correction of constipation and other causes of toxæmia, the removal of septic foci and especially to a diet with adequate vitamin content. In thyroid deficiency small doses of this gland can work wonders. Massage, which improves the circulation and the nutrition of the hair papillæ, is a most important therapeutic measure. The massage must not be perfunctory, but accompanied by movement of the scalp, as described in the section on the care of the hair (p. 47). Oily applications to the hair, and massage of the scalp with oil, make grey hair look darker and postpone the appearance of ageing for a time. Exposure to the mercury vapour lamp certainly appears to darken grey hair, though apparently only for a short time, a few hours or days. This effect may be due to the action of the ultra-violet rays upon the oil of the hair. Exposure, half an hour per week, to strong heat appears to improve the colour of grey hair for a time. On the other hand, Sabouraud mentioned that some of the adventurers on Polar expeditions regained colour in their hair ; but this might be due to improved health. Of drugs, pilocarpine appears to have a definite darkening effect on the hair of certain patients ; this is discussed on page 41. However, recent work on the effect of Vitamin B therapy (discussed in the paragraph on Aetiology) may, if confirmed, revolutionize the treatment of canities. Dyes can be advised only in special circumstances; see Chapter XIX.

## Altered Colour of the Hair.

In canities the colour of the hair is diminished or lost. The reverse process, the restoration of the colour of hair, can also occur. After an illness such as typhoid fever, where there is a profuse fall of hair, the new hair sometimes comes in darker than the old growth. Occasionally this phenomenon occurs after epilation by X-ray, and after keeping the hair shaved for a time. In old people with white hair there is sometimes a return of colour in a number of hairs of the scalp ; I have reliable accounts of several such cases, from both friends and patients, and see the case of Dr. Isdell quoted on page 27. I knew one lady who at fifty-nine had white hair except over the occipital region, where she had a quantity of very dark brown hair ; originally her hair had all been fair. The white hairs of alopecia areata become repigmented. The feathers of birds often change from light to dark or vice versa ; the cause of this alteration in colour has been found in some cases to be due to the lacunæ becoming filled with a reddish oily fluid. When those feathers were dried the colour was bleached, and then these lacunæ were found to be filled with air.

G. W. Griffiths [1] reported the case of a fire engineer aged sixty-five. He was exposed while on duty to exceeding cold—north wind and the spray from his hose blowing on his helmet—so that the eyebrows and whiskers were frozen stiff. Next day he was exhausted, and in the afternoon his hair turned black. Dr. Griffiths had known the man for forty years and could vouch that he had had white hair for three years, and before that time, eight years of grey hair following a life with blond hair. The hair, at the time of the report, remained black and oily. In his article Griffiths quotes several cases of altered colour of the hair which had been published in medical papers. In one lady the hair whitened in six days after three weeks of fever, began to darken again on the seventh day and returned to its original colour by the end of the week.

Jackson's case is referred to on page 28 ; here the return of colour took place several times. Many observers have reported alterations of colour, usually to a lighter shade, occurring during periods of acute mental outbreaks and during acute illness.

Pautier and Woringer [2] had a patient with multiple tumours on the scalp which had been improved by treatment with X-ray. It was

---

[1] *J. Cutan. and Genito-Urin. Dis.*, 1895, **13**, 376.
[2] *Bull. soc. franç. de derm. et syph.*, 1933, **40**, 1535.

uncertain whether the swellings were sarcomatous. Much of the hair over the tumours had fallen out, and of that remaining much had been grey. Although the patient was aged sixty-two, some months after the treatment with X-ray considerable re-growth of hair had occurred, and was no longer grey, but deep chestnut in colour. Dr. Smyly [1] narrated the case of a child who at the age of four months developed paralysis of the left side of the face and palate together with exophthalmos, consequent upon suppuration of the left temporal bone. One morning the hair on the right side of the scalp and right eyebrow was seen to have changed from its usual mousey brown to a red-yellow colour. The skin of these parts and of the right hand was icteric and the pillow was stained yellow with the perspiration.

*Pilocarpine* aids the nutrition of the hair so that it becomes darker and thicker. The following case illustrates this point :

Prentiss [2] records the case of a lady aged twenty-five, to whom pilocarpine had been given for the condition of her kidney, in 1 cg. doses, increasing up to 2 cg. daily, between December 10, 1880, and February 22, 1881. The hair at the beginning of the course of treatment was light yellow. Darkening of the colour of the hair began to be noticed by December 28. By January 12 the hair was a chestnut-brown shade ; by May, it was thicker, coarser, almost pure black in colour. Some years later, in the reports of the International Medical Congress,[3] Dr. Prentiss again described this case and stated that the hair had remained dark brown.

Another similar case of darkening of the hair under the influence of the same drug was reported as having occurred in a lady aged seventy-two. The hair and eyebrows had been white for twenty years. She developed Bright's disease, and to relieve itching 20 to 30 drops of a fluid extract of jaborandi had been taken several times a day, from October, 1866, to February, 1888. By the autumn of 1887 the eyebrows and the hair of the head showed dark patches, and gradually became darker till, at the death of the patient, they were black. Microscopic examination of the dark hair proved that the colour was due to increase of the pigment of the hair and not to the application of a dye. Jackson gave a patient with white hair a lotion containing 20 gr. pilocarpine in 8 oz. of fluid. After a few weeks' use of the application the hair became dark near the scalp.

Exposure to strong sunlight often gives golden tints to dark hair.

[1] *The Medical Press and Circular*, N.S. **35**, 184.
[2] *Philad. Med. Times*, 1880–1881, **11**, 609.
[3] *Internat. Nat. Congress*, Berlin, 1890, **4**, Abt. XIII, 24.

Grey hair sometimes darkens temporarily under exposure to sunlight, natural or artificial.

The use of ammonia in hair lotions makes greying hair after a short time look more grey ; but dark hair in the young may with the same lotion take on bright chestnut tints.

Alterations of colour of the hair have occurred in workers with copper, indigo, cobalt and other metals. Copper-workers may have bright green hair, due to the deposit of a fine dust of copper crystals. Workers dealing with cobalt and indigo may develop blue hair, and it is obvious that coal and soot depositing on the hair make it look black. In argyria, the silver in the hair in some cases lends to it a silvery sheen.

Alterations of colour may occur with drugs employed during the treatment of certain conditions of the scalp. Thus, for example, it is well known that the use of resorcin in hair lotions can turn fair hair and white hair to various shades of yellow. If bicarbonate of soda is used, in local applications to the scalp, dark hair in time turns auburn or brown. Tar lotions used on white hair have sometimes given the hair a golden shade. (See p. 33.) Hairdressers add a blue colouring powder to the ingredients used when washing grey and white hair. Naphthol gives a bright yellow hue to white hair. Chlorine bleaches the hair ; chrysarobin turns it red-brown. When ringworm is treated with ointments containing copper, the hair takes on a bright blue-green shade. Billi [1] reported a case in which a lotion of bichloride of mercury was followed by an ointment of yellow oxide of mercury ; the hair became vivid green. Certain methods of permanent waving darken grey hair. This has also occurred after mercurial lotions have been in use before the waving process.

The subject of hair dyes is dealt with in Chapter XIX.

[1] *Ann. de derm. et syph.*, 1872, **4**, 138.

# CHAPTER III

# CARE OF THE HAIR

Brushing and combing—Massage—Cutting and singeing—Washing and cleaning—Artificial curling and waving—Formulæ.

**Brushing and Combing the Hair.** Correct use of the HAIR BRUSH plays an important part in the health of the scalp as well as the appearance of the hair. A brush should have firm and well-spaced groups of bristles. The bristles should vary in length and should be graded so that the longest are in the centre of every group. This arrangement of the bristles permits more even and deep penetration of the brush through the hair to the scalp. Some nylon brushes abrade the scalp and can break long and dry hair. Wire brushes may be used with short hair, but tend to cause tangling of long hairs and injury to the scalp. The frame may be of wood, vulcanite, ivory or metal ; the material of the frame ought to be able to resist the cleaning which is frequently necessary. Metal frames, which are unaffected by ordinary washing, are more useful than wood, which is readily stained by careless methods of cleaning. Sometimes the bristles are set in a resilient layer of rubber attached to a frame.

An ordinary hair brush can be washed in soap and water. The bottom of a wide basin is covered with hot water to such a depth that when the brush is plunged into it, with the bristles downwards, the fluid scarcely reaches the level of the frame. If the water is too deep, it comes in contact with the frame and loosens the glue which attaches the bristles to the frame. The water must not be boiling ; too high a temperature spoils the bristles. A soapy foam is made by stirring in soap or soap flakes ; then the brush is vigorously beaten up and down in the basin. If the water becomes very dirty, a second quantity of soapy water must be used, and the process repeated until the brush looks clean. The soap must then be removed from the bristles by rinsing the brush in cold water. If the wooden frame has become marked by its immersion in the water some form of oil polish can be rubbed in. If brushes are too frequently wet with water the bristles become softened ; boiling water for washing is not permissible except in the case of a wire brush. The process of drying should not be hurried ; the brush can be exposed to the sun, or laid on a towel not too near hot pipes or a fire. Some clean their brushes with special spirit and sulphonated oil preparations.

A brush should be reserved for the use of a single individual. If it has been used by several people or by any person with dandruff or other disease, disinfection must be carried out by plunging the brush into boiling water. This is easy only in the case of a metal brush. Brushes should therefore be used solely by their owners ; in this case the frame of the brush may consist of ivory or other decorative material. It is not widely enough known that even dandruff can be conveyed to those who use brushes and combs belonging to individuals whose scalp harbours the malady. It is safer never to lend brushes and combs, because even when no definite disease of the hair and scalp is visible to casual inspection, dandruff or early ringworm may be present. A brush which has been lent to anyone should be thoroughly cleaned before being used again by its owner.

Hairdressers should employ freshly cleaned brushes and combs for every client ; no exception to this rule should ever be permitted. For this reason they should use only a type of brush which can be easily and thoroughly cleansed. Brushes of metal, with wire bristles, can be quickly cleaned in boiling water, and they dry rapidly when the water is shaken off. Hence metal brushes are preferable when frequent washing is necessary, as in hairdressing establishments. When disease of the scalp is suspected, the metal brush can be easily sterilized. However, as wire brushes are inadvisable with long hair and a diseased scalp, far the safest plan is that all clients should take their own brushes and combs when they visit the barber or the hairdresser.

When it becomes known that a brush has been used on a scalp with a disease so serious as ringworm, the brush should be destroyed. The hairdresser dare not run the risk of using such a brush again. A clean towel or paper must always be placed on the back of the chair for the head to lean upon. Hairdressers should wash the fingers in water and a disinfectant soap before every new visitor.

For the adequate care of the scalp and the arrangement of the hair a COMB is a tool as essential as a brush. The comb is required also for the purpose of arranging a straight parting of the hair. Combs are made of horn, vulcanite, wood, ivory, tortoiseshell and metal. Horn frequently breaks, leaving a jagged edge which frays or even breaks the hair. The teeth of a comb should be evenly spaced, not too close together, and their free ends must be blunt and smooth. Too pointed teeth may scratch the scalp ; they have caused wounds, which became septic and led to boils and carbuncles. Teeth of uneven length may cause tearing and tangling of the hair. All precautions against infection must be taken with the comb as with the brush. Dandruff is due to a micro-organism (see p. 162) and can be conveyed by a comb as well as by a brush. The comb must be frequently washed in hot soft water and soap. With a coarse, hard, short brush, such as a nail brush, it can be freed from the thick deposit of grease, dust, soot and scales which soon collect on its teeth. Scrubbing with a weak solution of ammonia or with spirit is also effective.

*Brushing the hair* achieves several desirable results. The individual hairs lie more smoothly. The natural oil is distributed more evenly, and as light is reflected from regularly arranged hair the coiffure looks more glossy than does unbrushed, untidy hair. Still more important is the fact that the circulation of the scalp is stimulated by vigorous brushing with firm bristles. When the scalp is brushed, the bristles should create a warm, tingling sensation on the skin. After the scalp has received vigorous brushing, the hair has to be treated with care.

The method of brushing the hair requires consideration :—Force must never be used when brushing or combing. When the hair is very long or very thick, when it is tangled, when it has become too dry, as with certain methods of " permanent waving," and when it is falling profusely, the brush should not be drawn rapidly down in one long stroke from the scalp to the hair ends. Instead, the following method of combing or brushing should be carried out. With the comb and fingers the hair is divided into several strands. Then while the left hand holds a lock of hair a few inches above its free end, the right hand sweeps the brush downwards from just below the left hand. When the free end is thus smoothed out, the left hand grasps the tresses a few inches higher up and this fresh part is brushed downward till it is smooth. The process is repeated till at length the scalp is reached, when the brush can make a long, deliberate sweep down the whole length of the hair. If the usual modern method is adopted in cases of tangled hair, the brush being brought quickly down all the way from the scalp, without any preliminary smoothing of the free ends, tearing and breaking of the individual hairs is caused ; knots are formed which can never be unravelled, but must be cut out ; and when there is hairfall, the fall is precipitated, even the young hairs being torn out by the roots.

The same criticism holds in regard to the method of *combing the hair.* The average assistant in the hairdressing establishment attacks the tangled hair from the scalp. With a strong jerking motion she forces the comb from the scalp a few inches downward ; then on encountering an obstacle or a knot, she jerks the comb upward and outward ; again drags the instrument down a further two inches, and again jerks it away. After several such forcible attacks she succeeds in dragging the comb down to the free end, filled with broken and knotted strands of hair. Tearing out and breaking long hair can be avoided by adopting the correct method of combing which the modern hairdresser has little opportunity to learn in these days of short or shingled hair. The comb should be used gently in the same way as the brush. With the left hand holding a tress 2 inches above the free end, the right hand combs carefully and slowly down till the tress is quite smooth. Then the tress is grasped 2 inches higher up, and the process is repeated, and so on until at length the comb can be passed all the way down from the scalp to the waist, if the hair is long, without encountering any obstacle.

Combing some of the hair upward, from the free ends, is sometimes carried out in order to convey an appearance of more abundant hair. This method used to be called " French combing." It is in itself harmless, but care must be taken lest the hair be tangled or broken when it has again to be smoothed downward.

In Victorian times girls were taught to give every night a hundred strokes of the brush, from the scalp to the free ends of their long tresses ; in frosty weather the hair stood out like a halo and crackled with the electricity induced. The hair can also with advantage be brushed at such an angle that the stroke draws the hair from the scalp. This conveys a stimulating glow and causes the individual hairs to separate and stand out. The ordinary method of brushing downward, in the direction of the hair, causes the hair shafts to lie close together, flat on the scalp, whereas the separation of the hairs caused by brushing away from the scalp gives an impression of abundant hair. For patients who are pessimistic about their hair this method of brushing restores hope. The apparent luxuriance has no basis in fact, but the average individual is more concerned with the appearance than the reality.

I sum up this section by quoting the opinion of Erasmus Wilson. Since his day (1853) little that is new has been discovered concerning the subject of hair brushing. He writes : " There are two purposes to be obtained by brushing ; firstly, to give health to the skin of the head, and strength and vigour to the hair ; for which end you cannot brush too much or use brushes too penetrating or too hard, such as will produce active friction of the skin ; secondly, to smooth the hair, or perhaps go to the length of freeing it from dust, for which object your brushes may be as soft as you please and your hand as light as is agreeable." He quotes with approval the hairdresser who said : " You cannot brush the head too much, or the hair too little." With the fashion of short hair prevalent to-day, the hard, coarse brush, which makes the scalp tingle, is rightly in high favour. With long hair, if such a brush is drawn rapidly down the tresses, the hair is apt to be stretched, torn and tangled. Coarse, hard bristles and wire brushes may abrade a healthy scalp and have caused extension of an existing dermatitis (Adamson).

**Massage of the scalp** is of supreme importance for the preservation of the circulation on which the hair papilla depends. This subject is dealt with at length in the section on Diffuse Hairfall (p. 91). Suffice it to state here that the scalp should be massaged over the skull, and thus kept freely movable, at least once a day. Even two minutes a day will make a marked difference to the health of the hair.

**Cutting the Hair.** I have been unable to find any scientific proof of the popular idea that the hair of children and women is strengthened by cutting it short. Many mothers have told me that when a child has been delicate and had a poor head of hair, the hair was cut and kept short for several years; and that when allowed to grow again, it was greatly improved; in some cases it had even grown in curly. The same phenomenon has been observed after epilation with X-ray; thin straight hair has returned black and curly, but usually the curls do not remain long. After X-ray epilation I have also seen the reverse occur; no adequate explanation for these diverse facts is at present available. In a large family of children it is impossible to devote the time and care necessary to brush and otherwise care for the head with poor hair, in the hope of ensuring a stronger growth. For the past twenty-five years busy women have complained that they have not time to brush and comb long hair. To such women, though sceptical as to the real reason of the preference for short hair, I reply that it is better to cut the hair; as this simplifies the care of the scalp, the growth of the hair would be given every chance of improving in the future.

It is often said that cutting the hair hastens growth. Pincus carried out careful experiments on healthy subjects. He cut off circles of hair on the scalps of men and measured the rate of growth of hair on the shorn and the unshorn neighbouring areas. He found that the hair grew less rapidly on the shorn areas. Recent research bears out this observation (see remarks on this subject in Chapter I, p. 18). Erasmus Wilson had interesting theories on the best method of hair cutting. Long hairs, he said, which have split ends, should be cut. Where there are many hairs in poor condition an excellent result is obtained by treating the head and pruning the hair as a gardener does his roses—cutting some, like the strong branches, near the ends; others, which are weakly, near the scalp; and plucking out the very poor ones by the roots.

**Singeing the Hair.** I can find no scientific proof of the value of this popular procedure. Split hair points are better cut than singed. The heat of singeing tends to dry the hair shaft higher up. The public are told that singeing the hair seals up the cut ends and " prevents the juices of the hair from running out." I have made many microscopical examinations, with low- and high-power lenses, of cut and of singed ends of hair taken from the heads of both young and old people. The examinations were carried out immediately after the hair had been cut or singed, two to four days, two, five, six, seven and nine weeks, and six months later ; the results are described below.

MICROSCOPICAL APPEARANCE OF CUT HAIR : If the scissors are sharp, and the cut is made rapidly and cleanly, the severed part, within half an hour of the operation, usually looks straight or oblique. However, some cut hairs show a jagged edge with a few frayed ends of the cortex and

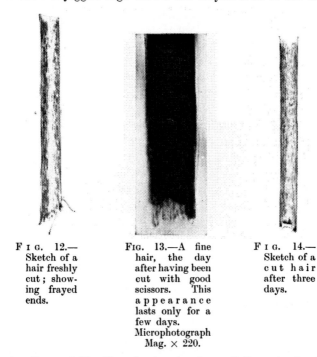

F I G. 12.— Sketch of a hair freshly cut ; showing frayed ends.

FIG. 13.—A fine hair, the day after having been cut with good scissors. This appearance lasts only for a few days. Microphotograph Mag. × 220.

F I G. 14.— Sketch of a cut hair after three days.

cuticle standing out like threads straying beyond the cut edge (Fig. 12). If these cut ends are examined two or three days later, the majority show several square-topped lines jutting out from the free cut end of the hair, like small towers along a wall (Fig. 13). At a first glance the impression is that the lines (cortex longitudinal cells) are growing out, trying to join and form a new point. On examination one, three and five weeks later, one sees that these uneven lines of cortex cells have disappeared ; the cuticle and the outer layers of the cortex appear to have fallen inwards, as if the cells were folding over the cut ends ; the medulla remains unaltered. Exactly the same rounded-off ends were seen in a tress of hair which had been cut six months previously. The microscopic picture no longer showed an irregular angularity, with thin, straying threads, but a hair terminal which gently curved inwards, and in the majority of cases remained flat in the middle (Fig. 15). No attempt to grow again to a point was visible in any hair, but in quite a number the newly formed end had a completely rounded termination. After examining many hairs from different women, I could distinguish clearly the freshly cut ends and the distal ends which had been cut weeks and months before.

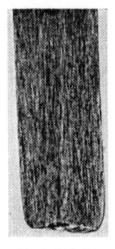 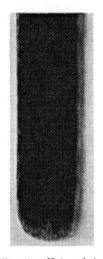

FIG. 15.—A thick hair end four weeks after having been cut. Many show this appearance in a week, and some show a similar appearance months later. Microphotograph Mag. × 220.

FIG. 16.—Hair end six months after being cut. Only a few hairs show such a completely rounded-off rejuvenated end. Microphotograph Mag. × 220.

In only a few hairs, cut four and six months previously, did I see the distal ends with a blunt nose, rounded like a bullet (Fig. 16).

For this experiment all the hairs were cut with the same pair of scissors, of the type used by hospital nurses ; such an instrument has wide, but sharp blades. For the purpose of comparison, other hairs were cut with very sharp manicure scissors ; when cut by such delicate blades, the hairs showed a much less frayed outline. Indeed, in the case of a girl of thirteen, whose hairs were of exceptionally fine diameter, it was difficult to distinguish the freshly-cut parts from the tips which had been severed three weeks previously.

Figs. 12 to 15 were taken from hairs which had never been permanently waved, curled or twisted. The hairs of Fig. 16 had had a permanent wave six months before, but this may have no bearing on their appearance.

Microscopical Appearance of Singed Hair. A grey-haired woman allowed me to cut an inch off the end of the hair on one side of the head ; the hair on the other side was singed. Grey hair was chosen because the absence of pigment allowed a clear view of the burnt portions of hair. Specimens of the singed hair were taken at varying intervals. Fig. 17 shows the immediate charring, which extends a considerable distance up the shaft. This hair was cut off ¾ inch above its singed end, placed in Canada balsam and photographed within a quarter of an hour of the singeing. Fig. 18 shows the charred condition of an adjacent hair

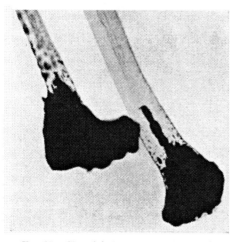

Fig. 17.—Singed hair twenty minutes after.
Microphotograph Mag. × 100.

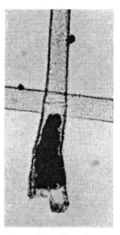

Fig. 18.—Singed grey hair fifteen days later. A typical picture, showing how the charred portion extends into the substance of the hair, with distension of the cortex. Microphotograph Mag. × about 60.

end fifteen days later : there are bubbles of gas among the black particles, the hair shaft is distended, and the free end broken up. Fig. 19 shows the condition of adjacent hair twenty-eight days after singeing ; there are still charred particles and gas cavities, and the free end is swollen and broken. Fig. 20 shows an unusual picture of a hair thirty-six days after singeing ; the charred portion extends up the medulla, whilst the cortex and medulla remain clear. This feature of clear cortex and cuticle was seen in only a few of the hairs examined ; the picture suggests that the gas evolved during the singeing has pushed up some of the scorched dead particles along the loose structure of the medulla. By the fifth week, it was noticeable that many of the hairs on the singed side of the head had split ends and in contrast, decidedly fewer hairs of the other side of the head, where the hairs had been cut, showed split ends. By the sixth and seventh week, the picture of the majority of the singed hairs which had not split resembled that seen after twenty-eight days, except that there were fewer charred particles. By the ninth week, the charred portions had separated off; the terminals still showed a distended swollen condition (see Fig. 21).

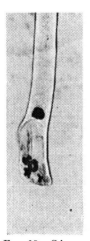 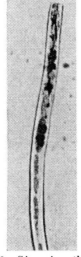 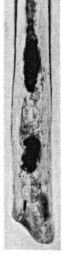

FIG. 19.—S i n g e d grey hair twenty-eight days after. Shows gas bubbles and healing of charred hair end. Microphotograph Mag. × 60.

FIG. 20.—S i n g e i n g thirty-six days later. In this picture the hair shows a large medulla. The gas evolved in singeing has pushed the charred portions up the channel of loose medullary cells. Hence there is less distension of the cortex, and the hair does not break up. Microphotograph Mag. × 60.

FIG. 21.—Singed hair after more t h a n  t h r e e months. Note healed rounded end and extension up medulla of the c h a r r e d portions, or of gas. Microphotograph Mag. × 120.

After three months, many of the singed ends presented an appearance exactly like that of six weeks before. However, another feature was noticed : the ends of hairs cut from the singed side of the head showed several black blotches, at varying intervals, in a colourless medulla. These extended up to 1 and 1½ inches from the singed tip ; at a distance higher than 2 inches they were not seen in any of the hairs. On the other side of the head, on which no hairs had been singed, no similar black spots were visible. As the dark spots in no way resembled the small patches of pigment often seen lying in a clear medulla, I believed that they were carbon particles absorbed from the singed ends. But, on examining the hairs after they had lain for four days in a somewhat fluid Canada balsam, to my surprise I could not see a single remaining black spot; this proved that the unusual appearance had been due not to carbon, but to gas.

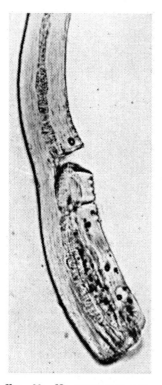

This phenomenon confirmed the opinion I had formed on examining the hairs a week after they had been singed, i.e. that in hairs with a wide medulla, bubbles of gas readily pass a certain distance up the loose cell structure. This feature is suggestive; research on the subject may shed light on the effect of local applications to the cut ends of hair shafts. Fig. 22 shows an unusual picture of a transverse break above a portion of hair with many gas bubbles. This hair had never been permanently waved, nor had it been touched with curling tongs or any local form of treatment.

Even in the case of singed hair, nature usually steps in and softens the original harsh outlines of the broadened ends which remain when the charred portion and the gas bubbles have fallen away or in part extended up the medullary canal. In three months these wide ends often show the healed, rounded-off appearance which follows ordinary cutting (see Fig. 21).

Fig. 22.—No permanent wave nor any curling process had ever been carried out on this hair. Singed hair (after three and a half months) showing transverse fracture (very rare) and gas bubbles extending upwards. Microphotograph Mag. × 200.

**Washing the Hair.** One is often questioned on this subject. Should the hair be frequently washed? at how long intervals? and what is the best method of cleansing the hair?

In this country one is accustomed to see men washing their heads practically every morning; women wash their head on an average between once a week and once a month. In modern days women tend to have their hair washed when their " wave " requires attention from the hairdresser. If the hair is well brushed and combed, and the brush and comb kept scrupulously clean, frequent washing is not so necessary as is usually supposed. In Southern climes, where the hair of women is remarkable for its luxuriance, length and gloss, washing is but rarely performed ; in many cases not more than once in many years. I have first-hand information concerning two ladies whose beautiful hair has never been washed since girlhood. It is injurious to have the hair constantly moist ; this has been proved by the recent work on animal hairs and textile fabrics. If, however, the hair is properly dried, no harm accrues. I heard of a lady whose long hair was washed every day ; after many years it remains in excellent condition.

When the hair is thin and very oily, it is necessary to cleanse it more often than when the scalp is dry and the hair coarse. Unless the hair is very thick there is no reason why it should not be washed at home. Some hairdressers concentrate on cleaning the hair and deal only perfunctorily with the skin of the scalp. In smoky towns, women who have fair or white hair find that they usually wash more often than those who have dark hair which does not show the blackening effect of dust and smoke. On the other hand, I observed for many years a lady who lived in London, and whose hair remained exquisitely white and the scalp spotlessly clean ; she never washed the head, but devoted considerable time daily to brushing, combing and rubbing the scalp and often used a lotion with phenol in spirit and water.

However, most women living and working in a dirty city atmosphere desire to cleanse the hair and scalp on an average once every month. For this purpose a lather of soap in plain hot water can be used. It is advisable to use a super-fatted soap, because it has no free alkali. Soap should not be used if the client has recently applied a remedy containing resorcin. It is often difficult to dress the hair after washing with soap and hard water. Soft water gives a different effect, because it leaves no deposit to be rinsed off. The removal of this deposit is aided by adding to the rinsing water a little dilute acetic acid or lemon juice. After rain-water washing, the hair has a beautiful gloss. Hebra's soap used to be a favourite shampoo ; it contained equal parts of soft soap, rectified spirit and spirit of lavender. To-day expense renders it impossible to use rectified spirit in such quantity ; surgical spirit or Lotio Sapo kalinus is ordered instead. The lotion is well rubbed into the scalp ; it does not make a good lather, but is a good cleanser. It is finally rinsed off, preferably in soft or rain water.

The " soapless shampoos " of modern manufacture are considered on page 54.

It has long been known that a *beaten-up egg* forms a cleansing substance which renders the hair particularly glossy. The egg can be poured over the scalp many times, then rinsed off with plain warm water. I prefer the use of the whole egg, but authorities differ, some advising only the yolk, others only the white of the egg. Pincus stated that the yolk of the egg was difficult to rinse off, and recommended therefore only the white of the egg. *Tincture of quillaia* (1 in 20) with water is an excellent shampoo, although it does not make a free lather. It is a natural soap obtained from tree bark. It is often the basis of the so-called " dry shampoo."

*The Dry Shampoo.* The so-called dry shampoo is not really dry, but its title is derived from the fact that no water is used in the composition of its liquid. The dry shampoo is a method of cleansing by means of spirit. Spirit has the advantage that after its use the hair dries rapidly. Provided that the dry shampoo is composed of good spirit and is correctly applied, it is an efficient cleanser of the hair and scalp. Various forms of spirit have been tested. Carbon tetrachloride had only a brief vogue ; its fumes caused some serious accidents. The inflammability of petrol vapour led to the discontinuance of that form of spirit. A smaller proportion of soap is used in the dry shampoo than in Soap spirit (B.P.C.), because when water is not employed, less soap is needed. The form of alcohol commonly used in the dry shampoo is Industrial spirit, which does not contain pyridine. The methylated spirit variety, which contains pyridine, is an irritant to the skin ; therefore it should never be used for the dry shampoo. Certain dry shampoos have caused irritation of the scalp. For effective cleansing the dry shampoo should be carried out only by experts. The success of the process depends upon the correct manner of massaging in the spirit, and the use of just the right amount of fluid. A hand skilled in the use of the towel is needed for the removal of the dirt and the drying of the hair.

*Shampoo powders* are much favoured in districts where the water is hard ; they contain ingredients for water softening, and hence enable the hair to be more readily cleansed than with plain hard water and soap. Shampoo powders used to consist of powdered soap and a small amount of alkalis and borax. Many powders had so much alkali that they injured dry hair. The best chemists endeavoured to remove this defect, with the result that some shampoo powders are beyond reproach in the matter of alkalinity.

*The soapless shampoo.* Recently, soap has been replaced by various cleansing agents, such as the sulphonated oils and the sulphonated higher fatty alcohols, especially lauryl, stearyl and cetyl alcohol. When used with hard water they do not leave a precipitate, as soap does, and their cleansing property is superior to that of soap. They have the disadvantage that they have a defatting action on the skin, less marked with the fatty alcohols than with the sulphonated oils. An experienced hair-dresser tells me that after their frequent use the skin of the scalp becomes scaly and the hair becomes sparse, as if new roots did not form. I agree about the scaling (see p. 161). Housewives confirm this experience after using sulphonated oil to clean their hands soiled with dust, dirt and garden mould. These cleansing agents are termed detergents ; cetavlon 2 to 5 per cent. is an effective type. A small amount of fluid is spread on the scalp, water is added till the hair is thoroughly soaked ; the scalp is well rubbed and all is rinsed off in clean water. There is not so much lather as with soap.

When *drying the hair*, use as little friction as possible, because moist hair in some cases is more readily broken than dry hair. Spread the hair out on a warm dry towel and expose it to the sun or to a warm lamp or the fire. A hot-air fan can be used when the instrument is at hand. Avoid great concentrated heat, as it is too drying.

*Powder* provides a method of cleansing the head without the use of fluid. Women who have very greasy or long hair often find that by the use of powder the tiresome process of frequent washing can be postponed. They dust over the scalp with crushed cold water starch or with plain talc ; then brush off the powder. The two ladies referred to on p. 53 had never washed their hair with water during their adult lives ; instead, they had used powder for cleansing.

Bathing in sea water is not injurious for the hair, but as salt water is sticky, after the bathe the salt water should be rinsed off with plain water.

**Artificial Curling of the Hair.** Throughout the ages we find a widespread preference for curly hair. Many of the ancient Greek and Roman statues show a regularly waved and curled coiffure which would do credit to the most fashionable modern woman. As a general rule, curling hair is more becoming, whilst to the plain face it provides a beauty which the features lack. A popular " anti-kink " method has been invented for straightening the fuzzy type of hair curl seen in black races, but this does not negative the fact that most women consider curly hair more beautiful than straight. Fortunate, therefore, are those who are born with curly hair. In the section on the anatomy of the hair (p. 1) it is stated that naturally curly hair has usually a flattened or oval form of hair shaft, whilst the straight hair is circular in diameter. It is not known how much the fact of curliness depends upon that feature. When the follicle of the hair has a twist, the cells growing up from the papilla probably push up more on one side than another ; this may lead to the formation of a shaft which, as it grows outward and upward, would tend to turn in a spiral wave. After acute illnesses with profuse hairfall, and after X-ray epilation, straight hair has sometimes grown in curly. As a rule, this alteration does not last ; the hair soon returns to its original straightness. This fact points to modification in the papilla or in the bulb rather than in the canal of the follicle, as the origin of the curling hair shaft.

Of the various methods employed in the attempt to produce the appearance of natural curls, the safest are those which bend the hair shaft when moist, and hold it in the induced position till it is dry. In order to understand the mechanism and the rationale underlying the production of artificial curls and waves the reader must study Chapter IV, which is written by Mr. W. T. Astbury. Here I shall only describe the means which women use ; I shall not attempt to explain their mode of action.

The most simple methods are those in which strands of hair are moistened with water and tightly bound round a metal pin, clamped in position and retained thus till the hair is dry. Or the hair may be bound round a strip of leather, or of lead covered with cotton fabric, the ends of the strip being twisted together. Notwithstanding the amusing appearance presented at bedtime by little rolls of tissue paper along the forehead, I believe that some women still prefer the old-fashioned curling-papers. After being unbound from these various devices, the hair springs free and retains its curl for a day. With straight hair the process must be repeated every night. The modern " water wave " has the same principle underlying its formation. The hair is moistened and, whilst still wet, is arranged with curved combs or metal " grips " pushed into position so as to form regular waves along the head. The hair is then dried rapidly, and after the removal of the combs, the waves remain. Such waves may not have the wayward and changeable charm of natural curls, but they present a formal regularity which has an attraction of its own.

Curling-tongs have their advocates. They act quickly and when care is taken not to use too great a degree of heat, they do no harm. The chief disadvantage of curling-tongs is the fact that it is difficult to ensure that the heat employed is not too great. A generation ago, Leftwich carried out clinical tests on the strength of hair which had been subjected to various methods of artificial curling, and, to his surprise, found that carefully used curling-tongs did not injure the hair. Artistic and skilled operators can wield the tongs to produce beautiful if short-lived waves for special social functions. But see pp. 22 and 73.

Hair of firm texture, abundant quantity and little oiliness responds well to all the above methods of producing artificial curls and waves. With the average woman these curls last from a day to a week. Hair absorbs moisture from the air and from the perspiration of the scalp, and therefore, in the case of fine straight hair, in damp weather the artificial curls produced by the above methods may vanish within a few hours. All manner of devices are resorted to in order to retain the position of the curl or wave. A common plan is to fix the curl under a fine net and attach it by means of almost invisible pins. In wet weather the application of a minute amount of oil prevents the atmospheric moisture from entering the hair, and thus helps to preserve a newly made curl. With hair which is naturally coarse and dry, the artificial curl or wave may be in part retained for a week or even a month when great care is spent on keeping the hair from pressure by the pillow, the hat and the brush. If the hair has some natural tendency to a wave or curl, the artificially produced wave may, with care, last several weeks.

Naturally greasy hair does not readily respond to these methods of producing curls. This may be due to the oily surface retaining the natural moisture within the hair. Spirit lotions are particularly useful for oily hair which clings together in dank tresses. Some of the oil is removed by applications of acetone, ether or rectified spirit. This allows the hairs to stand apart from each other and thus an impression of more abundant hair is conveyed, and the curls remain longer in position.

Since 1914 curling the hair by the method now known as " the permanent wave " has become popular. Women of all ages all over the civilized world have had their hair treated by this process, in spite of the fact that it entails the endurance of some hours of a monotonous, wearisome and often a painful operation. In the days when women wore their hair uncut, on wet and blustering days there were too often seen thin, unkempt strands of hair straying untidily over the brow, ears and neck. In the damp, windy climate of Britain, the permanent wave is useful for preserving a tidy coiffure. In the early days of the invention of permanent waving the hair was frequently damaged. To-day the operators are more skilled ; they alter the time of the application of heat, or the strength of the chemical solutions, to suit the individual hair. In consequence, complaints of burnt and broken hair are now comparatively rarely heard. The hair is not in truth given a " permanent wave," but its structure is altered more enduringly than by curling-tongs or by the cold-water waves already described. Several methods are employed for the production of this " permanent wave," some of which alter the hair structure more than others.

The process of producing a permanent wave used to occupy four hours ; the time has been somewhat reduced.  A head of short hair can now be treated in two and a half hours or less.  The head is first washed so that the hair is freed from dust, scurf and grease.  The hair is divided into thirty or forty strands, each of which is tightly twisted round a metal rod.  In some processes a paper or other material, soaked in an alkaline solution, is fixed round the coiled strands.  The operator often describes this solution as " oil " ; it is not oil, but it is viscous and therefore has the appearance of being an oily fluid.  Commonly used preparations contain 10 to 15 per cent. of bicarbonate of potassium in distilled water ; sometimes 10 per cent. of borax is added.  However, it should be mentioned here that in certain systems of permanent waving true oil is applied before the heating stage, in order to prevent too great drying and possible breaking of the hair.  The next procedure is the protection of the scalp with a clasp or flat ring of asbestos or other insulating material.  Then each coil of hair, with its central metal rod, is enclosed in a hollow metal cylinder ; in many cases these cylinders are suspended from the roof. The temperature of the cylinders is raised by means of an electric current which runs for about four to ten minutes, or even longer for some types of thick hair.  In other systems of treatment, as stated above, instead of using different times and degrees of heat, the strength of the chemical solution is graded according to the fineness or coarseness of the hair.  Or the heating is obtained from steam, which is generated by wetting a sachet containing a chemical, the hair being protected from contact with the ingredients employed to produce the necessary degree of heat.  In other methods, a cylindrical metal clip, previously heated by electricity, is fastened round the curl.

In the usual method of production of the human permanent wave, the moist hair in the cylinder is heated to the temperature of steam and the twisted shafts are bent into the form of a spiral curl.  When the cylinders and the enveloping papers are removed, the tight spiral curls are combed out and the hair is washed, so that all excess of chemical is removed.  Whilst the hair is still damp, the curls are combed out and are made to lie flat against the scalp ; then the hair is pushed into position with short curved side combs, in such a way that the whole coiffure is arranged in regular waves.  A net is placed over all, and whilst the hair is being dried with warm air, expert manipulation by the fingers of the hairdresser brings about the formation of regular waves.  The artificially produced waves, however, are not truly " permanent " ; they flatten out with time, and with the pressure of the pillow and the hat.  With a damp atmosphere, as in rainy weather, during the first few days or weeks the waves tend to resume the short spiral curls of the original shape produced by the heated cylinder, and hence look fuzzy. Every few days or so, a so-called " setting lotion " is sprayed on the hair to moisten it and enable the wearer to create new waves by manipulation with the fingers and short combs. Where time and expense count for little, the client visits the hairdresser before every social function, in order to have the fashionable, faultlessly proportioned waves and curls renewed.

Setting lotions vary greatly in composition, but the majority contain alkalis and borax, or gum substances, in spirit and water, tinted and scented to give æsthetic value. Redgrove gives the following formula of a good setting lotion : Gum tragacanth (powdered and finest quality) 0·1, Isopropyl alcohol 10·0, terpineol 0·25, water to 100. As the permanent-wave process has a drying effect on the hair, and renders it more fragile and easily broken, it is advisable to apply oil from time to time. This also gives to the coiffure a glossy sheen which has a beauty resembling that of well-brushed natural hair. With fine hair only a small quantity of oil must be used ; otherwise the hair cannot be readily moulded into waves. A home-made setting lotion consists of one part of the white of a fresh egg beaten up with twice the quantity of water ; this mixture is combed along the hair. The absence of the stray untidy wisps of hair so prevalent before 1916 is indeed an æsthetic advantage ; but, other things being equal, a well-kept natural head of hair conveys to the lover of beauty a greater sense of satisfaction.

Apart from the monotony of the almost architectural regularity of appearance of the fashionable coiffure, the permanent wave has several disadvantages. In the average case, as mentioned above, the waves have to be arranged every week or two by an expert hand, and this necessitates considerable time and frequent money-consuming visits to the hairdresser. If the hair is neglected even for only a few days, under the pressure of the hat, the pillow, the comb and the brush, its wave loses shape, becomes fuzzy and dry, without lustre, and the whole coiffure can appear as untidy as a badly kept natural head of hair. With fine hair, especially when bleached, the permanent-waving process must be most cautiously performed, and the wave created by many hairdressers is not very lasting. Unless the owner of such hair warns a new operator, so that the heating process may be arrested in good time, or a suitable chemical employed, the wave is obtained at the expense of the hair. In a few days the hair shafts break and split ; the unfortunate sufferer finds that her hair becomes of irregular lengths and keeps breaking off every day. Hairs thus damaged show, under the microscope, a loosening of the cuticle cells ; in one woman, the hair shaft looked as if it were a fur, so much did the individual cuticle cells stand out from the cortex (Fig. 23).

This patient used to soak her scalp with oil, and yet her hair remained dry and lustreless and " fuzzy." In such cases the appearance of the coiffure was spoiled until the hair had had time to grow in again. On the other hand, in the endeavour to avoid this catastrophe, I have seen the heating process arrested too soon, so that the permanent-wave effect did not endure for even a week.

There is a common belief that during pregnancy the ordinary permanent waving process does not always succeed. Apparently the truth is that there is more difficulty in waving the tip than the proximal end of the hair ; and during pregnancy the hair grows more slowly.

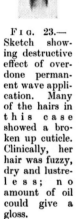

F I G. 23.— Sketch showing destructive effect of overdone permanent wave application. Many of the hairs in this case showed a broken up cuticle. Clinically, her hair was fuzzy, dry and lustreless; no amount of oil could give a gloss.

In good firms the modern work is usually performed with skill ; the hairdresser has so much experience that there is no excuse for injury by burning the scalp. But even in the case of the best establishments, the client must make certain that she is in the hands of a skilled operator ; for whilst it is unlikely that the scalp will be scorched, the hair itself may be overheated and therefore rendered so dry and brittle that it splits and breaks. When hair is thus waved, year after year, the shafts become injured. Their fragility is shown by the sharp bending of the shaft when a portion is removed for microscopical examination ; where the forceps have held the hair, a constriction and even breaking is visible. However, new hair grows in to replace the broken waved hair.

Another disadvantage of the permanent-waving process must be mentioned here. Many women postpone brushing and combing, lest this should destroy the regularity of their waves ; they also avoid the expense of frequent visits to the hairdresser. After a time of such neglect the scalp becomes unhealthy from lack of natural stimulation, and dandruff accumulates. Owing to the dislike of dislodging their waves and curls, brushing the hair has become so irregularly carried out by factory workers that pediculosis has become prevalent amongst them. With the average head of hair a normal amount of brushing and combing does not spoil the permanent wave, therefore there is no valid excuse for omitting due care of the scalp. A distressing feature of modern civilization is that the fashion of permanent waving has recently extended to men and to young children, in schools and even in the nursery.

Attention has been drawn by medical men to dangers which have been incurred during the lengthy operation of permanent waving. A certain number of women became ill when the process occupied four hours. For those with high blood-pressure, lung disease, severe anæmia or weak heart, there is a degree of risk, and especially when the process is painful. Injury was not uncommon in the early days, even in high-class establishments. Hairdressing firms endeavour to minimize the tedious aspect of the process by providing comfortable chairs, magazines and often even light refreshment.

THE COLD PERMANENT WAVE. In work not associated with permanent waving Goddard and Michaelis [1] described how thioglycholic acid could loosen the disulphide bonds of the keratin molecule. In 1936 Professor J. B. Speakman of Leeds University gave details of the process in connection with the waving of human hair. Research continued in Britain, but its application was held up during the war. In the meantime the method became popular in America, because its result depended upon chemical action ; no heating apparatus was required.

Various solutions are used in beauty parlours. In the early days a death occurred during the sitting ; expert medical examination proved that the fatality was due to acute poisoning by hydrogen sulphide.[2] In 1946 Lawrence Cotter [3] drew attention to the dangers, both local and systemic, caused by exposure to thioglycholic acid. Allergic and anæmic persons were especially liable to injury. Some developed dermatitis on entering a room which had thioglycholic acid fumes. In others serious damage to the blood, the liver and the nervous system followed too long or too frequent exposure, particularly when the solutions were strong. The effects were enduring ; recovery was slow, or did not occur. Locally, especially when the scalp was abraded or unhealthy, erythema, vesicles, papules, pustules and crusts appeared. The solution could penetrate into the follicle, and hairfall followed ; the bald areas lasted about six months. The operators suffered most, with lesions of the hands, fingers and nails ; even of the eyes when the face was touched by the affected hands. However, it is not necessary to employ thioglycholic acid as a reducing agent ; the best practice in Britain discountenanced its use. The safe reducing agent consists of hydrogen sulphite. Skilled operators vary the temperature for coarse and for fine hair ; and also grade the time of exposure and the strength of the solution for vertex, temples and occipital regions. Cohen [4] in 1949 confirmed Cotter's observations, and reported many cases of delayed, even widespread derma-

[1] Biol. Chem., 1934, 106, 605 ; and 1935, 112, 36.
[2] J.A.M.A., 1941, 116, 1515.          [3] Cotter, J.A.M.A., 1946, 131, 592.
[4] Cohen, Arch. Derm. and Syph., 1949, 60, 1, 14.

titis after the use of home outfits. Many scalps showed no evidence of injury until after several applications of such outfits. Then dermatitis might develop, or previous lesions, such as psoriasis, become aggravated. When the fingers and hands showed erythema, papules and vesicles, the association with a recent cold wave lotion is often long unsuspected ; instead, the dermatologist often tries patch tests for external irritants concerned in the patient's occupation. Biopsy showed acanthosis, thick hard follicles and obliterated papillæ of the interpapillary pegs.

Others report few injuries from the use of the cold wave, even of Home outfits. Controversy will continue, because the results are so various. Carey McCord [1] gives full details concerning the physical and the chemical changes brought about by the process. Many different formulæ are used : the majority contain thioglycholic acid and ammonium hydroxide as a neutralizer ; the best value had a $pH$ between 8·8 and 9·2. McNally and Scull [2] described the details of the process. After many experiments, they found that 6·5 per cent. solution of ammonium thioglycholate appeared to have no ill effects. Using a special home outfit preparation, Behrman and others [3] carried out careful experiments on 1,200 volunteers and on over 900 hospital patients and factory workers, some of whom had existing cutaneous lesions. They found no injurious effects when the process was properly performed. Examination of the blood and hepatic function tests were made on all the subjects. J. D. Downing [4] carried out tests with thioglycerol and ammonium thioglycolate lotions, and found that in those who had reactions the former caused more severe and more prolonged effects. Some individuals are sensitive to innumerable cosmetic applications.

The last word has not been spoken. That millions of people have had no injury is due to the fact that many of the home outfits with thioglycholic acid contain very weak solutions. The danger is less when skilled operators use the process, because the directions are more carefully followed, and the waving is not frequently performed. In my own experience I have seen cutaneous lesions, hairfall and baldness lasting six months in patients who have attended only the best hairdressing firms. Illustrations of temporary baldness after cold wave are given by Reiches and Clinton Lane. [5] What suits a young girl may not be advisable for middle-aged and delicate women. I have seen beautiful

[1] McCord, J., *Indust. Med.*, 1946, **15**, 669.
[2] McNally and Scull, *Arch. Derm. and Syph.*, 1948, **59**, 275.
[3] Behrman *et al.*, *J.A.M.A.*, 1949, **140**, 1208.
[4] *Arch. Derm. and Syph.*, 1951, **63**, 561.
[5] REICHES, A. J., and CLINTON LANE, *J.A.M.A.*, 1950, **144**, 305.

curls, made by the best firms, enduring only a few weeks ; in others the hair has become lank under two months. A skilled hairdresser of my acquaintance tells me that she has many clients with scalp lesions and long-lasting areas of baldness after applications of the cold wave by experienced operators in high-class establishments. She has observed that the worst effects have occurred in women who take too much alcohol ; this bears out the medical reports of the injury to the hepatic function. She is convinced that after frequent use of home outfits the hair shafts deteriorate and become what she describes as " spongy." She believes that the home outfits are dangerous, inasmuch as the girls who apply them often use them too often ; before a social function they are tempted to add to those curls which are losing the wave produced a short time previously. They keep no note of dates or methods ; and they continue to use the solutions when they are not in health. Many applications are often given with impunity, but after about three or four times trouble may begin. Bromate poisoning has occurred when the neutralizing solution (which resembles milk) has been ingested in error.

Professor J. B. Speakman tells me that certain firms in Britain supply reagents based on the sulphites for the production of the cold permanent wave. When thioglycholic acid is supplied, there are instructions recommending the use of rubber gloves by the operators. Home outfits as a rule have a reduced concentration of thioglycholic acid and the alkalinity of the solution ; this provides more safety, but necessitates longer times for treatment, which cannot be given in hairdressers' establishments.

" Oil " WAVING preparations contain often potassium carbonate and borax, 10 per cent. of each in distilled water. Ammonia softens keratin ; it is used in some of the permanent-waving solutions, e.g. ammonium carbonate $3\frac{1}{2}$ oz. ; borax $\frac{1}{2}$ oz., in 1 pint of water. Potassium carbonate is sometimes used instead of the borax.

Several preparations are employed for KEEPING THE HAIR IN POSITION ; the following prescription is an average example of their composition :

Pulv. Tragacanth 1 oz. ; Alcohol 90 per cent., 2 oz. Mix the tragacanth in the spirit ; add about 15 to 20 drops of oil to perfume it ; then add 24 oz. of boiling water ; shake well.

The ingredients employed in SETTING LOTIONS may be similar to those used in permanent wave solutions, but are usually in weaker proportion. Some setting lotions are alkaline (the proportion of alkali being about 3 per cent.), containing potassium carbonate, borax and ammonium carbonate in water. Some also contain alcohol, which in itself helps to fix hair in position, as it dries rapidly. Agar, gelatin, Irish moss, psyllium, linseed and quince seeds, tragacanth and acacia powder are used in different preparations ; some have quite a gummy consistence. The wave is set hard ; the hair is not brushed and is indeed scarcely touched for several days. The gummy material is then readily combed and brushed off the hair. These preparations can also be employed for damping the hair before adjusting curling-pins or other forms of wavers.

Those with fuzzy hair (e.g., negroes) use chemical HAIR-STRAIGHTENERS consisting of caustics, such as sodium or barium hydroxide, made up in a cream. The hair protein is converted into a protein " gel " which can be mechanically straightened, and the hair remains straight for a month. The skin of the face and scalp must be carefully protected before the application.

The following method for straightening woolly hair was given to me by Mr. J. E. Hackford, B.Sc., F.R.I.C. Treat the hair in sections ; moisten with a solution of ammonium thioglycollate having a $p$H value of 10 and a strength of approximately 10 per cent., which varies with the quality and fineness of the hair. Comb until the hair is relaxed, wetting the comb in the solution ; the process takes from a quarter to half an hour. Wash the hair in water. The neutralizing and oxidizing solution is made up thus : $1\frac{1}{2}$ vol. of a 50 per cent. solution of citric acid ; 1 vol. of 20 vol. $H_2O_2$ and $3\frac{1}{2}$ vol. of water. (The strength of the citric acid is thus 15 per cent.) Then shampoo and set the hair.

# CHAPTER IV

# THE MOLECULAR STRUCTURE AND ELASTIC PROPERTIES OF HAIR

By W. T. Astbury, M.A., Sc.D., F.Inst.P., F.R.S.

Professor of Biomolecular Structure and Honorary Reader in Textile Physics, University of Leeds.

Mammalian hair is built in the main from *keratin*, a protein of outstanding stability and unusually high sulphur content. The study of the molecular structure and elastic properties of hair is therefore largely the study of the constitution and properties of keratin, but it is only in recent years that real progress has been possible. Our present knowledge of the keratin molecule—and probably for the moment we understand more about keratin than about any other protein—rests essentially on the findings of X-ray analysis,[1] through which we have been permitted to catch a glimpse of its actual shape and dimensions.

Fig. 24a is an X-ray diffraction photograph of a small parallel bundle of *unstretched* human hairs. Such a photograph, though it bears no relation or resemblance to anything that can be seen by the human eye even when aided by the most powerful microscope, is none the less an indirect portrait of the form and mutual arrangement of the invisible molecules, a portrait which is susceptible of mathematical analysis and capable of yielding information of the most fundamental significance. In what follows we shall, of course, omit the analytical details, both theoretical and practical, and confine ourselves to the general conclusions.

The first conclusion to be drawn from the X-ray examination of hair, etc., is that all mammalian hairs, nails, hooves, spines, horn, and whalebone are similarly constituted : though there are obvious morphological differences, these differences are more of degree than of kind, for the building substance is always keratin. All give what is substantially the same X-ray photograph (Fig. 24a), that of keratin, and, whatever else is in question, all are endowed with certain common properties, those

---

[1] X-ray analysis, one of the major tools of modern physical research into the structure of matter, should not be confused with the radiography of medical practice. Radiography gives us only " shadow photographs " of objects of macroscopic dimensions ; but X-ray analysis gives us the " diffraction patterns " formed by objects of sub-microscopic dimensions—in fact, by the atoms and molecules themselves. The relevant parts of photographs such as Figs. 24a and 24b are the dark parts : the white spot merely marks the centre of the photograph.

of keratin. Though nominally we are concerned here with the molecular behaviour of human hair, most of what follows applies equally well to wool or horn, for instance. A horn or nail can be stretched and " permanently set " just as well as a hair.

The second conclusion is simply part of a general principle that has gradually revealed itself in the X-ray study of natural fibres as a whole— that to a first approximation they may be thought of as *molecular yarns* : in other words, as a yarn or sliver is constructed from visible fibres, so each individual fibre is constructed from invisible molecules. The molecules from which fibres are built are " fibre molecules" in a double sense, for they are also " molecular fibres " : in the world of molecules they are

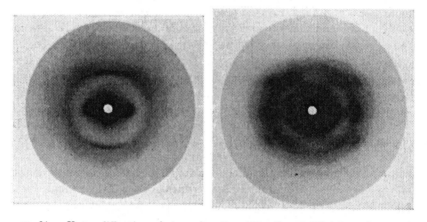

FIG. 24a.—X-ray diffraction photograph of a small parallel bundle of unstretched human hairs (α-keratin).

FIG. 24b.—X-ray diffraction photograph of a small parallel bundle of human hairs stretched in steam to twice their original length (" steam-set " β-keratin).

characterized by the fact that they may be hundreds of times as long as they are thick, and in a hair, for example, they lie all roughly parallel to the fibre length. Their thickness is of the order of one ten-millionth of a centimetre, and they are grouped into long, thin bundles, of varying size and perfection, which are no other than sub-microscopic crystallites of keratin lying, of course, also roughly parallel to the fibre length. This, then, is the first broad mental picture to be conjured up of the invisible interior of a hair : we must think of it as made up of long chain-molecules lying in the body of the fibre as fibres lie in the body of a yarn ; that is to say, all pointing roughly along the length of the fibre, but in addition aggregated into ill-defined bundles. Such a picture explains at once those properties of a hair which it shares with other natural fibres, that of splitting lengthways, for instance, and that of swelling, when wetted, very much more sideways than lengthways. It will be clear that absorption of water (and other reagents) into the fibre substance must take place by separating the molecular chains or chain-bundles, and since even the latter are much longer than they are thick the percentage lateral swelling will be proportionately greater than the percentage longitudinal swelling. Human hair, taken from complete dryness to saturation with water, swells sideways by about 14 per cent. of its dry thickness, but extends lengthways by only 1–2 per cent. of its dry length.

The molecular chains which form the basis of keratin are " polypeptide chains," the common basis of all proteins. A polypeptide chain may be represented by the general formula :

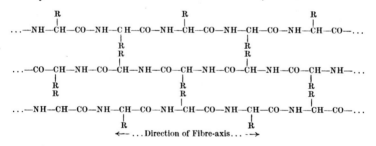

in which R′, R″, R‴, etc., stand for various univalent radicles, such as —H, —CH₃, —CH₂—CH₂—COOH, etc.—only about two dozen types are used in the whole of protein chemistry—which function as " side-chains " to the " main-chains " and serve to distinguish one protein from another. Such polypeptide chains, probably hundreds of times as long as they are thick, lie along the length of the hair fibre and attach themselves to one another by combinations between their side-chains, thus :

$$...{-}NH{-}CH{-}CO{-}NH{-}CH{-}CO{-}NH{-}CH{-}CO{-}NH{-}CH{-}CO{-}NH{-}CH{-}CO{-}...$$

thereby building up what may be called polypeptide " grids."

Now X-rays show that these keratin grids are not normally flat (though for convenience they have been so represented above), but in ordinary unstretched hair are " buckled " so as to accommodate the numerous interactions between the side-chains : and the buckling takes the form of a regular folding of the main-chains, as illustrated in Fig. 25(α), which is a skeleton model of short lengths of two neighbouring main-chains only, linked by their ladder of side-chains (the R-groups in the general scheme given above). When hair is *stretched*, however, the X-ray diffraction photograph changes : it is gradually replaced, as the extension increases, by a photograph rather like Fig. 24*b*, which is characteristic of a *flat* polypeptide grid. And when the hair is allowed to contract once more, Fig. 24*a* returns—and we can go through this interchange of photographs as many times as we care to stretch the hair and let it go. We have here a very remarkable phenomenon in the mechanics of molecules, an intramolecular transformation from a short to a long molecule merely by the act of pulling ! Hair is specially distinguished by its beautiful long-range elasticity—indiarubber is the only other common example—and this is the explanation as revealed by X-ray analysis. The keratin molecule in normal unstretched hair (α-keratin) is formed from regularly

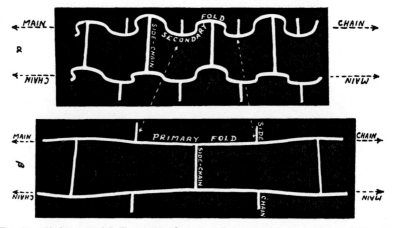

Fig. 25.—Skeleton models illustrating the essential structural features of α- and β-keratin, and the change which takes place during the transition from one form to the other when hair is stretched. Short lengths of two neighbouring main-chains only are shown.

folded polypeptide chains, but when the hair is stretched, these chains are pulled out practically straight to form a molecule roughly twice as long (β-keratin), which always strives to return to its stable folded form when the stretching force is removed. Corresponding to Fig. 25 (α), the skeleton model of β-keratin is shown in Fig. 25 (β) : it will be clear that the principal change brought about by the transformation from α- to β-keratin is simply an elongation of the molecule arising out of the straightening of the main-chains ; in other respects the form of the " grid " remains very much the same. When we stretch a hair the keratin grids are smoothed out : when we let it contract they buckle again. There appears to be practically no slipping of the grids over one another, for in the presence of water at ordinary temperatures the fibre always makes a perfect recovery to its original unstretched length—a most valuable asset, both biological and industrial. Natural silk and fibres of vegetable origin are deficient in this respect : unlike keratin, the chain-molecules from which they are built are naturally straight, so that when the fibres are stretched unduly, extension takes place by a process of internal slipping, an irreversible sliding of the chain-bundles over one another, with consequent permanent elongation. Anyone who has washed artificial silk garments will vouch for the fact that they must be treated with respect.

The part played by water in the elasticity of hair is fundamental ; it is almost as important as that played by the keratin itself. In all the processes of life the proteins and water act in collaboration, and in a general way the elastic properties of hair tell us why. It is because many of the protein side-chains are so active that they must even be protected from one another. In the complete absence of water certain parts of the keratin molecule cling so tightly together that the whole structure " seizes up," so to speak : the possibility of intramolecular rearrangement, such as is demanded by the transformation from $\alpha$- to $\beta$-keratin or the reverse, is practically eliminated, and the fibre can neither be stretched nor contracted. When water molecules are present, however—themselves highly active little bodies, oppositely charged on two opposite sides—the situation is much less rigid : they serve to engage the attention of the side-chains and soften their attractions for one another. To drop the metaphor, the process is one of intramolecular lubrication, or incipient solution.

This is the simplest aspect of the action of water on hair. As its water-content is increased, hair stretches both more easily and farther, till at complete saturation, when it holds an amount of water almost equal to one-third of its weight when dry, it can be stretched quite quickly to about one and a half times its normal length, and even to almost one and three-quarters if the fibre is uniform and the stretching is carried out slowly. Similarly, the tendency of a stretched hair to return to its unstretched length also goes up with the water-content : a hair that has been stretched and then dried while still in the stretched state hardly contracts at all ; but once it is wetted again it contracts with amazing speed.

The æsthetic value to the animal world of such a property must be considerable. In the rough and tumble of life the hair fibres, built as they are from highly deformable molecules, must inevitably suffer deformation of one sort or another—to become so tousled that their collective beauty is destroyed. But this does not matter much, for the keratin molecule always returns to its natural α-form in the presence of water, and the first shower of rain, or even a " cat-lick," is sufficient. We all know that however disreputable we may look on first rising in the morning, at least we can get our hair back into shape by moistening it.

On the other hand, we know too that we can *keep* it in shape by drying it again. As just pointed out, the keratin molecule is easily stretched [1] or otherwise deformed when water is present, but it remains in the stretched or deformed state if the water is dried off before elastic recovery can take place. This is the scientific basis of the familiar " water-waving " : it depends on what may conveniently be described as " cohesive set " (to distinguish it from " temporary " and " permanent set " —see below), that property of keratin of " seizing up " in the absence of water. And the moral is this : if you have naturally curly hair, don't be afraid of wetting it ; but beware if you have not ! [2]

Apart from the rather-to-be expected effects we have just considered, water reacts with *strained* hair also in a special and more deep-seated manner. It is an experimental fact that the normal keratin grid is in equilibrium in the folded, or α-, configuration illustrated by Fig. 25 (α), from which it follows that when it is forcibly stretched into the β-configuration illustrated by Fig. 25 (β), stresses are set up which try to burst the internal linkages of the molecule. When quite dry the latter holds out—within reasonable limits—against this disruptive tendency, but it fails when water or certain other reagents are present, for the active molecules of such substances now only serve to complete the breakdown initiated by mechanical deformation. Where the actual breakdown occurs is revealed directly by X-ray analysis under the extreme conditions which obtain when a hair is stretched in steam, hot water, or cold dilute caustic alkali, for instance ; but it can be shown conclusively that it takes place even in water at ordinary temperatures, given sufficient time. Fig. 24*b* is an X-ray diffraction photograph of human hair stretched in steam : it differs from the photograph which is given by hair stretched in cold water by certain small peculiarities only which prove, on geometrical analysis, that the action of the steam is confined almost exclusively to one

[1] The reader may be reminded that when a hair is bent it is stretched on the convex side ; or if a curly hair is pulled straight, it is stretched on what was initially the concave side.

[2] The visible curls or waves in hair must not be confused with, or ascribed to, the invisible " waves " in the normal form (α) of the keratin molecule. The molecules of all hair, whether curly or not, are normally in the α-form, the stable configuration to which they always strive to return after deformation. Naturally curly hair thus returns to its curly outlines when wetted, while naturally straight hair becomes straight once more. Natural waves in hair are the result of rhythmic and differential growth processes in the follicle.

direction—in fact, that direction parallel to which the side-chains lie (Fig. 25). It is evident what happens : as α-keratin is pulled out into the β-configuration stresses pile up in the linked side-chains and thus accumulate energy for the spontaneous contraction which takes place when the stretched fibre is afterwards released in water. This driving force is dissipated beforehand, however, if it should happen that the cross-linkages collapse under the stress—and X-rays show definitely that they do so collapse under the continued action of water, and at a rate which increases as the temperature of the water is raised, or if it is made alkaline, for example. As just mentioned, it is easy enough to demonstrate the effect even in cold water, if a hair is held stretched and kept wet for a sufficient length of time. Any time the hair is let go during such treatment it is found to contract more and more slowly the longer the time it has been held stretched in the wet state : it gradually loses its " kick."

This is the phenomenon of " relaxation," the breakdown of cross-linkages under stress ; but it appears to be followed almost immediately by another phenomenon, the formation of new, but relatively unstable, linkages which tend to hold the stretched grid in the extended form ; and here we have now " temporary set," so called to distinguish it from the " cohesive set " already explained and the true " permanent set " which we are about to consider. Temporary set is produced whenever a stretched hair is treated with cold dilute alkalis or water that is not too hot. It shows itself in the fact that if the stretched hair is afterwards released in *cold* water (after first washing out the alkali if cold dilute alkali has been used instead of warm water), it contracts only part of the way back to its original unstretched length. So long then as a temporarily set hair is submitted to cold water it never recovers entirely ; but if, while free to contract, it is treated with cold dilute alkali or with sufficiently hot water, it forthwith completes its postponed contraction and may even finally become *shorter* than its original unstretched length (see below). Temporary set produced by treating stretched hair with warm water or cold dilute alkalis thus somewhat resembles cohesive set— though only superficially—in that it can be reversed by re-treatment with water, provided the temperature of the latter is high enough. And the longer the stretched hair has been held stretched in hot water, or the higher the temperature of this " setting water," as we may call it, the less readily is the temporary set subsequently reversed in hot water, for it requires longer and longer times, or higher and higher temperatures.

The natural outcome of all this is that there comes a stage in hot water treatment at which temporary set passes into true permanent set, in the sense that it can no more be reversed even by the action of steam on the freed fibre. This stage is reached as the temperature of the " setting water " approaches boiling ; and in the end, to put it briefly, it is found that if a stretched hair has been exposed for a certain time to steam or to water at, or near, the temperature of steam, then it is afterwards little affected by warm water and even steam makes it contract only part of the way back to its original unstretched length : for all practical purposes it is indeed " set."

The reason for this appears to be twofold : if we use hotter and hotter water, not only does the process of " relaxation " become quicker and more complete, but also the new linkages tending to stabilize the grid in the extended configuration pass over into a stable, steam-resisting, form. Both these effects have been demonstrated separately in the laboratory and their progress analysed, and we may now feel fairly confident that the principles underlying the setting of hair are established. Below, we shall say a few words about recent practice in the setting of hair at ordinary temperatures, but for the moment it will be more instructive to continue along the present line of thought, because not only were the experiments just described those from which the principles were derived, but also they are fundamental for the understanding of any process of setting keratin—the low temperature process is indeed simply a logical development. Summarizing, then, the steps in the argument so far, we may say that :

(1) The continued action of water or alkalis on the strained keratin molecule leads to hydrolytic breakdown in the cross-linkages between the main-chains ("relaxation "), which dissipates the stresses that are the driving force of elastic recovery in cold water.

(2) New, but relatively unstable, linkages then build up which tend to fix the molecule in the stretched state ("temporary set ").

(3) On raising the temperature of the water in which the fibre is held stretched, relaxation is accelerated and the new linkages become more and more stable ("permanent set ").

(4) The degree of permanence of set depends on the temperature of the water in which the fibre was held stretched, the time for which it was held stretched, and the temperature of the water to which it is afterwards submitted in order to reverse the set.

These generalizations have been arrived at largely from the study of " straight-stretched " hair ; that is to say, hair that has been extended by simple pulling : but experiments on " bent-stretched " (waved) hair give little or no cause to doubt that similar principles hold however the deformation is produced. The important points brought out by X-ray analysis are : (a) that the keratin molecule is above all things a *deformable* molecule—in fact, a polypeptide grid the equilibrium configuration of which is a function of the nature and distribution of its cross-linkages ; (b) that when it is deformed in the presence of water or alkalis certain of the strained cross-linkages break down to relieve the intramolecular stresses ; and (c) that the broken cross-linkages can be replaced in the presence of steam or hot water by new, unstressed, linkages which hold the molecule in the deformed state. Thus we should expect that hair whose convex borders have been stretched by bending should show *at least* the setting phenomena that are shown by hair that has been stretched by simple pulling—we say " at least," because other types of deformation, compression on the concave sides for example, are introduced by the act of bending, especially bending a non-homogeneous cylinder such as a hair fibre—and, indeed, that is just what is found by experiment : the setting properties of bent-stretched hairs are similar to those of straight-stretched hairs, but with secondary effects added.

As is well known, hairdressers when steam-setting hair in " permanent waves " do not confine themselves to the use of steam or hot water only— the process would take too long : they avail themselves of the fact that " relaxation " is accelerated in the presence of alkalis. Before steam- ing, the hair is therefore usually damped with some mild alkaline solu- tion or other, but it is very important to remember that strong alkalis, or too long periods of steaming, are to be avoided. Strong alkalis not only break down the side-chain linkages, but also hydrolyse the protein main-chains and so lead to serious disruption of the molecules. Waving by means of hot irons is not open to this objectionable possibility, but it, too, has a danger of its own, that of having the irons too hot and so burning the hair : 130° C. or so is probably as high a temperature as may be permitted with safety. The method is based on the fact that even undamped hair always contains at ordinary atmospheric humidities sufficient water to be used for setting purposes if its temperature is raised : for reasons implied above, the degree of permanence so obtained, however, is not in general very high, though undoubtedly satisfactory over modest periods.

" Permanent waving " as an art depends in reality not on permanent set alone, but on a skilful combination of permanent set with cohesive set, for it is clear that in practice the final waves developed are rarely just as left by the steam. Obviously the attainment of such an ideal is hardly practicable, even were it desirable. What the hairdresser does is to set the hair in a series of fairly close spirals and use the curvature of these as a sort of main-spring to his own efforts. The closely curled hair is damped, combed out, rearranged, and then finally reset by drying; that is, *by cohesive set.* Just such an amount—with additional distortions superimposed—of the original excessive curvature is retained to bring about the desired effect. The whole point of the process is this, that whereas straight hair set by cohesive set alone tends to unwave (see above), hair set permanently in sharper curves than those in which it is temporarily held by cohesive set naturally tends to retain the waves, and even, on moistening, to become wavier still. The underlying principle is in both cases the same, that the keratin molecule in the presence of water tries to recover from deformation; but whereas unstrained keratin is normally α-keratin, after permanent set the intramolecular breakdown and rebuilding processes have effectively evolved a new unstrained conformation, and it is to this that the cohesively set molecule now tries to return. Thus we have the explanation of why permanently waved hair falls into small curls on wetting: the artistic cohesive set is released, the original permanent spirals return, and then, as is well known, the hairdresser can again reset the hair according to taste.

Nothing has been said above about the influence of the type of hair or of its variable chemical constitution, though of course these aspects of hairdressing practice are also of first-rate importance. Hairdressers have certain empirical rules to guide them when dealing with different heads of hair or with different regions of the same head, but it cannot be said that current practice rests on precise scientific knowledge, for the reason that such knowledge is not yet available. Complete chemical analyses of keratin present very great difficulties—and yet its complex physical properties, and the innumerable variations on the main theme of these properties, cannot be correlated with its constitution until this gigantic labour has been accomplished. At the present moment it is perhaps not an exaggeration to say that in some respects physical interpretation is definitely in advance of chemical: the general principles of the keratin " machine " have been brought to light, and we have a rough plan of the arrangement of the atoms; but we still cannot say exactly where each atom is. Nevertheless, recent chemical advances— by Speakman, for example—are distinctly encouraging. They show that the intramolecular breakdown occurring during " relaxation " is concerned at least in part with –S—S– linkages between neighbouring main-chains, and that the rebuilding process involves both the breakdown products of these linkages and the terminal $–NH_2$ groups of basic side-chains.

Owing to the War, few people knew of the British discovery of processes for imparting a permanent wave to women's hair at ordinary temperatures. As indicated above, these processes are a logical outcome of the principles laid bare in the X-ray and physico-chemical study of setting by steam or hot water ; namely, that it is necessary first to break down the stressed cross-linkages and then to re-build them in new, unstressed configurations. Full details of the new processes are to be found in papers by Professor J. B. Speakman, of the Department of Textile Industries, Leeds University.[1] They depend on treating the hair (1) with a reducing agent to break down the disulphide bonds and cause relaxation in the fibres while they are wound on a curler, and (2) with either an oxidizing agent, a metal salt, or an organic compound containing two or more reactive halogen atoms, in order to re-form cross-linkages between the peptide chains and so fix the hair in the curled condition. A wide variety of reducing agents and cross-linking agents has been used. In America, during the war, " permanent waving " at ordinary temperatures became very popular, though apparently methods were used that do not conform with the best practice that was discovered and has since been applied in Britain, and is now also adopted in America.

All lines of investigation go to prove that the practice of " permanent waving " is inseparable from irreversible changes in the keratin molecule, changes that must be described, however reluctantly, as damage. In careful hands the molecular degeneration may be kept down to a minimum, and probably would be looked upon by many as trifling when weighed against the improved appearance of the hair ; but it is there all the same, and ignorance or lack of skill can easily cause serious harm. There is a simple laboratory experiment which is rather extreme, no doubt, but which serves to emphasize this point. If a hair is stretched by about 50 per cent., say, and steamed while stretched for several hours, the scale-sheath often breaks up into short cylindrical sections which are so loose that they can be slid along the cortex like rings on a curtain-rod ! (See Figs. 26a and b.)

We cannot close this brief account of the exceedingly beautiful elastic properties of hair without some mention of the phenomenon of " super-contraction," that was first brought to light in hair. Everyone knows that hair can be stretched, but it has now been shown that it can also be *contracted* to much shorter than its normal unstretched length. That this should be possible is, however, no more than a fair deduction from the structural principles set out above ; for between the stage of side-chain breakdown (" relaxation ") and that of side-chain re-combination

[1] *J. Soc. Dyers and Colourists*, 1936, **52**, 423 ; 1941, **57**, 73 ; British Patent 453, 700 ; 453, 701.

("permanent set") there must be an intermediate stage during which the keratin main-chains are in a particularly unhampered state, and then we might expect them to fold up even more than they do when contracting to the α-configuration. Experiments shows that this prediction is sound. One of the simplest ways of inducing the "supercontracting" state follows directly from the reasoning given above. The hair must be stretched and steamed *for a short time only*—just so long as to cause intramolecular breakdown and yet inappreciable re-combination. On leaving it then to contract freely in the steam it overshoots its origin,

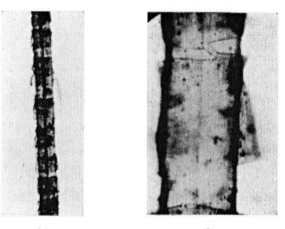

(a)                                    (b)

Fig. 26.—Human hair showing loosened cuticle after steaming for 6 hours at 50% extension. (a) Mag. × c. 70. (b) Another example Mag. × c. 300. (*Photographs by H. J. Woods, University of Leeds.*)

so to speak, and finally takes up a length which, under optimum conditions, is no more than about two-thirds of its length at the commencement of the experiment. Perhaps a more amusing method of demonstrating supercontraction is by means of the photo-chemical action of soft X-rays, for these rays have the power of modifying the side-chain linkages even without previously stretching the hair. All that one has to do in this case is to expose the hair for several hours to the X-ray beam, and then to expose it to steam. The resulting contraction is truly amazing.

*Note on the fibrous proteins of the keratin-myosin group.*—X-ray and related investigations that have developed out of the original studies of hair (summarized above) have shown that the question of the structure of keratin is only one aspect of a much wider problem, that of the structure and properties of a great family of fibrous proteins that we have called the keratin-myosin group. The same general type of X-ray diffraction diagram is given not only by all the many kinds of mammalian hairs, spines, horn, etc., but also by the fibrous proteins of the epidermis, by myosin, and even by fibrinogen and fibrin. (Fibrinogen is the constituent of the blood which changes to fibrin when clotting takes place, while myosin is the principal protein constituent of muscle tissue and the seat of its elastic properties.) In all these the molecules are constructed to a common pattern, and they are all endowed with substantially similar long-range elastic properties based on the $\alpha$-$\beta$ intramolecular transformation—the contraction of muscle, for instance, appears to be the counterpart of the supercontraction of hair. Their chemical constitutions in terms of amino acids vary considerably, however, and it is an urgent task of protein chemistry to resolve this paradox. The biogenetic implications of the keratin-myosin group strike deep. All its members are probably adaptations of a single root idea, an idea that must be one of the great co-ordinating principles in molecular biology.

## REFERENCES

W. T. ASTBURY. " Fundamentals of Fibre Structure." (Oxford University Press, 1933.)

W. T. ASTBURY and H. J. WOODS. " X-ray Studies of the Structure of Hair, Wool, and Related Fibres," *Phil. Trans. Roy. Soc.*, 1933, A, **232**, 333 ; see also W. T. ASTBURY and W. A. SISSON, *Proc. Roy. Soc.*, 1935, A. **150**, 533 ; H. J. WOODS, *Proc. Roy. Soc.*, 1938, A, **166**, 76 ; I. MACARTHUR, *Nature*, 1943, **152**, 36.

H. J. WOODS. " Supercontraction and Set in Animal Hairs," *Nature*, 1933, **132**, 709.

W. T. ASTBURY and S. DICKINSON. " X-ray Studies of the Molecular Structure of Myosin," *Proc. Roy. Soc.*, 1940, B, **129**, 307.

K. BAILEY, W. T. ASTBURY and K. M. RUDALL. " Fibrinogen and Fibrin as Members of the Keratin-Myosin Group, and the Nature of the Clotting of Blood," *Nature*, 1943, **151**, 716.

W. T. ASTBURY. " X-rays and the Stoichiometry of the Proteins, with Special Reference to the Structure of the Keratin-Myosin Group," *J. Chem Soc.*, 1942, 337.

W. T. ASTBURY. " X-rays and the Stoichiometry of the Proteins " (*Advances in Enzymology*, Vol. III, New York, 1943).

W. T. ASTBURY. " The Forms of Biological Molecules." (*Essays on Growth and Form presented to D'Arcy Wentworth Thompson*, Oxford University Press, 1945).

W. T. ASTBURY. " The Molecular Structure of Skin, Hair and Related Tissues," *Brit. J. Derm. and Syph.*, 1950, **62**, I.

# CHAPTER V

## COMMON DISORDERS OF THE HAIR

Before describing definite diseases of the hair and scalp, it is advisable to consider a few conditions which patients frequently mention.

**Dull Hair.** *The patient complains that the hair is* DULL AND LIFELESS. The condition may be due to one of the following causes, mentioned as far as possible in order of frequency of occurrence :

1. Dull hair is often a sign of lack of adequate CARE OF THE SCALP. With insufficient brushing and combing the natural oil is not evenly spread along the hair ; and thus no glossy surface is possible. Every housekeeper knows how dull is the wooden surface of furniture which is not well rubbed. Quite apart from the benefit of the mechanical effect of the brush and comb upon the hair shafts, there is the benefit of the stimulus to the nutrition of the hair bulbs which is brought about by the resultant quickening of the circulation of the scalp. This subject is dealt with in the sections dealing with the care of the hair (p. 43) and the treatment of diffuse hairfall (p. 89).

2. Dull, lifeless hair often accompanies DISEASE OF THE SCALP. Undoubtedly the most common of these is dandruff. This is usually known to the patient by the shedding of the scales on to the face and clothing. Apart from the trouble these cause in dressing the hair, the æsthetic discomfort is a source of annoyance to sensitive people. However, it is astonishing how many people suffer from dandruff and remain quite unaware of the fact. This ignorance is due sometimes to timidity in the use of the brush and the comb, for fear of dislodging the position and shape of fragile permanent or water waves and curls. In other cases the presence of dandruff is concealed by an excess of oiliness of the scalp, which retains the scales massed on the surface of the skin ; the patient complains only of oily hair and is unaware of the underlying dandruff. Other scaly diseases of the scalp (p. 157) lead to lack of lustre of the hair ; in such cases the patient would not seek advice on account of dullness of the hair, but for some more prominent symptom.

3. A dull and lifeless appearance of the hair may be due to POOR HEALTH. It is remarkable how, in certain people, hair with a natural gloss assumes a dull, drab appearance, even with transient ill-health of a few days' duration. In medical literature there is little reference to the subject of the effect of the general health upon the appearance of

the hair. Yet many women have told me that their hair lacks gloss and " looks dead " when they feel out of health. Since World War II this lustreless appearance of the hair, even in young women, has become common. A generation ago, novelists frequently alluded to the glossy hair seen with health and the lack of lustre accompanying low vitality. In the medical writings of the same epoch, when the physician brought less science but more art to the practice of his profession, one finds shrewd observations about the effect of the general health upon the hair. Erasmus Wilson's explanation of the cause of dull, lifeless hair cannot receive acceptance to-day, but every woman who has long hair will recognize the correctness of his description of the facts : " In a state of perfect health the hair may be full, glossy and rich in its hues, in consequence of the absorption from the blood of a nutritive juice, containing its proper proportion of oily and albuminous elements. In persons out of health it may lose its brilliancy of hue, and become lank and straight from the imbibition of juices imperfect in composition and ill-elaborated ; while, in a third group, there may be total lack of such nutritive juice, and the hair, as a consequence, looks dry, faded and as indeed is the case dead."

4. It is difficult to dissociate truth from fancy when so many factors are concerned in altering the appearance of the hair. Climate, a dry or a moisture-laden atmosphere, inadequate ventilation, heavy and tight-fitting head-gear, the presence of perspiration in hot weather, the neglect of brushing and combing, all play a part in bringing about a lifeless appearance of the hair. Many patients have told me that their hair became stiff and impossible to dress artistically just before or just after the menstrual period, and during minor illnesses, such as a " sore throat," or a " cold in the head." In some people I have found that this alteration is due to the degree of oiliness present. Observations made by intelligent women patients have convinced me that this secretion varies in amount and character with the health, often with the menstrual periods ; and hence influences the appearance of the coiffure, rendering it dull or glossy, (p. 81).

5. A few days after the hair has been set by a " PERMANENT WAVE " it often begins to look dull and lacking in gloss. It is astonishing how often an inexpert assistant fails to inform a new client of this possibility, and forgets to advise the use of some oily application in the event of the hair becoming very dry, as is frequent after a hot wave process. This is explained by the fact that most women return every ten days or so to have the hair reset, and the hairdresser then applies oil or brilliantine. Some women, however, never complain, but never return ; owing to the

lustreless appearance of their coiffure, they fear that the natural texture of their hair has been irremediably altered. This is indeed the case when the process of permanent waving has been carried too far. Microphotographs show the loosened cuticle cells (see Chapter IV and Fig. 23).

6. Dull hair may be due to the use of UNSUITABLE LOTIONS. For example, if normal hair is washed with rain water and brushed till there is a fine gloss, then damped with a lotion containing too much alkali, gum tragacanth or glycerine, on the following day the coiffure has lost its sheen and the hair appears dull and unmanageable. When a CLEANSING POWDER has not been thoroughly brushed out the hair looks dull.

**Dry Hair.** Patients often complain that their HAIR IS DRY, but on examination one usually finds they are in error. In the case of a young man who complained of loss of hair and dryness I found an oily scalp and abundant microbacilli. He had allowed the hair to grow long, so that it could be brushed over to conceal the baldness of the temples. In order to keep the long fine hairs tidily in position he had found that it was necessary to apply an oily brilliantine ; from this fact he had drawn the mistaken deduction that his hair was dry. Dryness may be complained of when the hair is thick and curly, yet the scalp may not show any abnormal dryness. The most common cause of a dry appearance is the use of alkalis and pure spirit in lotions, and when a hot permanent wave application has been overdone, or oil has not been applied after the process. Many scaly conditions of the scalp seen to-day are due to the use of cleansing detergents. These have a strong degreasing effect which in some people leads to flaking of the epidermis of the scalp. When the hair is too dry it may show greyish nodes (trichorrhexis nodosa) or breaking and splitting at the free ends (trichoclasia and trichoptilosis). (See Chapter XVI.) In childhood it is rare to see the hair broken or split except when fungus invades the shafts. In young and adult women, on the other hand, it is common to find the hairs short, broken and split, especially round the brow, when the hair has been subjected to all manner of lotions and cosmetic devices, with hot tongs or twisted metal used for the production of waves and curls.

**Oily Hair.** *The patient may complain of* GREASINESS *or* OILINESS *of the scalp* and consequent difficulty in arranging the hair. It is of the utmost importance to discover whether this symptom is due to " seborrhœa oleosa." If there is *hairfall*, and the microbacillus is found in scrapings made from the scalp, the prognosis is so serious that vigorous treatment must be instituted at once. As the patient, in the more serious type of oiliness, usually complains of hairfall, this form of oiliness is dealt with in the section dealing with hairfall and oiliness (p. 101).

If, on the other hand, the oiliness of the scalp is *unaccompanied by hairfall*, and after several examinations no microbacilli are found in the scrapings from the scalp, the prognosis is good. I am convinced of the fact that there is a form of oiliness of the scalp which has no bad effect upon the hair. Many women have told me that they notice increased oiliness near the menstrual period, and when they " feel out-of-sorts." This oiliness is not uncommon in women with excellent thick hair. I have watched two such women for over twenty years. Their hair is not noticeably thinner, nor has the oiliness ever diminished appreciably. One of these, a most intelligent observer, had greasy hair all her life ; I gave her various lotions when she was in her teens, over thirty years ago. She replied to my inquiries at the end of 1932 : " My hair is still normally thick and healthy, but still greasy. Perhaps the greasiness is a little less. 1 have used all sorts of remedies, even at one time two hair lotions daily ; but *nothing ever made any difference except good health.*[1] I think it is a constitutional matter ; as if I feel a bit seedy my hair gets greasy more quickly. My hair was better during pregnancy ; lactation made no difference. The hair is less greasy just before menstruation, more greasy just after." The other woman had hair with less natural curl, so that with the pre-war style of hairdressing her coiffure never looked neat. With short hair and waves she concealed the oiliness better ; she did not lose much hair, but began to turn grey in her early forties.

There are apparently two types of oiliness without hairfall ; one is associated with normal health and good hair, the other develops during a period of ill health. The patient, usually a young woman whose hair is not normally oily, complains that she has noticed her hair becoming steadily more oily for a few months or a year ; yet there is no hairfall. No microbacilli are found on microscopical investigation. Treatment of the general health may result in steady cure.

**Hyperidrosis** or excessive perspiration is often mistaken for oiliness by the patient and even by the physician, especially as it is in many cases accompanied by excessive oiliness. Increased perspiration on the scalp and forehead is frequently seen with those conditions which lead to undue perspiration on the body, the palms or soles. Thus it occurs with weakness during convalescence, during states of pyrexia, and also in nervous individuals. It is associated with certain forms of dyspepsia. Unilateral sweating accompanies some organic and some functional nervous maladies. It must not be forgotten also that in hot and humid

---

[1] Italics are mine.—A. S.

weather there may be so much perspiration on the scalp that brushing the hair makes it damp and removes any wave or artificial curl ; this appearance is often mistaken by the patient for a condition of oiliness.

**Hairfall.** Perhaps the most common symptom for which patients of any age consult the physician is HAIRFALL. It is not difficult to diagnose loss of hair, but it is essential to discover the cause before one can prescribe effective treatment.

Hairfall occurring over a limited period of time is so common an experience that few seek the advice of a physician unless the hair becomes so thin that the skin of the scalp shines through the hair, or the fall is so acute or so prolonged that they fear the possible onset of baldness. A marked degree of hairfall is a malady dreaded alike by young and old, and by both men and women.

When we consider this subject we enter a new domain. We pass from DISORDERS to DISEASE, and so begin a new chapter.

# CHAPTER VI

# DIFFUSE HAIRFALL : A. WITHOUT DISEASE OF THE SCALP

Two main causes play their part in conditions with profuse loss of hair. Hairfall may be due to (A) general or blood conditions, which interfere with the nutrition of the hair root, or to (B) local disease of the scalp. Both causes may be in operation together.

CLINICAL INVESTIGATION. When a patient seeks advice regarding a heavy loss of hair, we should at the first glance notice (1) whether the hair is so thin that the skin of the scalp shows through it over a large part of the head, and yet the scalp itself shows no disease ; (2) if there is complete baldness over a large area of the scalp ; or (3) the baldness occurs in patches. It is the first of these conditions which we have to discuss here.

Examine, next, the situation and the type of the hairs which remain, and any characteristic feature of the *skin of the scalp* : whether it is oily, scaly or erythematous. If such lesions are found, consult the chapters in which these signs are dealt with—VIII and XI to XV. The *age* of the patient, whether a child or an adult, provides the clue to certain forms of baldness. Inquire carefully into the *mode of the onset* of the loss of hair, whether it was gradual or sudden, and if the fall were localized or all over the scalp. Inquire into the *past history* : whether the fall began after some generalized rash, such as the eruptive fevers or secondary syphilis ; whether X-ray or thallium acetate has been administered ; whether and how long ago the patient suffered from acute illness, or had an accident, a shock, an operation, or bore a child. The history of onset prevents one fallacy in diagnosis : thus, if one did not learn that the baldness had begun in patches, as in *alopecia areata*, many of which had joined to form one large bald area or even a completely bald scalp, a mistaken diagnosis might easily be made. Since World War II loss of hair has become very common. Even now (1950) frequent reports are published concerning hairfall with accompanying signs of dietary and vitamin deficiency, often associated with endocrine dysfunction. The *family history* may shed important light on the origin of congenital conditions of loss of hair.

The presence of KERATOSIS and other scaly conditions of the scalp lead us to make further investigations concerning the bald appearance which is accompanied by those cutaneous signs (see pp. 144 and 180, and Chapter IX).

BALDNESS occurring in PATCHES is discussed in Chapter IX. Complete or almost COMPLETE BALDNESS is an uncommon condition, which is considered in Chapter VII.

(A) Here we now have to deal with the various causes of **diffuse hairfall without** apparent **disease of the scalp.**

From time to time almost everyone has a noticeable degree of hairfall which continues for a few days or weeks. Except by the sufferer, this hairfall is regarded as insignificant. It has been observed that diet has some influence on the hair ; this is mentioned in the section dealing with the sulphur-content of the hair, p. 90. This was certainly the case during and after World War II. *Transitory hairfall* is frequent after passing conditions of lowered health. I have frequently seen a period of hairfall occur after a short illness such as tonsillitis, in which the temperature lasted only two days and never rose above 99·4° F. Many women lose hair during months of prolonged ill-health due to obscure toxæmia and worry, and the fall has ceased during periods of improved health. In both these forms of hairfall I have examined many scalp scrapings, and been unable to find anything suggestive of seborrhœa ; an occasional microbacillus on a film does not indicate the presence of seborrhœic infection. In the undoubted cases of hairfall due to seborrhœa, the microbacilli are present in teeming numbers ; the slide appears covered with a film of these minute bacilli (see p. 105, Fig. 28).

However, a physician is rarely consulted for a moderate degree of hairfall. Hence we must start by defining clearly what condition constitutes DIFFUSE HAIRFALL, the *defluvium capillorum* of the ancient writers.

*Definition.* Some confine the term *Defluvium Capillorum* to the severe loss of hair all over the scalp which takes place rapidly, within a few days, setting in about a fortnight after a great nervous shock. The condition then resembles alopecia totalis, but the hair returns in one to three months. In diffuse hairfall, a general thinning of the hair occurs all over the scalp ; in time the skin shows through the long hair. The hairs fall out in large numbers every day : the brush and comb bring out hundreds. The patient often brings to show the doctor a paper bag with a large wad of hairs which have fallen within twenty-four hours. This fact is of supreme importance ; the hair comes out from *every part of the scalp.* If one pulls gently at the hair of the temples, behind the ears or on the vertex, the fingers bring away hairs in large quantity. The same type of rapid and diffuse hairfall is seen after the *erythema dose of X-ray* or the dose of *thallium acetate* which is administered expressly for the purpose of denuding the scalp of hair. The hairfall after X-ray treatment begins ten days after the application and continues for three to six weeks.

*Ætiology.* Six to eight weeks after any cause of high fever, diffuse hairfall follows ; the hair papillæ suffer in consequence of the acute toxæmia. Diffuse hairfall occurs after pneumonia, and in particular after influenza and typhoid fever the amount of hairfall is truly alarming. It is also seen after the *eruptive fevers*, especially erysipelas, measles and scarlet fever. After illnesses in which the temperature has exceeded 103° F. the hair begins to fall about two to six weeks after the onset of the fever ; in some patients it is most marked two to two and a half months after the illness. If untreated, the fall continues for about six weeks. The scalp never becomes quite bald ; some long hairs always remain. With the exact logic so characteristic of the French, Sabouraud observed that the temperature which led to hairfall is between 39° and 39·5° C. (i.e. 103° F.), that even a prolonged fever did not cause diffuse hairfall, provided the temperature did not rise above 39° C. On the other hand, where the illness involves shock, such as accompanies peritonitis, diffuse hairfall is usual. J. D. Rolleston told me that the average case of scarlet fever has become so mild a malady that it is not nowadays followed by much hairfall, and that the hairfall which follows the other specific fevers usually begins before the patient leaves the building, i.e. within a month of the onset of the fever. This agrees with my experience, that after any acute rise in temperature, however brief, there is usually a comparatively insignificant amount of hairfall which begins in two to six weeks from the time of the fever ; the severe diffuse hairfall is noticed rather later. The patient rarely notices the association, having forgotten a brief, acute illness.

Owing to the severity of the influenza epidemic which occurred just after the war of 1914–18, many cases of diffuse hairfall were met with. H. H. Hazen [1] reported fifty cases, forty-seven of whom were women ; all were young. Only five of these had had fever under 102·5° F. The hair fell between two weeks and three months after the subsidence of the fever. The average time between the onset of fever and the beginning of hairfall was nine weeks. In all these cases the hair returned rapidly. The chief method of treatment consisted in massaging the scalp twice a day until it glowed, and rubbing in vegetable oil.

About the same time Augustus Simpson [2] found that six patients who had been massaging the scalp and using remedies for seborrhœic dermatitis were those who escaped with only a slight degree of hairfall. He therefore emphasized the importance of keeping up good circulation in the scalp as a preventive of hairfall after fever.

After *childbirth* the loss of hair may be as severe as after high fever, and at the same interval, two to two and a half months later. It often

[1] *J. Amer. Med. Assoc.*, 1919, **77**, 1452.  [2] *Med. Rec.*, 1919, **95**, 402.

also follows *miscarriage.* I have heard of and known many cases in whom the hairfall after miscarriage and after pregnancy was so slight that the patient was quite unaware of it. Sabouraud noted that when the infant was breast-fed the mother did not lose hair; but if lactation was stopped, especially if suddenly, there might be loss of hair after the usual interval, eight to ten weeks. When hairfall follows a severe *operation, accident* or other cause of *shock*, it may occur after the same period of time, or it may come on within a fortnight, and is then more severe, even a total baldness. However, severe surgical operations and childbirth are not necessarily succeeded by any loss of hair. The state of the general health, and in particular of the thyroid gland, has probably much influence on the preservation of the hair in such cases. In the secondary stage of *syphilis*, the onset is more gradual, and the hair falls in a characteristic manner with irregular patches; it is described under bald patches in Chapter IX, p. 132.

During the course of *chronic maladies,* such as anæmia, leukæmia, diabetes, Graves' disease or any other cause of lowered vitality or general malnutrition, hairfall may continue, in more or less marked degree, over a period of many years. I have seen it continuing for years in women who suffered from a mild form of Graves' disease. With chronic toxæmia, such as occurs with a septic focus (teeth, tonsils, appendix) there may be a heavy daily loss of hair long before the local source of poison becomes manifest. It is astonishing how long a moderate degree of hairfall may endure without any noticeable baldness. New hairs apparently grow in soon after the fall of the old; this delays the appearance of baldness. If the hair is worn long, the patient observes that the average length of the hair becomes shorter. In cases of *malnutrition* and of *wasting disease,* such as cancer or tuberculosis, with frequent brief rises of temperature, the hair may fall profusely; on the other hand, the hair may remain quite thick. Sabouraud maintained that in the latter type the fever does not rise over 38° C.; where there was hairfall, there had been many bouts of high fever, over 39° C.

Diffuse hairfall may accompany *skin diseases* affecting the scalp, such as acute eczema or dermatitis due to many causes. *Exfoliative dermatitis* is usually associated with profuse loss of hair. This is seen with the dermatitis which sometimes follows the administration of metallic salts of thallium, bismuth, arsenic and gold, also with mecaprine dermatitis.

Excess of *Vitamin A* has caused loss of hair; [1] I have seen this when

[1] WOLLBACH and BESSY discuss effects of excess and of deficiency of vitamins. *Physiol. Rev.*, 1942, **22**, 233. See also *Nature*, 1949, **164**, 530; and *Lancet*, 1951, **1**. 394.

keratosis and other signs of its *deficiency* were present. With deficiency of *Vitamin B* there is ample evidence of the evil effect on the hair ; equally successful are the reports of benefit when the whole complex of that vitamin is administered.

Many degrees of loss of hair accompany the various *endocrine disorders.* With *myxœdema* there is characteristic dry, brittle, lustreless and scanty hair. With *hypothyroidism* the loss of hair is more often seen along the margin of the scalp than on the vertex ; especially common is the frontal band of baldness. With *hypopituitarism* the hair on the body becomes fine and scanty ; the hair on the scalp may be similarly affected, but it often undergoes no change. In the later stages of *acromegaly*, when the pituitary hyperactivity dies down, there may be baldness on the vertex. In many of the diseases which cause *hypertrichosis*, and with *virilism*, the hair on the scalp assumes the male type of baldness. This topic is discussed on page 288 in the chapter on hypertrichosis. In young women with *male pattern baldness* there is usually seborrhœa oleosa (page 104) or an endocrine cause in operation. *Parathyroid* deficiency can cause scanty hair as well as defects in the nails and teeth. *Ovarian* deficiency would, one expects, cause loss of hair ; but this subject presents contradictory features, for other endocrine factors are involved at the time of life when the ovarian function declines. After the *menopause* there is some loss of hair. This is first seen on the vertex, and is usually noticed between the fifty-fifth and the sixtieth year, but when the hereditary lifetime is long, this may be delayed till the seventieth year. Usually a woman notices first that the partings are thin ; later, towards the posterior region of the vertex, she becomes troubled by the sight of an oval-shaped bald patch. In *old age*, in both sexes, the hair roots share the general atrophy of the tissues; as the shafts of the hairs become finer and shorter, the scalp presents the appearance of being only thinly covered with hairs. The follicles may disappear, and the skin become glossy.

*Diagnosis.* The diffuse hairfall now under consideration has certain features which differentiate it from *seborrhœa oleosa*, the common cause of hairfall and baldness, especially in men. Seborrhœa oleosa may complicate the condition and confuse the prognosis. Sabouraud stated that for all practical purposes one can say, when one is consulted about severe loss of hair, that in nine cases out of ten one finds seborrhœa oleosa (see Chapter VIII) ; one in ten has had acute fever, shock or operation ; and one in a hundred has secondary syphilis. I add malnutrition since World War I. Note whether the scalp is greasy. Then pull the hairs behind the ears, and find if they come away easily ; this denotes infection or operative shock. Next examine the cervical glands and seek for other signs of syphilis ; inquire into the history of recent illness and dietary habits. Examination of the fallen hair roots rarely yields information of any value as to the cause of diffuse hairfall. Once the hair bulb has separated from the papilla, before it falls out, it passes through definite and progressive stages of decay ; these various stages are described and illustrated in Chapter I, Figs. 6, 7 and 8*a*.

*Prognosis.* Except after severe and prolonged fever, such as typhoid fever, the prognosis of *rapid* and profuse hairfall is excellent. The downy regrowth is usually seen even before all the loose hairs have fallen out. Even in marked cases, provided local treatment is adopted in good time, all the hair should return. If active treatment is begun early, the fall often seems to be arrested. If the scalp is left for months or years without any treatment, in people who have bad health, and when local causes such as seborrhœa complicate matters, permanent thinning of the hair may remain. Later on, the scalp develops a glossy appearance ; examination with a lens reveals the absence of hair follicles, even atrophy of the skin. The prognosis is then serious. If the patient is young and healthy, and the follicles remain visible, the prognosis is very hopeful. Encourage these patients ; they have every reason to hope, for regrowth of the fallen hair is usual, even after the most serious illness and a prolonged period of thin hair. When treatment is undertaken it must be persevered with until there is regrowth of the hair.

As regards *chronic* diffuse hairfall, in cases where there is chronic toxæmia, and nutrition is deficient, the outlook is unfavourable. The fall is slow, but steady, and may continue for years. The cause may not be discovered until extensive damage has occurred. Frequently local maladies, in particular pityriasis (Chapter XI) and seborrhœa (Chapter VIII), complicate the case. Even if the cause is a general toxæmia and has been discovered early, it may not be possible to remove it. Or the nervous factor may be present ; many patients cannot rest, or will not allow themselves any repose, cannot escape financial or domestic worry, cannot give up work in unsuitable climatic or other harmful surroundings ; the general health of such individuals never reaches a normal standard. Again, when sufferers from more or less chronic invalidism are harassed by care or obliged to continue their work, they are too weary to carry out the energetic local measures which are necessary to delay progressive hairfall and to stimulate a regrowth of hair.

*Endocrine cases.*—Hairfall due to simple anæmia and uncomplicated thyroid deficiency responds satisfactorily to iron and to thyroid gland. After the menopause, when the hair on the vertex is much thinner, the outlook is serious, as regards return of the hair, unless the health is good and the patient can be relied on to persevere with local applications. At, and just after the menopause, provided the general health is good, the tendency to thinning of the hair can be arrested with correct local treatment. Sometimes in later life, when a woman is well over sixty years of age, I have seen a degree of regrowth of hair without any or with only a mild form of local treatment. Sabouraud noticed the same phenomenon in men. The outlook for young women with the male pattern baldness is serious, see p. 104.

Pityriasis or seborrhœa, or both, may co-exist with diffuse hairfall due to one or other of the general causes above mentioned. This fact must never be forgotten when the lines of treatment are being decided. One must also remember that both forms of local malady may be much aggravated by the systemic toxæmia which leads to diffuse hairfall.

*Treatment.* The TREATMENT OF DIFFUSE HAIRFALL, in the absence of local disease of the scalp and hair, aims at improving the circulation of the scalp. This can be achieved by four main methods—(1) measures directed to the improvement of the general health, including the use of endocrine glands ; (2) certain drugs, which have been found to stimulate the hair follicles ; (3) mechanical means ; and (4) certain electrical agents.

(1) Treatment directed to the IMPROVEMENT OF THE GENERAL HEALTH is necessary when the patient shows lowered vitality. The administration of small doses of thyroid, even when the patient shows no signs of athyroidism, is of undoubted benefit in many cases of hairfall. A combination of endocrine glands can be prescribed ; especially after the menopause is this advisable. Ovarian preparations are especially useful for women of fifty to sixty years of age. Experimental feeding of animals with the anterior lobe of the pituitary has led to hair growth.[1] Parathyroid gland has also aided some patients. In toxæmic cases, the individual case is treated with appropriate endocrine preparations, according to the signs of glandular deficiency which are present. Septic foci must be dealt with. The diet must be properly balanced, with abundant vitamin content. Where protein is deficient in the diet an adequate supply of vitamin B should be ensured. Lime is usually advisable also.

(2) Certain DRUGS have been recommended as capable of encouraging hair growth, (*a*) when given internally ; and (*b*) in local applications.

(*a*) Pilocarpine has long been credited with having a specific action upon the hair follicles. Pilocarpine has made hair grow even in myxœdematous patients ; it was used before there was any knowledge of the value of thyroid in these cases. Samuel West described a case in whom

---

[1] E. GOETSCH, " Influence of Pituitary feeding upon growth and Sex Development," *Bull. Johns Hopkins Hosp.*, 1916, **27**, 29.

the scalp was bald ; after pilocarpine gr. $\frac{1}{6}$ had been taken thrice daily for months, the hair became fairly thick.[1] I find the drawback to its use in young subjects is that it causes perspiration and often profuse salivation. Humagsolan was once much in vogue ; I never found it succeed where other measures had failed.  Max Joseph expressed a similar opinion.

The rationale underlying treatment with humagsolan merits mention here. Several observers in Germany were convinced of the value of a water-soluble keratin preparation, named humagsolan, made by Zuntz by hydrolysis with sulphuric acid.  Saalfield, Punner, Blaschko and others testified to its value in many types of cases of hairfall.  Local dosage with ultra-violet light appeared, they said, to aid its action.  Where the hair roots had been destroyed, it was ineffective.  Laboratory experiments on animals show that hair is adversely affected when the diet is poor in quantity or quality of protein.  Keratin, the main constituent in hair and nails, has a high sulphur content, the sulphur being present as an amino-acid cystine.  Certain American workers considered that as sulphur was important for the hair, the administration of keratin or of sulphur might be useful in cases with loss of hair.  Cystine being expensive, they used hydrolysed wool, prepared as a solution containing a high proportion of cystine.  Given by mouth, it aided growth of hair in rabbits fed on a diet poor in cystine.  H. Brown and Klauder [2] tested the value of hydrolysed wool given during one to three months to forty patients suffering from loss of hair due to various causes. Marked success followed in only two cases, patients with alopecia totalis. In most cases the result of the experiment was doubtful or negative.  Hydrolysed wool therapy appeared to increase the sulphur content of the hair, but it did not lead to increased hair growth except in cases in whom the sulphur content of the hair was low.  Hence they concluded that it is inadvisable to give hydrolysed wool or similar preparations as a routine measure for hairfall ; they should be reserved for cases with low sulphur hair content.

(b) Drugs recommended for use in *local applications*.  Pilocarpine is useful in ointments and lotions.  Tincture of jaborandi is a time-honoured favourite in hair lotions.  Quinine, potassium nitrate and perchloride of mercury are also reputed to have a specific local action upon the hair follicles.  Sulphur has stood the test of time as an application which encourages hair growth.  It can be given in oil, which penetrates into the hair follicles better than when used in a lotion with spirit and water. In the colloidal state it may be still more efficacious.  Oil of cade was recommended by Sabouraud, who believed that it had a specific effect upon the hair ; he prescribed it, in vasolanolin, for many conditions of the hair and scalp.  The most well known drugs which apparently stimulate hair growth are : cantharides, ammonia, terebinth, camphor, acetic

[1] *St. Bart's Hosp. Repts.*, 1884, **20**, 125.
[2] HERBERT BROWN and JOSEPH KLAUDER, "Sulphur content of hair and nails in abnormal states," *Archiv. Derm. and Syph.*, 1933, **27**, 584.

acid, capsicum and other rubefacients. Cholesterin preparations had favour, especially with German writers. Some maintain that it has a specific effect upon the sebaceous glands ; others believe that as cholesterin is a fat solvent it acts by enabling other remedies to penetrate better into the follicles. Another explanation is that benefit obtained from its employment is due to the friction and massage during its application. This remedy is dealt with under seborrhœa (p. 108). Widely advertised " Hair Tonics " usually contain perchloride of mercury, salicylic acid, sulphur and/or betanaphthol.

Erasmus Wilson gave a list of no fewer than ninety substances which from time to time have been credited with success in the production of fresh hair growth. This acute observer pointed out that all of these substances acted either as stimulants or as fats, and that the application of grease, oil or fats, was preceded by friction of the scalp. This leads us to the consideration of the benefit obtained by massage and vibration, and on this subject Erasmus Wilson again spoke with authority.

(3) *Mechanical means.* MASSAGE and VIBRATION of the scalp are most important means of improving the local circulation and hence stimulating a growth of hair. After youth is passed, in many people the scalp is found to be stretched so tightly over the skull that it is difficult to move the skin over the bone. The patient should be shown how to grip the head on both sides, over the ears, then how to move the scalp vigorously with the fingers and thumbs. This is a tiring process and the average man feels too bored to continue it daily for the necessary ten to twenty minutes. If he is told he may read during the process, he will find that time will pass quickly. With a book before him he can rest his elbows on a table and automatically continue the movements on the scalp. Later, when the scalp has become more loose, he can knead and pinch it.

Erasmus Wilson wrote in 1853 : " I pointed out the principle of local treatment of falling hair, weak hair, and baldness ; and showed that the principle was simply *excitation or stimulation of the skin.* I do not mean that mere local stimulation will effect all that is required, without the aid of constitutional treatment, but so far as local treatment alone is concerned, the principle, as I before stated, is stimulation ; the manner of effecting stimulation may be, and is, multifarious. An old lady who practises the art of hair-producing in London, gets, as I am informed, her patient between her knees, and then begins a system of pommelling, pinching, rubbing and shampooing the skin of the head, until she stimulates every part of it effectually."

Beating the scalp with a hairbrush till the flesh tingles is a useful prescription. The brush should have long firm bristles ; some are made of whalebone, some are set in resilient frames (see p. 42). Another most successful method of stimulating the circulation is hard combing, using a comb with blunt, but firm teeth. The skin must not be abraded ; but, short of this degree of traumatism, the comb can scarcely be used too vigorously. For those who can afford it the services of an assistant should be obtained ; nothing can surpass the beneficial effect obtained from vibration and massage when performed by the skilled hand which lifts the scalp from the skull and kneads the flesh in the direction of the blood-vessels and nerves. Friction, massage and kneading by the fingers when using lotions or ointments is always advisable ; thus one can ensure improvement of the local circulation even if the ingredients in the application employed are of little value. It is advisable also to massage the muscles of the back of the neck and the shoulders, especially in older subjects suffering from stiffness and the nodules of so-called fibrositis. Vibration with electrically driven apparatus communicates a fine glow to the scalp, but it is less pleasant and not more efficacious than vibrations given by the fingers of a skilled operator. One objection to the use of an electrically driven vibrator is that long hair is apt to get tangled and caught in parts of the apparatus.

The " *oil shampoo*," or the oil cure, merits brief reference. For this shampoo, oil of vegetable origin is preferable to a mineral oil. The vegetable oil penetrates better, and any excess is more easily removed ; almond and castor oil are excellent for this purpose. Most operators heat the oil in a water bath before use. The scalp also should be warmed, either with hot towels, an infra-red or a radiant heat lamp. The hair is divided into many partings and a little oil well rubbed into the scalp with the fingers or a minute brush. Then the scalp is carefully and methodically massaged, usually in circles, from brow to neck, with the tips of the fingers, which must be lifted up carefully, so that there is no tangling of the hair. In the case of scanty or fine hair, which looks very dark and dank after the use of even the smallest quantity of oil, the oil must be removed from the hair shafts by washing it off with soap and water or the dry shampoo. In some cases scalp massage with oil may be advantageously carried out once a week or so for several months. The oil improves the appearance of the hair, and although it probably does not by itself aid the regrowth of hair, the massage of the scalp, which is carried out during the process of oiling, is certainly useful for this purpose. Possibly one factor in the therapeutic value of oil is the fact that by retaining the skin warmth it may aid the subcutaneous circulation, and hence improve the nutrition of the hair follicles.

(4) ELECTRICAL METHODS. Many forms of electricity are of proved

value.   Ultra-violet light administered to the scalp and to the whole body certainly aids some patients; this powerful agent must not be used without medical supervision, especially when there are septic foci, kidney or lung disease.   It is particularly valuable in convalescence after acute maladies. When an exposure has been followed by sleeplessness and exhaustion there has been overdosage ; after a correct dose there is a sense of exhilaration and the sleep is sound.   The stimulating property of the high-frequency vacuum tubes, introduced about 1905, was so pronounced that innumerable imitations of this instrument have been made.   Small, portable " high-frequency " machines can be obtained in many forms and sizes.   They have undoubtedly a sphere of usefulness, but their effect cannot be compared with that of the Oudin resonator of a large high-frequency machine.   This apparatus is no longer manufactured ; it and the static machine may return to favour.   After turning on the current the operator should hold the flat of the tube in the hand and gently slide it on to the scalp of the patient.   Some people are extremely nervous ; for such patients it is helpful at the first application if the operator holds one finger on the tube, thus ensuring that only a mild degree of tingling is conveyed to the scalp.   When an operator moves the tube about over the scalp in a jerky, quick and unrhythmical manner, the patient is rendered so nervous that the beneficial general effect of the treatment is, in delicate or sensitive patients, entirely lost.   For this reason conversation should be forbidden when a nurse gives treatment ; it distracts her attention and causes her to move the tube irregularly.   The tube should slide with a steady rhythm, smoothly and slowly all over the vertex, then more rapidly over the temples, on which regions the glowing sensation is apt to become painful.   The occiput usually requires little treatment. When the current is of correct strength, it can rarely be borne for more than ten minutes ; then the whole scalp seems to be afire, and the shower of fine sparks which come from the surface of the glass applicator can no longer be endured.   When the scalp is brushed or combed even as long as six to eight hours after the treatment, there is felt a pleasant tingling or tender sensation.   The treatment may be given three times a week ; from ten to twenty treatments are required for the average case.   When the scalp has been neglected for years, even after prolonged treatment with lotions and a moderate amount of hand friction, it remains pale and unresponsive.   This is especially true in the case of elderly people.   Even after several of the strongest of the high-frequency applications, the colour of the skin may remain pale ; but as a rule, within a fortnight (six applications) the reaction improves and on removing the tube, the formerly white skin is seen to be rosy red.   This effect is especially marked on the vertex. As the course of treatment progresses, the skin of the scalp becomes quite red almost immediately after the application has started.

The general health benefits from applications of the vacuum tube. Patients say that however weary they may feel before, they feel alert after the treatment ; this sensation of well-being endures for a varying period of time.

Of recent years many employ the vacuum tube taken from a diathermy machine ; this conveys a sensation of warmth, but it is not so stimulating as the tube activated by the current obtained from the Oudin resonator (now not manufactured). The high-frequency apparatus of former days was activated by a coil, had a single spark gap, was of high voltage and low amperage. The high frequency of to-day is of lower voltage and greater amperage than the older apparatus ; it is a form of diathermy. In nervous conditions, and with high blood-pressure, the use of the high voltage tube on the scalp is inadvisable. Vacuum tubes used with the static machine cause a gentle glow ; fine sparks descend in a profuse but painless shower. The good local effect of the static machine is increased by its bracing effect upon the whole body. Owing to our damp climate the static machine is hard to start up ; hence in these days of crowded clinics, its use has been abandoned.

*Radiant heat* has much value, but it is used less than would be expected because the lamp dries the hair too much, and the heat soon becomes intolerable on the head.

*Ultra-violet light* has achieved popularity with both lay and scientific circles. It can be used on the same day as the high-frequency application. I prefer it to be administered after the scalp has become reddened by the vacuum tube. Or it may be given after the scalp has become flushed by exposure to infra-red rays, or to radiant heat. Ultra-violet light from the average mercury vapour lamp can be given in small doses of gradually increasing duration. Some operators aim at an erythema dose every time. The face, brow and neck must be carefully protected. There are many methods by which the necessary protection from the rays can be obtained, but none are more efficient than a simple square of dark cloth in which a hole has been cut in order to allow full exposure of the vertex. When the hair is extremely thin, and when there is a completely bald area, an expert may give the ultra-violet light with the burner held at a short distance, so that a marked reaction is produced. In other cases success follows only after the whole body has been treated with ultra-violet light. The Kromayer lamp is usually reserved for local bald patches, and is therefore mentioned in the section dealing with alopecia areata.

The above-mentioned electrical modalities have displaced the galvanic and faradic currents which had certain grave drawbacks. The amount of current which could be employed was so small as to have an almost negligible effect. Only those who were thoroughly accustomed to the apparatus could be trusted to use it without giving unpleasant, even dangerous shocks to the patient. No one except an expert in electro-therapeutics should venture to pass a galvanic current through the brain ; sensations as of flashes of light and giddiness may be caused by quite modest doses.

Small divided doses of *X-ray* used to be given with the object of promoting growth of hair, but this method is so uncertain, and except in expert hands, so dangerous, that it was never popular. An epilation dose of X-ray is being re-introduced for alopecia areata ; before the introduction of ultra-violet light appeared, we frequently employed an erythema dose of X-ray for this disease.

When, in place of malaria therapy, short wave currents were administered through the brain to patients with general paralysis, it was noted that on bald heads there was regrowth of hair. This raised hopes that a new cure had been discovered, but when the treatment ceased the hairs fell out again. I have had similar experience after strong applications of high frequency.

# CHAPTER VII

## LARGE AREAS OF BALDNESS

The hair may be absent over all or a large part of the scalp, or over an area which is too extensive to be described as a patch. Apart from the baldness due to seborrhœa oleosa, and the diffuse loss of hair dealt with in the preceding chapter, such baldness is rare and can be discussed under comparatively few headings.

CLINICAL INVESTIGATION. All important for diagnosis are the *age* of the patient and the *history of the onset* of the baldness. Make certain that none of the causes of DIFFUSE HAIRFALL described in Chapter VI have recently been in operation. More or less complete baldness may follow acute fever or the other causes mentioned in the section dealing with diffuse hairfall, especially if convalescence has been slow and no local treatment given to the scalp. This has happened especially after typhoid fever, even in quite young adults. Long-neglected hairfall due to chronic constitutional disease, extending over many years, especially in those over forty, often results in widespread baldness, especially over the temples and vertex, and sometimes the sides of the head. The colour and appearance of the patient give the clue to the diagnosis ; examination of the blood and all the organs should be carried out in obscure cases. Some of the causes of CICATRICIAL ALOPECIA which are dealt with in Chapter IX, may, after the lapse of time, lead to baldness over all or most of the scalp, with here and there a few sparse islets of hair ; in these cases the atrophied condition of the skin settles the diagnosis. When these causes have been excluded, the diseases in the list given below should be considered.

One *source of fallacy* must be mentioned here. An infant may be brought by an anxious mother who believes that her child is going bald, because the original hair has fallen out after the first month of life, as is normal ; or because her two- or three-months-old infant has hair which lies flat, or is short and thin on the occiput or on one side of the head. The baby who lies always in the same position rubs the same part of the head on the pillow, and pressure prevents the hair growing freely on that part. On examination some of the hairs are found to be entirely absent ; some are short, but normal, and others are broken off. No local treatment, other than oiling the region, should be required. Stimulants must never be rubbed into the scalp of an infant. R. Bowers found similar bald areas in adults who rubbed the scalp too vigorously when trying to gain regrowth of hair.[1]

Large areas of baldness may be due to :

I   Seborrhœa oleosa.
II   Baldness after X-ray in therapeutic epilation dose.
III   Baldness after the administration of thallium.
IV   Congenital atrichia.
V   Total alopecia from various causes.
VI   Ichthyosis follicularis.
VII   Ichthyosis.
VIII   Several of the causes of baldness with atrophy which are discussed in Chapter IX.

I. SEBORRHŒA OLEOSA. Diffuse hairfall may begin between the seventeenth and the twentieth year and by the thirtieth year may often extend over almost the whole of the scalp. A ring of hair is left over the ears and the occipital region. This disease is fully discussed in Chapter VIII under hairfall with oiliness. This is undoubtedly the chief cause, in adult males, of large areas of baldness.

II and III. BALDNESS FOLLOWING X-RAY OR THALLIUM ACETATE which have been given with the object of causing the hair to fall, does not usually give rise to difficulty in diagnosis. However, as mentioned on p. 96, in the paragraph on clinical investigation of bald patches, it is quite possible, especially in a busy out-patient clinic, that a young child may appear accompanied only by a small brother or sister who cannot give any clear history. If the epilation has been incomplete, the scalp may show downy hairs, together with a few sparsely scattered long and exclamation hairs ; and misleading papules or pustules may also be present. Provided one is on the outlook for such an occurrence, a mistake in diagnosis should not occur.

IV. *The patient is a child, who has been born without hair, or whose hair has never grown to be more than a slight down. The disease is* ATRICHIA CONGENITA—CONGENITAL ALOPECIA.

Atrichia Congenita. *Definition.* A congenital ectodermal defect is the term used to denote a condition with defective development of the epidermis or its appendages. Congenital atrichosis or atrichia is a condition in which the hair is absent or very scanty. Only a few cases have been recorded. Complete absence of all hair is very rare. The infants are born without hair on the scalp, eyelids or eyebrows, or there may be present a very few, fine hairs, which after prolonged treatment may grow to be an inch long. P. Ziegler [2] reported the case of a girl who was bald

---

[1] *Brit. J. Derm. and Syph.*, 1950, **62**, 262.
[2] P. ZIEGLER, *Arch. Dermat. und Syph.*, 1897, **39**, 213.

until thirteen ; then a tuft of hair grew in on the occiput at the time of the menstrual periods ; this fell out again. No hair was seen anywhere except a slight down on the cheeks and forearms ; her teeth and nails were normal. A microscopic examination revealed many hair papillæ, but complete absence of hair and hair follicles, due apparently to defective growth of the external root sheath ; the sebaceous glands and arrector pili muscles were normal. Balzar and Barthelmy [1] described a healthy man of forty-two, with very few, but firm hairs, on the scalp and eyebrows, good teeth, a smooth skin, but striated nails. His mother, sister and only daughter were similarly affected. Cockayne [2] studied the subject from the point of view of the inheritance of ectodermal dystrophies.

Hyde [3] classified congenital atrichia under several headings : (1) Complete absence of hair, due to defective intrauterine development. (2) The hair with which the infant is born falls out and is replaced only by down, or the hair which is present at birth does not fall, but remains scanty for life. (3) There are circumscribed patches of hair with deeply pigmented nævi, but downy hairs elsewhere on the scalp. Or the circumscribed patches of hair may appear on the occiput, middle line or posterior fontanelle. (4) Cases with circumscribed patches, who in later life become normal. (5) Cases belonging to any of the above groups, with, in addition, defective teeth and nails. Other causes have been studied by the Mayo Clinic.[4]

Sabouraud described a **congenital triangular absence of hair** on the temporal region on one or both sides. The skin was normal. Other cases have been reported ; some have been mistaken for commencing alopecia.

A rare condition, of which only about thirty cases have been recorded, is described by Touraine.[5] The hairs of the head are scanty and fine. The hairs of the beard and moustache may be good, but those of the eyebrows, eyelashes, armpits, pubis and the body are absent or atrophic. The patients never perspire, owing to absence of the sweat glands ; this leads to illness in warm weather. Most of the sebaceous glands are absent ; there are few and defective teeth ; the nails and the features show various deformities ; the intellect is usually below par and sometimes abnormal.

A case of congenital and familial absence of hair was reported in 1936.[6] The patient, one of a long-lived Burmese family, was healthy ; perspiration was normal and there was no endocrine defect. His two elder brothers suffered from the same condition of absence of hair.

---

[1] BALZAR and BARTHELMY, *Bull. Soc. Franç. Derm. et Syph.* 1914, **25**, 321.

[2] E. A. COCKAYNE, "Inherited Abnormalities of the Skin." London, 1933, Oxford Univ. Press.

[3] HYDE, *J. Cutaneous Diseases*, 1909, **27**, 1.

[4] UPSHAW and MONTGOMERY, *Arch. Derm. and Syph.*, 1949, **60**, 1170.

[5] TOURAINE, *Bull. Soc. Franç. Derm. et Syph.*, 1935, **42**, 1929.

[6] MIN SEIN, *Lancet*, 1936, ii, 564.

*Ætiology.* The causes are alluded to in the above description of the various types of cases. Males are affected twice as often as females. The disease has appeared in several members of a family and in several generations, sometimes associated with defects of the teeth and nails. Sabouraud reminded us that we ought to consider the possibility of congenital syphilis. Some cases have been associated with epidermolysis bullosa (Chapter XV), and with injury at birth due to forceps ; with this type there is usually atrophy of the skin (p. 148). And see cases described in V below.

*Prognosis.* The outlook is serious. The hair may be induced to grow a little, then falls out again and again. When there has been a fine down from infancy, there is some hope that it may grow in longer after puberty.

**V.** *The patient may be a child or an adult. He has had normal hair, but it has fallen out, from the scalp, eyebrows and eyelids, and sometimes also from the body. The condition is* ALOPECIA TOTALIS ET UNIVERSALIS.

**Universal alopecia** (Syn. Alopecia totalis et universalis) is a condition in which not only the hairs of the scalp, but the hairs of the eyebrows, eyelashes and even those of the body, fall out. It is sometimes a development of alopecia areata. In time the skin loses its tone and the scalp can be picked up in folds ; such cases are not likely to recover. **Total alopecia,** in which the entire scalp is bald, has occurred in cases of children and young adults with CONGENITAL SYPHILIS. W. J. O'Donovan has usefully put on record three cases, all members of one family, who were thus affected ; yet in only one of them was present the syphilitic sign of notched incisor (Hutchinson's) teeth. Sabouraud believed that most of the cases of so-called congenital absence of hair had a syphilitic background, and advised that treatment on these lines should be persistently carried out. Antisyphilitic treatment is sometimes successful, even where no clear history is obtainable ; hence the importance of bearing in mind the

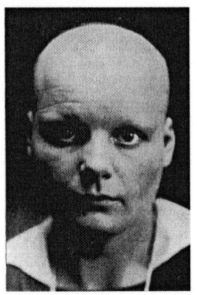

FIG. 27. — Alopecia Universalis. (*Photograph kindly lent by Dr. H. W. Barber.*)

possibility of syphilis as a causal agent in these uncommon cases of total and congenital alopecia.

Total alopecia can follow any form of generalized ERYTHRODERMIA. The physician may not see the case till the initial erythema has passed away. Here the history is all important (see Chapter XIII, p. 205).

VI. **Ichthyosis Follicularis** is a congenital and usually familial malady, so rare that few dermatologists have seen a case. The child may have normal hair at birth, but within a few months to two years the scalp begins to show the keratosis pilaris which eventually destroys the hair. There is considerable baldness, the skin being rough to the touch, due to pin-head-sized, horny cones, at the openings of the hair follicles on the scalp. A few follicles retain weak hairs, others show fine atrophy. The eyebrows and eyelashes were absent in several of the recorded cases,[1] and the skin of the body was dry, as in Xerodermia. ULERYTHEMA OPHRYOGENES (pp. 146 and 183) is probably an advanced stage of this disease. Sections showed hyperkeratosis of the follicles, which extended farther down than it does in lichen pilaris. In a lengthy study of congenital alopecia, Gilbert and Oliver [2] described the congenital baldness of two brothers, who appear to belong, clinically, to this type. Keratosis pilaris was present on the scalp and on some parts of the body. The cases underwent a minute and searching investigation, but nothing abnormal was found except that it was difficult to induce perspiration in them. Three years later, much improvement was noticed. The elder patient, a lad then of about twenty, ascribed his progress to the fact that he had vigorously and regularly scrubbed his scalp, thus removing the keratosis ; " this," he said, " allowed the hairs to come through." Cases described by Brocq, Lesser, MacLeod and Chalmers Watson, all had keratosis pilaris connected with their baldness.

VII. ICHTHYOSIS is considered under scales, its prominent diagnostic feature (see Chapter XI). The hair is scanty, dry and short ; the patient is a child, whose first hair has fallen out and has not again grown in properly.

TREATMENT OF LARGE AREAS OF BALDNESS. In every form, all the local methods described on pages 89 to 95 should be perseveringly given. General treatment, especially antisyphilitic remedies, should be given a trial in cases of congenital and total alopecia. For congenital atrichia the outlook is more serious ; large doses of lime and repeated courses of exposure to ultra violet light administered to the scalp and to the whole body have succeeded in obstinate cases. Endocrine treatment should be tried, especially thyroid. Where keratosis is present, wash frequently and use an ointment with salicylic acid, gr. 10 to 30 to the oz. Keratosis is considered to be one manifestation of deficiency of vitamin A ; it is aided by large doses of this vitamin. Other experiments tend to prove that keratosis may also be due to Vitamin C deficiency.

---

[1] J. M. H. MacLEOD, *Brit. Journ. Dermat.*, 1909, **21**, 165. This paper contains a very complete study of follicular diseases, with a bibliography.

[2] *Arch. Derm. and Syph.*, 1926, **13**, 359.

## CHAPTER VIII

# DIFFUSE HAIRFALL: B. WITH DISEASE OF THE SCALP, HAIRFALL AND OILINESS

Hairfall, diffused over the whole or a large part of the scalp, or localized to definite patches, accompanies quite a number of diseases of the scalp. Thus, for example, it is seen when there is generalized *erythrodermia*, also with local *folliculitis* ; but in such cases the patient does not consult the physician on account of hairfall, but for other symptoms which hold a more prominent place amongst the causes of his distress. Hairfall, when occurring together with some other characteristic or prominent sign of disease of the scalp, is discussed in the several sections dealing with that particular distinctive sign, in Chapters IX to XVIII.

We have now to consider the cases in which hairfall, without constitutional disorder, is the chief condition of the scalp for which advice is sought. Here we meet perhaps the most common complaint of all— *hairfall with oiliness*.

## I. HAIRFALL WITH OILINESS

*The patient is young, usually a man in the late teens or early twenties, who complains of loss of hair on temples and vertex and oiliness of the scalp. The most common causal condition is* SEBORRHŒA OLEOSA.

**Seborrhœa Oleosa.** *Introductory remarks and definition.* Dermatology is often blamed for its involved nomenclature. In no department is this reproach more justified than in that which concerns the ordinary baldness of men. Confusion long existed between the two terms, oiliness (seborrhœa oleosa) and dry seborrhœa (seborrhœa sicca), because it was once believed that the oily sebum became solidified on the scalp as in a comedo. The names originate quite simply : a dermatologist holds a certain theory, to which all the facts observed by him appear to conform. He selects a Latin name descriptive of the cause or main symptom ; this name is understood by the profession all over the world. However, the selected name is, after the passage of years, found to be inadequate ; it includes not all, but only a part of the truth. A new name is launched from the camp of the specialists, and this in its turn becomes outworn. But the previous name remains for a generation the popular title with the medical world outside the circle of dermatologists of one country.

101

Hence the name *Seborrhœa* does not convey the same meaning to every medical reader. As the word implies excess of oily secretion, the name *Seborrhœa sicca* (dry seborrhœa) contains within it a contradiction. Yet the title seborrhœa sicca was for long applied to the common condition of scaliness, popularly called dandruff, correctly named pityriasis sicca. (See pages 157 to 167, where this sign is considered at length.) The term seborrhœa oleosa, strictly speaking, indicates the presence of an excessive flow of sebum from the sebaceous glands. But the name is usually employed to denote disease—this too is a confusion of terms. Certain scalps show an excessive degree of oiliness throughout life, and yet there is no disease, only discomfort for æsthetic reasons (p. 81). However, the term seborrhœa is now used to denote greasiness of the skin, i.e. excess of sebaceous secretion ; closely associated is the term SEBORRHŒA OLEOSA, which denotes *oiliness of the scalp accompanied by hairfall.*

In seborrhœa oleosa the hairfall usually begins when the patient is quite young, about the age of puberty. It begins first on the temples, then affects the tonsure area and finally the whole vertex. Thus seborrhœa oleosa is in truth the baldness so common in men.

*Course and Prognosis of Seborrhœa Oleosa.* In a case of severe seborrhœa oleosa the usual course is at first a rapid, and then a gradual, march towards the complete baldness, with a stretched, glossy skin, which is so frequently seen in men. The affection begins in early youth. Heredity plays an important rôle ; marked baldness tends to run in families. The usual history of a typical case has been admirably described by Sabouraud. At first the young man has dandruff, i.e. *pityriasis sicca,* with bottle bacilli in the scurf scales (p. 163) ; he may show signs of this before puberty. A few years later, at the age of fifteen to seventeen, the scales tend to become sticky and thick, with a mild serous exudation—*pityriasis steatoides,* with staphylococcus albus infection, has set in. Later still, at any time between seventeen and twenty, oiliness, true *seborrhœa oleosa,* begins. The microbacillus of the seborrhœic gland infection displaces the bottle bacillus of pityriasis sicca and the polymorphous coccus of pityriasis steatoides (p. 162). With the onset of true seborrhœa the hair begins to fall. Since World War II I have been impressed by the fact that many cases of Male Pattern baldness in both men and women have had no oiliness. This may be due to the increased use of cleansing detergents, which certainly cause dryness. Hairdressers also tell me that they have noticed less oiliness ; they ascribed this to deficiency of fats in the diet. The oiliness varies in amount ; it may be moderate or it may be very marked, especially in hot weather. Often seborrhœa at the same time appears on the face, especially around the nose and chin, and on the middle line of the back and the front of the chest. Acne vulgaris is frequently associated with the onset of seborrhœa oleosa ; the same microbacillus is found in the comedo contents.[1]

Seborrhœa begins on the temporal regions and on the posterior region of the vertex. Hair begins to fall from the temples and from the posterior part of the vertex, and not diffusely, all over the scalp, as in the hairfall which follows fevers or operations (p. 85). In severe cases, when the infection first sets in, many hundred hairs may fall every day. This profuse hairfall continues for several months, and is succeeded by a time when comparatively few hairs fall, only between thirty and fifty a day. There are then periods of exemption, when the sufferer begins to hope that he will have no further loss of hair. In some of these intervals of respite there may be even a little regrowth of fine hairs. But the loss of hair returns, and in the intervals when there is no fall, the regrowth becomes less, and the individual hairs which return are finer and shorter. After the thirtieth year there is a decrease in the rate and amount of the hairfall. Sabouraud stated that in the really severe cases of baldness, with glossy skin all over the top of the head, which is seen so frequently in middle-aged men, the loss of hair has been marked by the age of thirty. He went so far as to say that if a man has not lost half of his hair by the time he is thirty years old, he will never develop the extreme type of baldness.

From the above description of the usual course of seborrhœa oleosa in men, it might be gathered that when once seborrhœa begins on the scalp, there is no hope for a young man ; that sooner or later his scalp must become entirely bald, with the exception of the ring of hair which even in the worst cases appears to be left at the occiput and above the ears. However, treatment can do much to arrest the progress of the

---

[1] The nomenclature is so involved that although the association of seborrhœa, pityriasis and "seborrhœic dermatitis" is discussed at length in the section on pityriasis (p. 159), it is advisable to add a footnote here. On the greasy-skinned individual one sees the large openings of the sebaceous glands down the middle line of the chest, back and front, and on the nasolabial folds and chin. A characteristic circinate eruption, with scales, on a fawn pink base, is apt to occur on these areas, wrongly named seborrhœic dermatitis. To this group of associated symptoms Darier gave the name *Kerose* ; H. W. Barber describes these, with the accompanying metabolic errors, as the "seborrhœic state" (p. 163). It must be clearly understood that this rash is not associated with microbacilli nor with hairfall. Instead, it shows the flora of pityriasis ; therefore Sabouraud's names, pityriasis circinata or eczematized pityriasis steatoides, have always appealed to me, as being less confusing and more descriptive.

hairfall. The fall usually decreases in rate after the age of thirty. The knowledge of this normal decrease in the activity of the hairfall after the age of thirty conveys much comfort to a patient in the early twenties and to his friends, who usually believe that the natural course of the affliction involves a steady march, throughout the whole of a lifetime, towards complete baldness.

Baldness of the male type used to be very rare in women. Not infrequently there is seen a condition of excessive oiliness of the scalp, which endures for years, yet is not associated with hairfall (see p. 81) ; in these cases, in women, I have found few or no microbacilli present. Before 1914 I had collected a considerable number of cases of true seborrhœa oleosa in women ; they had over the vertex, and in some cases also on the temples, a profuse hairfall, accompanied by excessive oiliness. Abundant microbacilli were found in the scalp scrapings of all these cases. Since 1936 I have seen a number of such cases, often without oiliness ; possibly this is due to the shorter hair and more frequent washing which now prevails. Recent research places emphasis on the rôle played by excess of the male hormone in the production of acne, seborrhœa oleosa and male pattern baldness in both men and women (see Ætiology, p. 106). This knowledge of the endocrine factor has displaced the predominance of the Sabouraud microbacillus as a cause of baldness. Nevertheless, the association of the microbacillus with seborrhœa oleosa is still worthy of consideration. In the majority of women with male pattern baldness the oiliness and hairfall develops rather rapidly. Before 1914, owing to the fact that women wore long hair and that there was no method of permanent wave, the natural state of the scalp and the thinning hair could not be concealed except by wearing pads and false hair. In some of these cases the oiliness had developed when the general health was normal ; in others it had appeared after a definite period of chronic illness. Often the oiliness had been preceded by pityriasis ; the oiliness gave the scales the greasy, crusted appearance of pityriasis steatoides. It is of interest that in these cases it is rare to see seborrhœic dermatitis, either on the scalp or the body.

*Diagnosis.* When there is doubt as to the diagnosis and therefore the prognosis of hairfall with oiliness or scales, whether the condition is one of seborrhœa alone, of pityriasis with secondary staphylococcal infection, or of pityriasis with underlying oily secretion, the microscope reveals with which we have to deal. First cleanse a small area of the scalp with a swab of cotton-wool dipped in either ether or absolute alcohol, then press the scalp with the edge of a glass slide and push it firmly along the skin, so that the sebum and epidermal scales are squeezed on to the slide. Stain with methylene blue or gentian violet. With seborrhœa oleosa, micro-bacilli are seen in teeming numbers (Fig. 28). If the less serious condition is present, there will be seen many cocci and bottle bacilli, but comparatively few or no microbacilli. In some of the most serious conditions of seborrhœa oleosa, with micro-bacilli teeming in the scalp scrapings, the hair roots showed few or no microbacilli. This finding is in marked contrast to that occurring in some types of alopecia areata, and is referred

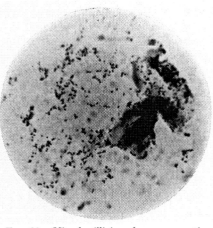

Fig. 28.—Microbacilli in sebaceous secretion. Microphotograph mag. × 800.

to in the section dealing with that disease (see p. 117).

*Ætiology.* The cause of the ordinary baldness of men has been debated for centuries. Before any discussion of modern theories on its endocrine origin, I summarize some of the more popular old hypotheses. First of all, baldness, or the opposite condition, the retention of a thick head of hair till the fifth decade, is a hereditary matter. Even to-day, the chief exponent of the endocrine origin of baldness allows the import-ance of the hereditary factor. Formerly, it was argued that the habit of frequent or daily washing of the scalp, indulged in by many town-dwellers, was one cause of baldness. The wearing of tight, unventilated hats was next regarded as the chief culprit. I do not know whether the modern fashion of loose and light hats has improved the hair of men ; but I am certain that women lose their hair when they adopt the tight caps which in certain uniforms are essential headgear. Cutting the hair short is said to be harmful because of the absence of the natural stimu-lation of long hair when permitted to grow.

Painstaking research on this subject was carried out over a period of over forty years by the great Parisian dermatologist, Sabouraud. He described the microbacillus always present with acne and with seborrhœa of the scalp, and believed that it played a prominent part in the production of baldness. Although Sabouraud laid emphasis upon the microbacillus, many readers have overlooked his careful observations on other contribu-tory causes of seborrhœa. He found microbacilli always present ; oiliness usually present ; the associated constitutional factors varied with the individual.    In 1902 Sabouraud stated : [1]  " Seborrhœa is a microbic malady, but develops only under certain conditions of age and of the general health." This statement disproves the widespread belief that he regarded the microbacillus as the cause of seborrhœa. He drew attention to the fact that baldness is rare in peasants who have hard physical work in the open air, and that it is common in sedentary and city workers. Sabouraud also observed the usefulness of large doses of phosphoric acid in cases of hairfall with seborrhœa. With this medicamentation remarkable benefit was obtained in the asthenic state which often accompanies the seborrhœic loss of hair. Sulphur and iodine taken by mouth, he also noted, were of much value in certain cases. " We have observed too often," he proceeded, " the association of excessive hyperacidity of the urine with baldness in quite young people not to attribute to the general condition, and to the gastric condition which it implies, an active part in the severity of the seborrhœic loss of hair.    Even if this colossal urinary hyperacidity is only a chance coincidence in cases of seborrhœa of the scalp, the physician should do all he can to counteract what is at least an anomaly.    Correct general alkaline treatment, and attention to the digestion, has given in several cases results which the local treatment alone would probably not have affected." H. W. Barber [2] has written much on the " seborrhœic state." At puberty the sebaceous glands become normally more active. With deficient exercise and dietetic errors their secretion is so altered that it permits the seborrhœic triad of organisms to gain a footing—the bottle bacillus (which causes dandruff), the microbacillus and certain cocci. Large doses of alkalis he found very beneficial ; this I can confirm.

It has long been believed that there was a connection between the endocrine glands and baldness.    In elderly men who have been bald there is sometimes a regrowth of fine hair at the decline of sexual life. Young women with seborrhœa oleosa and hairfall often develop masculine hair growth on the face and elsewhere.    At the menopause there is often hirsuties on the face, male pattern hairfall on the scalp, sometimes oily skin and acne.    Sabouraud conducted an enquiry in the East and stated that eunuchs never became bald ; the same coincidence was noted by Aristotle and other writers in antiquity.    Sabouraud noted (and quoted Leopold Levi as another observer) that when a woman with seborrhœa becomes pregnant, the hairfall ceases before the third month and recom-

---

[1] *Maladies du Cuir Chevelu*, Vol. I, Maladies Seborrhéiques.    Paris, 1902, p. 283.
[2] H. W. Barber, the *Lancet*, 1929, ii, 483, 591, and chapter on " Diseases of the Skin," in *Medical Diseases of the War*, by Arthur Hurst.    London, Edward Arnold, 1944 ; also " Modern Trends of Dermatology," 1948.

mences two to two and a half months after childbirth. In Levi's case this was seen in a woman who had borne twelve children. Male pattern baldness in women is arrested about the third month of pregnancy; other seborrhœic symptoms, such as acne, also disappear at that time. This is due to the rise of œstrogen in the blood stream which occurs during pregnancy.

It is now an accepted theory that the main factor in the development of seborrhœa, of acne vulgaris and of male baldness is the endocrine constitution of the individual. The more active the male hormone (androgen) the greater the production of the various manifestations of seborrhœa; and therefore the earlier the appearance of male baldness. The changes in the sebaceous glands which show hyperkeratosis of the mouths of the follicles, comedones and acne, are due to androgen stimulation of the skin; œstrogens counteract this process. Ovarian deficiency is not uncommon in women, but it alone does not lead to baldness. Thus the chief factors in male loss of hair are : excess of male hormone ; deficiency of œstrone, with relative preponderance of adrenal androgen ; increased adrenal androgen, such as occurs with adrenal cortex hyperplasia, adenoma or malignant disease, and also with increase of the adrenotropic hormone of the pituitary. Œstrone is curative in ovarian deficiency when uncomplicated by adrenal involvement ; here the male hormone becomes predominant. Hairfall accompanies many diseases of the pituitary ; see the chapter on hypertrichosis, with discussion of the causes of masculine distribution of hair growth and fall. Hamilton's research on 104 eunuchs and eunochoids has definitely established the fact that there is a relationship between the testes and baldness.[1] His paper must be studied by those who desire to understand the association of seborrhœa, acne vulgaris and male type baldness with the condition of the testes. With appropriate dosage of testosterone propionate given to sexually immature men he produced sexual maturity ; with this there developed male type baldness. However, he states that although normal testicular secretion promotes baldness in many men, *there are other factors concerned.* There is, he says, no conclusive proof that baldness is due only to excessive amount or unusual type of androgen ; " In normal men androgens form a link in a family of indirect causes which induce baldness." One important cause is a hereditary predisposition to baldness. In his experimental research, androgen therapy produced baldness only in the men who had a family tendency to baldness. Where such pedigree tendency was absent, even intensive androgen therapy did not cause baldness. The androgen which induces loss of hair comes from

[1] JAMES HAMILTON, *Amer. J. Anat.*, 1942, **71**, 451.

the ovaries, the testes and the adrenals.  The androgenic secretion is diminished by œstrogens, but they do not act as true substitutes.  Dr. H. W. Barber [1] summarizes thus the effect of sex hormones on the scalp : Androgens stimulate surface epithelium and sebaceous glands, tending to produce hyperkeratosis and seborrhœa ; œstrogens diminish keratinization and sebaceous activity.  He believes that the organisms found on seborrhœic skin are not the cause of primary seborrhœa.  With this I do not entirely agree.

Other theories on the subject of baldness merit brief mention here.  Work in Germany ran on such entirely different lines that even before 1939 they made no mention of Sabouraud !  Max Joseph [2] stated that baldness is a sex character of men and occurs where there is a seborrhœic soil.  It is preceded by the formation of scales, due to an abnormal process of cornification in which the superficial horny cells retain their nucleus and remain soft.  Some German workers maintained that there was a connection between the growth of the hair and the metabolism of cholesterin.[3]  In health the secretion from the sebaceous glands contains a high cholesterol content.  When, owing to constitutional disease, there is a decreased amount of cholesterol in the sebaceous gland secretion, there occur in the follicles certain changes which lead to an unhealthy appearance of the hair and eventually to hairfall.  When the hyperkeratosis affects the outer root sheath, the hair falls out.  This abnormal cornification process is supposed to be due to deficiency of cholesterol.  During pregnancy there is an increase of cholesterol content in the blood, with improvement in the hair as regards both its appearance and the arrest of hairfall.  Many German teachers restored the old conception of the association of pityriasis sicca with seborrhœa ; for both conditions cholesterol was rubbed well into the scalp.  The record of successful cases certainly reads convincingly ; but it is difficult to gather whether the writers are describing serborrhœa oleosa ; often they appear to be giving details of pityriasis steatoides.  Sabouraud gave preparations of cholestrol a fair test, but had no success.

Cederberg [4] believed that in severe cases of hairfall, seborrhœa and an infective parakeratosis (pityriasis) alternate after an initial specific microbacillus infection.  He maintained that there was an underlying general toxæmia—chronic, such as alcoholism or syphilis, and various local infections (as of the bile passages, oral sepsis and genito-urinary infections) ; or acute, such as influenza, typhus, erysipelas or acute local infections.  The male endocrine factor was also important.

*Treatment.*  Endocrine treatment is considered on p. 111.  To deal first with local methods : The treatment of seborrhœa oleosa is one of the

---

[1] " Modern Trends in Dermatology," Butterworth, 1948, p. 113.

[2] MAX JOSEPH, *Therapie der Gegenwart*, 1927, **68**, 207.

[3] RUDOLF JAFFÉ, *Klin. Woch.*, 1926, **5**, 507 ; ALFRED ELIASSOW, *Derm. Woch.*, 1926, **83**, 1463 ; HABERMANN, *Deut. Med. Woch.*, 1928, **54**, 1560 ; KRICHEL, *Deut. Med. Woch.*, 1929, **55**, 275.    [4] CEDERBERG, *Derm. Woch.*, 1932, **94**, 272.

most difficult problems in dermatology. The main recommendations are (1) washing and removal of oiliness, (2) the use of grease dissolvents ; and (3) sulphur applications ; others advise cholesterol. (4) I wish to emphasize the importance of a fourth factor : attention to the general health. (See remarks on this subject on pp. 111 et seq.) When the seborrhœa is complicated by pityriasis, tar is usually advised ; I prefer mercury. The treatment requires perseverance and regularity in its daily performance. In severe cases this demands an amount of time and a degree of patience which are rarely devoted to the treatment by any sufferer.

1. When scaliness is present as well as oiliness, it is essential to dismiss from the mind of the patient the popular idea that a scaly scalp is a dry scalp and therefore should not often be washed. WASHING must be frequent and thorough. Ordinary soap contains a soda salt. Soap and water remove scales and dissolve grease ; hence good soap and soft water cleanse the scalp and allow penetration of local remedies. Modern sulphonated oil and other applications for cleansing and washing are considered on page 53. Hebra's soap was in common use before 1914 : soft soap, one part, to two parts of rectified spirit ; perfumed with spirit of lavender. Spirit soap B.P.C. has replaced it. Washing is easily carried out with any ordinary good soap ; soft is preferable to hard water. With men, with very oily scalps, it may be essential to wash the scalp every day.

When patients have much hairfall, they notice that washing at first seems to bring away a great number of hairs ; they rarely observe that this initial increase is soon followed by a decrease which lasts for a varying number of days. Explain to the patient that it is not the washing which has caused the temporary apparent increase of hairfall. What has happened is that the washing, and the friction of drying, has hastened the fall of those hairs which were already loosened from their roots and soon about to fall. A second washing is indicated to be necessary as soon as an increased rate of hairfall follows the improvement noticed after the previous washing. By close observation the individual soon learns how to regulate the intervals between washing. Again, one must impress upon the patient the fact that it is the scalp which requires careful washing, not the whole length of the hair. Whilst the scalp requires to be washed every few days, or even every day in severe cases of pityriasis and seborrhœa, long hair, especially at the free end, would become dry and brittle if washed so often. The entire length of long hair requires to be brushed daily, but can be washed much less frequently (cp. p. 52). To rinse away the soap from the scalp, soft or distilled water is better than hard water ; clean rain water is excellent. For certain types of fine hair, it is better to wash with an egg, well-beaten, whole, or only the yolk. Sabouraud recommended a decoction of quillaia, which must be well rinsed off afterwards.

2. GREASE DISSOLVENTS. The scalp must be kept free from oil, especially in the case of the rapid development of baldness in young men. Various forms of spirit preparations are used to dissolve the grease before applying remedial drugs ; ether and absolute alcohol formed the basis of most lotions before 1914. These are nowadays very expensive to use for a malady which requires a lengthy period of treatment (see Formulæ, p. 303). Modern cleansing agents are discussed in the section on Washing the Hair, p. 52. Acetone and ether are cheaper than rectified spirit, and are sometimes added to the lotions used for an oily scalp. Ether should not be used alone, as it is inflammable ; the patient should be warned of this fact. Petrol is still more dangerous.

3. SULPHUR can be used in lotions, ointments and powders. It must never be forgotten that a few individuals react with violent dermatitis to the mildest applications of sulphur. Apparently, so far as its efficacy is concerned, the variety of sulphur matters little. For women, especially when the hair is long, it is frequently ordered in a powdered form ; the hair is divided into many partings and the powder rubbed in for a quarter of an hour. A muslin or other cap is worn at night to keep the powder from the pillow and the face. The latter precaution is especially important in the case of those who develop dermatitis if sulphur falls on the face and neck. The powder can be brushed out of the hair in the morning, and the scalp washed several times a week. When patients object to powder, lotions containing sulphur may be given ; 1 part of sulphur to 10 to 14 parts of spirit and water is a usual proportion. Colloidal preparations of sulphur may be used instead of precipitated sulphur, both in lotions and in salves. Astringent drugs, tannic acid and chloral hydrate, have also long been favoured, in spirit lotions, for the treatment of seborrhœa oleosa.

In the severe cases met with in men, treatment consists in the use of sulphur preparations every night and thorough washing in the morning, then friction with a hard brush moistened with a lotion containing a stimulant such as pilocarpine or quinine. Sabouraud first introduced carbon bisulphide as the most effective form of sulphur and spirit. The trouble involved in its use led to its neglect ; but one recent patient tells me that he found it more valuable than any other lotion (see page 304).

In ancient days pityriasis was treated by rubbing soda on the scalp. It is interesting that Pincus employed the same drug for arresting hairfall, probably of seborrhœic origin. He prescribed 1 drachm of bicarbonate of soda in 3 oz. of distilled water ; ½ oz. of the mixture was rubbed into the scalp on two consecutive days of the week, for two or five minutes. Oil was applied on one of the other days. This treatment was continued for five, twelve, or even eighteen months, until the short hairs which fell numbered less than a fifth or a quarter of the total loss (p. 18). The hair was apt to acquire an auburn shade during the course of treatment.

4. I have always attributed great importance to the treatment of the GENERAL HEALTH.

Oiliness of the scalp, with acne of face and body, is greatly influenced by *diet, exercise* and *fresh air*. Avoid alcohol and chocolates, limit fats, starchy foods and sugar, take abundant vitamin content in food and, if necessary, in tablet and other preparations ; correct constipation, take sufficient daily exercise to keep the skin glowing and to induce healthy perspiration—all these factors count for much in delaying or arresting oiliness and hairfall.

*Endocrine therapy* has recently received increasing attention owing to the interest taken in the effect of hormones and vitamins on the presence and the absence of hair. See in particular Hamilton's article on the androgen stimulating properties in the sexually immature male, p. 107. In women with male pattern baldness this form of endocrine therapy holds promise. Barber advocates local applications of ointment containing œstrogen, to be given during the first half of the menstrual cycle. Œstrogens thus administered are more potent than when taken by mouth. In some cases this form of treatment restores hair growth, but for advanced types of male pattern baldness in women little can be done. This is also my experience. I have seen marked reactions on the face when the base in which the œstrogen is incorporated happens to be one to which the patient is sensitive. In 1943 Barber reported the case of a young married woman with male pattern baldness, no seborrhœa or hirsuties, but with palmar hyperkeratoses such as are sometimes seen at the climacteric. She responded to œstradiol given for several months. I have tried this form of therapy on older women, with apparent benefit. It must not be long continued ; uterine discharge and bleeding may ensue. I once saw a woman who had had oral œstrone therapy for over ten years after the menopause ; she then rather rapidly developed hirsuties with masculine distribution on the body, face and limbs, together with typical male baldness. In men with male pattern baldness œstrin therapy is not advisable. Overdosage leads to gynæcomastia and signs of female change of character. I tried it on an observant medical man, in small doses ; he was convinced that it arrested his progressive loss of hair. However, as he had been a vegetarian and took little exercise, normal diet and active exercise probably played a part in his improvement. Œstrogen (stilboestrol 1 mg. twice daily) I tested for severe acne vulgaris in several young men ; they benefited by the short course of treatment ; but not more than others who were attending hospital at the same time and enjoying ultra-violet light exposures.

Many years ago I published carefully taken notes of cases of seborrhœa oleosa in both men and women who had responded to treatment with diet and vaccines. When revising for this and the third edition I was tempted to omit these reports, but on re-reading them, I decided to retain a few. If we take these records together with Sabouraud's observations on the urinary hyperacidity, and the comparative freedom from baldness of the manual labourer, then consider the guarded conclusions of Hamilton as to the environmental and hereditary factors, surely we can conclude that the contributory causes of baldness are almost as important as the endocrine constitution in the average individual. With deeper knowledge we may find that with vitamin deficiency the endocrine glands also function wrongly. It has been maintained that hormones and vitamins are biological regulators of similar value ; that they both have a basic chemical reaction resembling an enzymic process.

Many years ago I tried an autogenous or, if unobtainable, a stock vaccine for the treatment of seborrhœa oleosa with hairfall.[1] The modern tendency to decry the usefulness of vaccine therapy is to me quite unconvincing. Many failures can be explained by faults in spacing and dosage and by hyper-sensitiveness after over-dosage. Whatever the rationale of the method, treatment of seborrhœa oleosa with vaccine is worthy of trial in women. In men it appeared only to delay or postpone the progress of baldness.

Case I. A young man, aged twenty-six, consulted me in April, 1911. The vertex was almost entirely bald, showing only a few long fine hairs and a scanty downiness. Greasiness of the scalp had started at the age of eighteen, and had developed gradually, together with profuse hairfall. He had lived in the East for six years, and had perspired profusely on the head after exercise and in hot weather. He had tried many kinds of local applications for several years, and latterly had been obliged to wash his head twice daily. No treatment had done any good, although evaporating lotions to some extent reduced the discomfort. He continued the use of evaporating lotions, and I tried vaccine treatment at once. Between April 19 and October 14 he had sixteen injections, increasing from 20 million to 300 million of the acne bacillus. It was found that he responded to a dose of 250 to 300 million and that the hair was distinctly drier for one day after, and later for three or four days

---

[1] *Practitioner*, 1911, **86**, 392, and 1912, **89**, 388. Notes on the Vaccine Treatment of Seborrhœa.

after the injection.    The hairfall began to decrease in July, and in September new hairs were found growing all over, and the hairfall was practically nil. He only required to wash the hair every few days, and that chiefly because, owing to the exceptionally hot summer, he perspired much.    The microbacillus was found in abundance on April 24 ; but only an occasional one could be detected by September, when he went abroad, and neglected to fulfil his promise to report.

CASE II.    In 1926 a young man of twenty-six consulted me with regard to his rapidly developing baldness.    He had an oily scalp, and hair receding from the temples ; microscopic examination revealed numerous microbacilli. He followed out the directions methodically and was cured.    He applied carbon bisulphide at night and washed every morning.    Between September 22 and November 30 he had weekly doses of a stock vaccine of acne bacillus increased from 100 to 250 million.    At the weekly visit I gave ultra-violet light from the concentrated tungsten arc lamp and also high-frequency tube applications.    The hairfall was arrested and downy hair appeared on the denuded areas.    He had no relapse until 1932 when he wrote to me from the East that oiliness and hairfall were returning.    I again ordered Sabouraud's carbon bisulphide lotion and renewed dietetic instructions.    By 1937 his hair had not receded farther than at his first visit in 1926.

Since the publication of the first edition of this book I have had more extensive experience of the treatment of baldness in men, and regret to admit that I have had many disappointments.    Some have made progress at first, even grown a fine crop of downy hair.    After a period of time without local treatment, these hairs usually fell out.    Nor did they grow longer in the comparatively few patients who had the necessary energy to persevere.    In many cases, however, I am quite certain that the baldness was prevented from becoming progressive, possibly due to the fact that these young men adopted a healthier mode of life and diet. One medical student with severe acne of the back and chest said that as these were always covered he did not object to the ugly papules. With the dietetic methods followed, together with wiser regulation of exercise and study, his acne was cured without endocrines or vaccines.

Several cases of women with commencing baldness and seborrhœa oleosa are of interest.    The bearing of the general health upon the local condition, and the effect of the vaccine upon the presence of the microbacillus are both apparent in these cases.

CASE III.    Miss A., aged twenty-eight, sought advice in August, 1906, for hairfall, which had been alarmingly profuse for over eight months.    She had always had a tendency to have a greasy scalp, but during the previous year the oiliness had greatly increased, necessitating more and more frequent washing of the head.    The hair was very thin on the vertex, and it was becoming more impossible to dress it neatly without washing the hair every second day.    A microscopic examination revealed the microbacillus in enormous numbers and no other germ except an occasional bottle bacillus. The patient was treated thoroughly with spirit lotions, frequent washing and ointments containing sulphur in varying proportions and forms, mercury, pyrogallic acid, formalin and other strong antiseptic and penetrating ingredients. After eight months of treatment carried out by the patient without any supervision, the scalp was found to be still oily ; the sebum oozing from the sebaceous follicles on the slightest pressure teemed with microbacilli. The patient went abroad for a year and continued the local treatment with more or less assiduity ; hairfall and oiliness decidedly improved. She relaxed treatment and the condition became as bad as ever in a few months. In August, 1909, microbacilli were still present and the hair began to fall profusely. A vaccine was made from a culture of the microbacillus sent to me from Paris by Dr. Sabouraud. Four injections were given, in doses varying from 100 to 300 million, on August 25, October 4, 19 and November 1. After each dose of vaccine there was a decrease of the oiliness of the scalp. Eleven months later she wrote from abroad to tell me that the improvement had continued, the oiliness had practically disappeared, the hairfall had ceased and there had been a regrowth of hair.

In this case local treatment had been tried for three years, with only slight improvement for short periods. The rapid and marked alteration for the better on the adoption of the vaccine treatment is strong presumptive proof that in this case the microbacillus played a prominent rôle.

Case IV. Mrs. F., aged thirty-two, came in May, 1912, with a history of six years' hairfall together with increasing greasiness of the scalp. Microbacilli were numerous. Previously, the scalp had been dry and scurfy. The general health was excellent. The hair had lost colour and was short and split at the free ends. For the first months I tried lotions without benefit. Between June and October she had eleven injections of a microbacillus vaccine, in doses from 100 to 300 million. Improvement began after the first dose ; the greasiness and the hairfall diminished with each injection until by the month of September the bright golden shade of the hair had returned and there were numerous young hairs springing up all over the scalp. By December she had neither greasiness nor hairfall, and no microbacillus could be found. Some six months later, she came back with a slight return of hairfall and oiliness and a history of several months of ill-health. With treatment of the general health the scalp became normal. There had not been found any microbacilli with the relapse, which apparently was due to the condition of the general health. Seventeen years later, she reported *no relapse*.

Case V. Miss M. E., aged twenty-eight, consulted me for oiliness and hairfall of an alarming degree which had lasted for one year. She had had oily hair all her life, but this had not been associated with hairfall till the year when the greasiness became marked. The hair was short, reaching only to the shoulders, and had split ends. The general health was poor. Nine weekly injections of microbacillus vaccine were given as soon as the microscopic examination revealed the presence of the germ in great abundance in the scalp scrapings. Improvement began with the first injection. After the second injection, she stated that the hair did not become as oily in ten days as it had formerly done in four days. After the ninth injection, very few microbacilli were found, and the improvement was maintained. In this case treatment was also directed to the general health.

The importance of attention to the general health was borne in upon me by the failure of treatment in Case VI, and the success in Case VII.

CASE VI. Miss B., aged twenty-nine, had had an oily scalp from the age of fifteen, but no hairfall till two years before she consulted me for increasing hairfall and oiliness. The hair was very thin over the vertex and microbacilli were very numerous. She was an artist, living a strenuous life with much expenditure of nervous energy. With the slightest excitement profuse perspiration broke out over the scalp. As she could not come regularly for injections, many lotions and powders were tried, without result, for two years. Then I gave injections of a microbacillus vaccine obtained from Paris, from Dr. Sabouraud. Great improvement followed the first three doses, the last of which amounted to 280 million. Then she was not seen for a month, when a dose of 100 million was given. Oiliness increased the next day, pointing to a miscalculation of dosage. After an interval, smaller doses were given, followed by considerable improvement, which lasted so long as she led a quiet country life. She reported later that the trouble returned when she came back to her exciting town life, which always had affected for the worse her general health.

CASE VII. In 1924, Miss R., aged twenty, consulted me for hairfall and oiliness. The hair was so thin over the vertex that the skin of the scalp gleamed through as is usual only in quite old women. The scalp showed much oiliness and a degree of pityriasis. There were also many grey hairs. The oiliness of the scalp began to be noticed at puberty, but the hair remained thick and in good condition till the age of sixteen. Then the oiliness began to increase and the hairfall had continued for four years. All kinds of treatment had been tried before she sought medical advice. A scalp scraping showed microbacilli in teeming numbers. The cæcum was loaded, the thyroid gland was slightly enlarged, the pulse average 96, and the hands were blue and cold even on a warm summer day. A diet was ordered which contained much fresh fruit and vegetables, fish and fresh meat, milk, butter and stoneground flour bread, marmite and a minimum of sugar, puddings and cakes. Locally, a lotion containing sulphur 1 part, alcohol 20, water 100 parts, was used in the morning, and at night a powder with 20 parts of sulph. præcip. to the ounce of talc and oxide of zinc. Acne bacillus vaccine was given, beginning with 90 million and increasing to 180 million, between the middle of October and end of December. The oiliness decreased ; by the end of January the scalp looked healthy, with plenty of young hairs. A stimulating lotion was then given, with tr. cantharides, camphor and alcohol āā 1 drachm to the ounce of distilled water. A year later there had been no relapse of the condition of the scalp and the general health was normal.

In this case the vaccine appeared to have hastened the cure, but no doubt the great improvement in the general health was also responsible for the restored condition of the hair.

On reading these case notes after forty years I believe that the main cause of success was probably due to the dietetic and other management of the general health. I was at that time interested in the treatment of intestinal toxæmia, and alive to the importance of fresh and raw food, with abundance of vegetables and fruit, and also of wholemeal bread and dairy products. I am still convinced of the importance of these measures. We now know that such a diet provides the essential vitamins which are deficient in long-cooked and over-refined articles of diet. We also are now aware of the importance of the vitamins and their action upon the endocrine glands.

This conclusion is borne out by the following instance : In 1937 a lad of 17 sought advice for hairfall and acne ; his hair was thin and of fine quality ; microbacilli were abundant on the temples. The family history was bad ; his father and a brother had been bald in the early thirties. Therefore I gave a bad prognosis, and advice on diet and exercise. A sulphur pomade and lotion were used whilst he continued at school. He joined the Army in 1940. I wrote to find out if he had lost more hair during the six years which had passed since his visit to me. He replied that he had found the treatment a success, that he had quite a good head of hair although, since he had joined the Forces, he could not devote any time to scalp drill. In the Army he obtained much meat, and therefore an adequate quantity of the Vitamin B which recent work suggests as playing a prominent rôle in maintaining the health of the hair.

# CHAPTER IX

## HAIRFALL WITH BALD PATCHES

After the diffuse hairfall which follows acute, and often accompanies chronic illness, and after hairfall with oiliness, perhaps the most common complaint is HAIRFALL WITH BALD PATCHES.

CLINICAL INVESTIGATION. When a patient complains of bald patches, before looking at the scalp, the observer gains some information merely by looking at the patient. Much can thus be learned regarding the *general health*, whether the patient has recently been ill, or is still suffering from some chronic malady, and whether there are signs of any hereditary malady such as syphilis. The *age* also gives valuable information ; certain diseases, such as ringworm, are more liable to attack children than adults, and vice versa. The *sex*, too : seborrhœa oleosa is common in men, rare in women.

Sometimes a mere glance at the bald patch will reveal to the expert eye that the area is not really bald, but is covered with the scales and broken hairs so characteristic of ringworm, or the yellow crusts of favus, so that a microscopic examination of the hairs is hardly required to clinch the diagnosis. Or again, the typical exclamation hairs (Fig. 50) at the margin of a patch of alopecia areata may be visible before the lens is requisitioned for close inspection. The crusts of impetigo and of other vesicles and pustules, or the presence of cysts or tumours, may at once reveal the cause of localized bald patches. The lens is required for investigating certain types of scales, such as the horny cones of keratosis. When the lens is turned on an apparently bald patch, which is sometimes very extensive, conical scales may be seen at the mouth of the follicles in monilethrix (p. 242) and ichthyosis follicularis (p. 100).

The *history of onset* is important. In the diffuse hairfall which follows fever, the rapid thinning of the hair may lead to the formation of irregular bald areas scattered over the scalp. Or there may be the history of an injury, a fall, a " cold perm " application or a burn, to account for the bald area which the patient believed was a disease, because a new method of hairdressing had revealed a bald patch of which she had hitherto lived in ignorance. Lesions on the face and neck may reveal the source of baldness in various pustular conditions, such as impetigo and chickenpox. The *shape* or angular margin of the patch may at once distinguish a traumatic alopecia. The *size* and *number* of the patches aid the diagnosis of a former herpes zoster, of chickenpox or pseudo-pelade. Again, it may be necessary

117

to *examine the whole body* in order to shed light on the cause of a bald patch. Thus, for example, a child may show bald areas suspiciously like those met with in adults suffering from secondary syphilis ; in that case, if the face were free from eruption, examination of the body is necessary in order to trace the corroborative evidence in the form of macules and papules. J. H. Sequeira reported a case in which the primary sore was found on the back of the neck of a very young child ; in this patient the infection had gained entrance through impetigo sores. It is a good clinical rule not to think of rareties until all common diagnoses have been excluded, but an extensive acquired baldness in a young person should make one consider the possibility of congenital syphilis when no simpler explanation can be found (see p. 99). Morphœa is so rare a cause of bald patches that in its early stage it could easily be mistaken unless other lesions were found on the body.

This is the place to mention the fact that after an *epilation dose* of X-ray and of thallium acetate, there should develop a complete baldness ; but when the doses have been inadequate, all the hairs do not fall out, and if the patient is a child who comes before the physician unaccompanied by a relative, a mistake in diagnosis is liable to happen (see also p. 96).

Conditions in which there is a bald area, larger than a patch, are dealt with in Chapter VII.

Examine the bald patch carefully, in order to decide whether the skin is normal, or whether there is atrophy or scarring. Sometimes it is difficult to decide whether the bald patch is permanently atrophied. No follicles may be visible ; the skin may appear glossy ; yet hair may return after several months. I have seen this occur after boils, severe impetigo and burns with permanent waving. Bald areas caused by the Cold Wave process may last as long as six months.

Cases where there is ATROPHY or SCARRING of the skin on the bald patch are dealt with on p. 136.

The following are the causes of BALD PATCHES WITHOUT ATROPHY or cicatricial condition of the skin, mentioned as far as possible in order of frequency of occurrence :

GROUP A.  BALD PATCHES WITHOUT ATROPHY

   I   Alopecia areata.
  II   Seborrhœa oleosa, especially common in men.
 III   Senile baldness in its early stage.
 IV   Pityriasis simplex capitis.
  V   Impetigo and other superficial pustular affections.
 VI   Secondary syphilis.
VII   Baldness over tumours, nævi, moles, etc.

VIII  Rare forms of ringworm.
IX  Trichotillomania.
X  Monilethrix.

The most common cause of bald patches without atrophy is ALOPECIA
AREATA. This disease is so commonly seen and is of so much importance
that it is dealt with at some length herewith.

I. *The patient complains of bald patches of rapid onset. Short hairs
like points of exclamation are seen at the circumference of the bald patches.
The disease is probably*
ALOPECIA AREATA.

One of the most serious causes of hairfall is **Alopecia Areata**. Except in a few rare cases, this disease has a definite appearance which renders it easy of diagnosis. Alopecia areata is characterized by patches of total baldness, at first of circular outline, which usually develop very quickly. The area of baldness spreads peripherally and the patch tends to assume an oval shape. The skin on the patch is pale, glossy, entirely bald. As a rule there is no itching; but sometimes a patient can foretell by a sensation of itching where a new patch

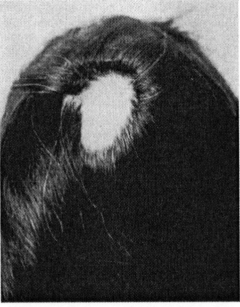

FIG. 29.—Typical early patch of alopecia areata.
Note oval shape, with finger of extension beginning.
(*Photograph kindly lent by Dr. Louis Forman.*)

is about to develop. Sometimes the hair follicles are visible on the smooth surface and in rapidly spreading cases black points may be seen where the hairs have broken off at skin-level. In mild cases the disease remains limited to one region, but in the majority of sufferers with alopecia areata several patches are seen on distant or adjacent parts of the scalp. Patches which develop close to the original one usually join it, slowly or rapidly, so that eventually there is formed an extensive bald area with a circinate outline. Whilst the areas first affected are becoming covered with new hair, fresh patches may be appearing and spreading. In extensively diseased cases only a few tufts of hair may be left on the vertex or the occiput, or the entire scalp may become completely bald. The disease originates usually on parts of the hairy scalp which appear to be in perfect health. The formation of the bald patch may develop so rapidly, within a day or two, that the patient is unaware of its existence till a friend calls attention to it. The fallen hairs are pale and atrophied at the proximal end, with shrunken white pointed bulbs. On close examination of a newly formed patch, a few short hairs are seen, about $\frac{1}{10}$ to $\frac{1}{8}$ inch in length, more numerous at the edges of the bald region, and sometimes also seen among the adjacent long hairs. These short hairs have a more or less characteristic shape which has been compared to an exclamation mark, because it is thick at the free end and atrophied near the scalp (Fig. 50). They usually measure about half a centimetre long; they are pale, having no pigment in the atrophied bulb and proximal portion; at the free end they are dark, thickened in appearance owing to dissociation of the shaft, and often broken as in trichorrhexis nodosa. When the patch is old, or is not spreading, these "exclamation" hairs are not seen at the margin of the bald patch nor in its vicinity. The presence of these short hairs round or near a patch indicates that the disease is spreading and that the region on which they are visible will soon become bald. On the areas where these short hairs appear in large numbers baldness rapidly follows. It is in those cases that one often sees black points in the follicles. These points are sometimes due to the roots of the fallen hairs broken off at scalp level, and usually indicate rapid extension of the disease. In other cases the points consist only of heaped-up cells and pigment; their contents are found when the scalp is scraped with a glass slide.

The long hairs around the bald areas may appear to be quite normal, but usually many come away in their entire length on being gently pulled. The roots of the hairs which come out so readily show various stages of atrophy. There is another type which I used to see quite frequently, in which the long hairs come away with part of the follicle attached to the root, so that the hair root has the appearance of being enclosed in a white glistening cap. In these adherent root sheaths, the microscope often revealed microbacilli filling the whole space. In Sabouraud's last study of alopecia he remarked on the fact that the microbacillus was seen in abundance in the follicles of an area affected by alopecia, whilst it might be absent in adjacent healthy regions. This association of the microbacillus with alopecia is said not to be found with alopecia occurring in children, but I have notes of several such cases (see p. 122).

There may be only one area affected throughout the entire course of a case of alopecia areata. There is no preference as to the site invaded. The bald patch may come on the vertex, the parietal, temporal or occipital region, but usually begins in the hairy scalp, not at its margin. The disease may be arrested by the removal of the cause, or it may steadily extend despite all treatment. On the other hand, it may become cured quite easily and rapidly. The first indications of the arrest of the disease are the absence of the short " exclamation " hairs and the fact that the long hairs in the vicinity of the patch cease to come out on being gently pulled.

In severe cases there are many patches of baldness, and the disease spreads to the whole scalp, the eyebrows, eyelids, moustache, and beard. Indeed, all the hairs of the body may fall (p. 99) ; this fact is often unnoticed by the patients ; the hairs in such cases become brittle and broken off. In rapidly spreading types the patient may complain of irritation, and a definite pink flush may be visible, especially at the border of the newly formed bald regions. Sometimes the alopecia may affect only the front of the legs, thighs, arms, or only the eyelashes or eyebrows. Sometimes dystrophy of the nails has accompanied alopecia areata.

One can distinguish from the above-described ordinary forms of alopecia areata a variety which was observed by Celsus in olden days, and called " ophiasis " because of its serpentine progress. Here the baldness begins at the occiput, with a band not more than two fingers' width, and progresses by two arms which advance above the ears and meet above the brow. The extension of this variety of alopecia is symmetrical. To-day, as in the time of Celsus, this type of " band " or " ribbon " alopecia is seen most frequently in childhood, but it also occurs in the adult and in old people. Such cases are very serious ; after the hair grows afresh the disease relapses and thus a final cure is rare. The hairs round these slowly advancing bald areas are very often not easily pulled out, nor is there any seborrhœa, and the hair follicles are not visible on the bald regions.

*Ætiology.* Alopecia areata affects both sexes. Sabouraud found 130 males in 200 cases ; Dr. Herbert Brown found 59 per cent. females . in his investigation of 135 cases (published in the *British Journal of Dermatology* in 1929). As regards the age incidence, Sabouraud found none under four years old and the majority between six and twelve ; Brown found 31 per cent. occurred in the first decade and 57 per cent. under twenty-one years. The disease has been seen in infants, even under a year old ; this is very rare. Certainly heredity plays a part in the causation of alopecia areata. Patients often remark that some of their relatives have had the disease and it often occurs in several members of a family in the same generation. Sabouraud traced a hereditary history of 20 per cent. of his 200 cases ; Brown found it in twenty-eight out of his 135 cases.

Thirty years ago one heard much about the *contagious* nature of the disease, but this theory of the causation of alopecia areata is now entirely abandoned. The epidemics which have occurred in schools and institutions have proved to be due to other local diseases, such as ringworm or artefacts (see p. 124). Yet even now, from time to time, one comes across cases occurring in families, or in friends living together, which lead one to suspect contagion from hat or brush. It was whilst searching for proofs of the contagious nature of alopecia areata that Sabouraud discovered the false foundation on which this long-cherished belief had been based. For some years Sabouraud considered that the microbacillus was the culprit. It was found in most of the follicles of the dead and dying hairs in adult cases of alopecia areata, whereas it was absent from adjacent healthy regions. However, Sabouraud found himself obliged to abandon the theory that the microbacillus played a causal rôle in the production of the average case of alopecia areata in children and in the ophiasis type of alopecia. I have notes of a case of a boy aged six ; the loose hairs round the alopecia patches had microbacilli teeming at the roots ; this was proved by culture. I have notes of many similar cases in young adults who yet had no seborrhœa oleosa of the scalp.

The association with the *nervous system* is manifested in a variety of ways. The disease is not infrequently associated with vitiligo and with scleroderma, two conditions which follow the area of distribution of nerves. The theory of reflex irritation has many advocates, because it has proved of practical value in the treatment of so many cases. Jacquet was its chief exponent. He regarded alopecia areata as only a symptom, and believed that in subjects affected with alopecia areata there was a general hypotony and a tendency to nervous disequilibrium. In such individuals some reflex irritation, acting through the sympathetic nervous system either from an adjacent or a distant source, was the chief precipitating cause of the alopecia areata. Any source of reflex irritation could set in motion the symptoms of alopecia areata, but the most usual exciting cause lay in the teeth. Often extraction of troublesome wisdom teeth or of diseased teeth has been followed by a cure or arrest of alopecia ; in other cases no success has resulted from the correction of such errors. Whitfield found success follow the correction of eye-strain. Barber and others have shown the relationship of some cases of alopecia areata with streptococcal foci in the teeth, tonsils, naso-pharynx and sinuses. One of my most stubborn cases was cured after antrum trouble was dealt with. In recent years I have found worry, fear and anxiety are potent causes of extensive alopecia. Another way in which the connection with the nervous system is shown is as the result of *traumatism*. Alopecia may develop near or adjacent to an injury to the scalp, as for example after operation on the mastoid, and after war wounds on the face or head. Sometimes the alopecia areata has appeared within a few days of the injury, sometimes not for about two months. In another type the alopecia comes on long after the accident, months or even years ; this is due to an ascending degeneration of the cord which at length has reached the sympathetic nerve centre in the spinal cord. In this type there are other signs of nerve involvement, such as glossy skin, vascular and perspiration changes. Again, the accident may bring about alopecia by its action upon the emotional factor.

Disturbance of the *endocrine glands* has proved to be in some cases the chief link in a chain of several causes. Alopecia areata occurs in a certain proportion of cases, with endocrine sympathetic disturbance, especially hyperthyroidism. Women have suffered from alopecia areata during pregnancy and had recurrence at the menopause. Such facts have been considered to show some relationship of alopecia areata with the thyroid, mammary and ovarian glands. A number of workers investigated the basal metabolism in cases of alopecia areata, but so contradictory were the reports that nothing of real value, pointing to any relationship, could be proved. Sabouraud's usual profound research led him to conclude that every observer could find a proportion of cases to confirm his own particular theory. Severe cases of alopecia areata have followed acute toxæmias, and some of these have proved resistant to every kind of treatment when the thyroid was affected; treatment directed to aid its function led to cure of the alopecia.

The relationship of *syphilis* to alopecia areata has been specially considered because of its importance in diagnosis and treatment. Sabouraud made an exhaustive investigation, and found evidence of congenital syphilis present in seven out of ten of the children affected with the ophiasis type of alopecia areata. In adult patients the two conditions may exist together and thus lead to difficulty in diagnosis and treatment. The prevalence of the history of congenital and acquired syphilis makes it hard to decide in certain individual cases whether the syphilis is only a contributory cause. On the other hand, Brown points out that in sixty cases only one had a positive Wasserman, and Orr, in a hundred cases, found evidence of syphilis in only one case.

Sabouraud criticized dispassionately his own findings as well as those of other workers, and considered that there is always a tendency towards conjecture and hypothesis : each observer finds the cause he desires to find, because alopecia areata appears in so many different types of individuals and can be preceded or accompanied by so many forms of toxæmia, or by reflex, endocrine and nervous manifestations. All of these, he concluded, have in turn, with insufficient proof, been regarded as playing the predominating rôle in the chain of causes.

Cederberg of Helsingfors [1] claimed that a spirilla was the main cause of infection, and that it entered the lymphatics by the route of diseased mucous membrane. The visible signs of unhealthy mucous membrane are seen in the mouth, but similar penetrable mucous membrane may exist in any part of the gastro-intestinal tract. The spirillæ were found in sections of early cases of alopecia areata, stained by the Levaditi process. They have a special affinity for the basal cell layer, and here they replace the normal pigment. In the follicle sheath they cause a toxic papillitis, which may bring about destruction of the hair and its follicle.

**Alopecia parvimaculata** is the name given to describe the epidemic form of alopecia which occasionally is seen in large institutions, especially in children, easily controlled with antiseptics locally, and arising without any apparent cause. Few dermatologists have seen such epidemics and great doubt has been cast on their occurrence. The baldness affects multiple small patches, oval, round or slightly angular ; the skin is smooth, white, sometimes studded over with black or broken-off hair roots, sometimes said to be atrophic. No ringworm fungi have ever been found. Haldin Davis [2] described an epidemic in an Institute containing 300 girls ; 174 were affected, also three adults. The epidemic was quickly arrested with simple antiseptics and the hair returned. Semon [3] had charge of a similar epidemic associated with scurfy, itching scalps. Davis agreed that those cases resembled his epidemic of some ten years previously. The admirable illustrations in Semon's paper show the familiar bald patches so frequently seen with pityriasis of the scalp. The lesions may be self-inflicted. However, Galewsky, Werther and other dermatologists have considered that they had to deal with an epidemic variety of alopecia of unknown but infectious cause.

Enough has been said to show that the causes to which alopecia areata has been attributed are legion. Probably this is due to the fact that in the majority of cases there is more than one cause in operation. There may be present together a degree of general toxæmia and a source of reflex irritation, and yet, until a third factor develops, alopecia may not develop. Or, again, the toxæmia produced by a septic focus may be unsuspected for years, when it causes no symptom beyond a readily

---

[1] *Derm. Woch.*, 1932, **94**, 539.
[2] HALDIN DAVIS, *Brit. J. Derm. and Syph.*, 1914, **26**, 207.
[3] H. C. SEMON, *Arch. Derm. and Syph.*, 1923, **8**, 785.

induced fatigue ; then some mental shock, financial or domestic strain, acute illness or prolonged chill, will precipitate the appearance of some apparently unrelated symptom, which symptom may be so far apart as a dilated heart, a duodenal ulcer or alopecia areata. Such an involved history has often preceded the appearance of alopecia areata. The same obscure, complicated history is found associated with widely varying conditions of disease.

The strange fact remains that alopecia areata often affects persons who seem free from disease. Puzzling cases are narrated in whom all the hair of the head and body has fallen out in the space of a few months or even days, and this has occurred in the case of individuals apparently in perfect health and without cause of mental strain.

*Diagnosis.* In the majority of cases there is no difficulty in the diagnosis of alopecia areata. The chief mistake in diagnosis occurs when a smooth bald patch is seen in a child, for ringworm in children occasionally resembles alopecia areata. In the uncommon " *bald ringworm* " careful examination, especially at the periphery, usually detects some broken hairs (p. 185). In *small-spored* ringworm the bald patch is scaly and the associated short broken hairs contain the fungus. Difficulty in diagnosis is caused by the " *black dot* " ringworm (p. 185) ; it has none of the scaliness seen with the common *M. audouini* infection, and there are black points in the follicles, due to the retention of broken-off hairs. When these are picked out and examined under the microscope the presence of the fungus decides the diagnosis. Ringworm is rare in adults ; alopecia areata is comparatively common. Sections of alopecia areata show normal epidermis and follicles, no sclerosis, sometimes moderate inflammatory changes. *Impetigo* in children has been mistaken for alopecia areata ; as the crusts fall, hairs entangled in it also fall, and therefore a few small bald areas are seen. These are slightly depressed and pink and do not enlarge ; the hairs grow in again at once. Similarly, the lesions following folliculitis, abscesses or carbuncles should cause no difficulty in diagnosis. Many types of *cicatricial baldness* occur ; these are described in the section of baldness with atrophy and scars (p. 144). In *folliculitis decalvans* and the *pseudo-pelade* of Brocq, there are many small areas of white, fine, atrophied tissue, not necessarily showing much depression. The patches in these cases are of slow development and join, forming a polycyclical border ; folliculitis decalvans shows reddened follicles of the loosened hairs which are about to fall. In *lupus erythematosus* the scar is not usually circular ; there is a history of preceding redness of the affected part and there may be patches present in other parts of the scalp or body which are still in the hyperæmic stage. The scars left by *gummata* may at first sight be mistaken for alopecia areata. No one ought to mistake the diffuse and widespread hairfall which occurs after certain *fevers*, after *X-ray*, and after the administration of *acetate of thallium* and other *mineral salts*. The hairfall after X-ray and thallium salts is rapid and extensive, all the hair falls off in a few days, the eyebrows are not affected, and a history of taking the drug is obtained. The completely bald scalp of an *alopecia totalis*, which has existed for some time, usually has a history of being preceded by alopecia areata occurring in round patches (see Chapter VII). This history and the absence of atrophy differentiate it from the complete baldness of an advanced case of *pseudopelade*. *Secondary syphilis* may cause difficulty in diagnosis, especially when, as Sabouraud pointed out, a patient with alopecia areata has contracted syphilis. The history is of importance, e.g. whether one or two patches have been present for a long time, and whether the recent diffuse hairfall has developed from the enlargement and coalescence of many new patches. Again, a patient with secondary syphilis may develop alopecia areata. If secondary syphilis is present, the other signs will also be seen—the eyebrows are affected as if cut with scissors, the mucous membrane of the throat and mouth show the characteristic grey " snail track " lesions, the glands in the groins and elsewhere will be enlarged, the serum reaction is usually positive.

*Course and Prognosis.* No one can at first foresee the course of any case of alopecia areata. The following facts should be considered before venturing to give any opinion as to the date of the regrowth of the hair. (1) In the mildest cases the baldness is not complete ; a slight down remains and begins to grow stronger in a few weeks. An average case begins to show regrowth of hair in the centre of the patch in two to three months. (2) If the short " exclamation " hairs are numerous, and many long hairs are easily pulled out in the neighbourhood or at the edge of the patch, one knows that the disease is rapidly spreading, but no one can say how long it will continue to do so. Nor can anyone tell whether fresh lesions will develop. As a rule, one patch remains alone for a month or six weeks. Then quite suddenly it enlarges, and several new patches appear, near and distant. There may follow a period of quiescence for four to six weeks, succeeded by another outbreak of many bald areas. The prognosis is grave when there are many patches ; the extension of a solitary patch is not so serious. The return to health is first shown by the appearance of a fine, often white down in the centre of the bare region ; this gradually strengthens, darkens in colour, and becomes strong hair. The down may not extend over the whole patch at once, but its appearance always heralds growth on that area to a healthy length.

As a rule the new hair comes in white and remains white for a considerable time before the natural colour of the hair returns.

The hair may be growing satisfactorily on the first patch and the outlook seem good, when, without any warning, several new lesions may appear in another part of the scalp ; the prognosis at once becomes grave. Many of the slighter forms tend to recur several times, at intervals of months or years. Some patients consult the physician when the follicles and hair roots have become so atrophied that recovery is impossible. When alopecia areata follows an acute illness, such as measles, it is often extensive and complete, affecting the whole body ; the prognosis is very serious. Some extensive cases appear to be incurable ; the hair grows in after strenuous treatment, only to fall out again. When a patient has a history of complete baldness extending over years, from childhood, the prognosis is very serious. Often in such cases the scalp is found to be so loose that the skin and underlying tissues can be picked up and pulled into folds, as in dermolysis.

Alopecia of the eyebrows may appear as one bald patch surrounded by normal hairs. This form often recovers. When the alopecia is diffuse and irregular, with total alopecia of the scalp, the outlook for recovery is not so good. Alopecia of the beard is very obstinate. Sabouraud considered that alopecia areata was cured when nature decided that it should be cured ; the physician might try every remedy, but no result would be achieved until nature steps in. He declared that the physician who has the patient in his charge at that moment obtains the credit for the successful result of the last method of treatment adopted, and that the honest medical man knows that he has not greatly influenced the course of the disease. In an exhaustive study of 230 cases, Walker and Rothman found that the prognosis was unfavourable if the disease began before puberty ; relapses were common, and Alopecia totalis might result.[1]

*Treatment.* Although the general health must receive careful attention, there is no doubt that in the majority of cases local treatment is of paramount importance. Almost any method which evokes local congestion does good. Every physician has a favourite method of local treatment. In early cases, I order the sulphur ointment of the British Pharmacopeia to be rubbed well into the patch and for at least an inch around it. All the loose, easily falling hairs round the patch should be pulled out at night and in the morning. Twice a week a strong preparation of iodine is applied over and around the patch. In *chronic* cases it is important to keep the long-standing patch in a continual state of irritation. Tincture of cantharides, ammonia and acetic acid are my

[1] *J. Invest. Derm.*, 1950 ; **14**, 403.

favourite applications. To bring about a strong local reaction I use liquor epispasticus rubbed in with a stiff brush. One must be careful to shake off all the excess of fluid before applying this strong lotion over and well around the patch, otherwise drops would run down where not desired and might flow on to the face with disastrous effect, causing erythema and blistering. The part is then exposed to the ultra-violet light at gradually decreasing distances ; or the dose is slowly increased once or twice a week ; give applications according to the degree of reaction and also the size of the surface to be treated. Modern lamps act rapidly ; it is essential therefore to obtain full instructions concerning the distance and the time of application. Tests for skin sensitivity should be made before embarking on any course of ultra-violet treatment. If bullæ form, they should be pricked and receive careful dressing. All active treatment is arrested until they dry up.

Certain cases of alopecia of *acute* onset have many hairs in the vicinity which are easily pulled out, with a glistening follicle sheath attached to the hair root, evidence probably of local inflammation. During several years of busy hospital clinics, in every one of these cases with the glistening sheath I stained the hair roots, and frequently, but by no means always, found the microbacillus in enormous numbers. When this was present, I had an autogenous vaccine prepared and injected it as soon as possible and increased the dose every fifth day. At the same time I applied iodine to the patch and for an inch round it, and drove it in with negative pole of the galvanic current. The results were satisfactory and rapid.

Sabouraud had a strong belief in oil of cade, which he ordered in equal parts of lanoline and vaseline. This ointment is well massaged in at night, so that the drug penetrates into the hair follicles ; in the morning the parts are cleansed with a solvent such as acetone or ether. He did not confine the application to the affected patch, but ordered it to be rubbed over the whole scalp, so as to delay or arrest the formation of new patches. Lee McCarthy reports success in the majority of his cases with Sabouraud's method. Most of his patients preferred a lotion to an ointment, and liked oil of cade in acetone, in the proportion of one in ten. Walker and Rothman found that when regrowth occurred during pregnancy, prolactin arrested the usual fall after delivery ; they applied it in ointment to the scalp. All the rules of massage and washing which are mentioned in the section dealing with the treatment of pityriasis sicca (p. 168), seborrhœa oleosa (p. 109), and stimulation of hair growth (p. 89), hold good for alopecia. Sabouraud stated that the nurses in the hospitals and the " old cronies " who have had frequent recurrences of alopecia areata told him that they preferred oil of cade to all other remedies.

I had the opportunity of trying the two methods on one extensively affected scalp. Sulphur and iodine were used on one side of the scalp and Sabouraud's prescription on the other ; both were equally successful. Sabouraud had no belief in iodine for alopecia areata ; for counter-irritation he liked chrysophanic acid. He pointed out that when he prescribed 0·20 centigrams of this drug in 20 grammes chloroform one received from the chemist two types of lotion—one which leaves a yellow powder on the skin, and one which is a clear brown fluid which colours the skin a brown mahogany but leaves no deposit. This latter is to be preferred. It can be used in the morning to wipe off the oil of cade ointment. However, chrysophanic acid cannot be employed by everyone, because it causes so intense an irritation of the skin ; then it is better to be diluted one in ten. Others tolerate it well, and no reaction occurs. Sabouraud found that the old-fashioned method of inducing vesication was satisfactory for the limited areas over which it could be employed ; it was dangerous to apply it to the whole scalp. There is a similar objection to the extensive use of the Kromayer lamp. Hair grows in over the areas exposed to strong doses of the ultra-violet light, but the regrowth is strictly limited to the irritated area and the result is not superior to that obtained by vesication. Of course ultra-violet treatment must be given before there is atrophy of the follicles. In my own experience the best results were obtained with local treatment by the Kromayer lamp, administered strongly enough to evoke a third degree reaction. In extensive cases the whole body also should be exposed to ultra-violet radiation twice a week for some months.

I used to place much reliance on the administration of a pastille dose of X-ray ; smaller doses were quite ineffective. Recently this dosage has been recommended by radiologists who believed that they had discovered a new method. Henry Corsi gave a cautious survey of the results obtained with treatment with Thorium X.[1] In those patients who already showed a tendency to recovery, Thorium X was beneficial ; but it was ineffective where the prognosis was serious, as in rapidly extending types. In several long-standing cases, half of the patch was painted with the Thorium X in varnish, 2,000 units to the cubic centimetre ; on the treated half the hair grew in. Pigmentation returns to the hairs almost at once after regrowth.

Reference may be made to methods of treatment too recent to have stood the test of time :

Mestchersky [2] wrote that he never despaired of bringing back hair by

---

[1] *Lancet*, 1943, ii, 346. See also P. Feeny, *Lancet*, 1947, ii, 506.

[2] *Revue Franç. de Dermat.*, 1930, **6**, 87.

systematic applications of ultra-violet light in doses sufficient to cause violent erythema.　Having noticed that hypertrichosis may appear near an area which has been exposed to traumatism and inflammation of the skin, he decided to try subcutaneous injections of sterile milk, and had a measure of success.　Djoritch [1] reported two cases cured with intradermal injections of sterile milk (Aolan).　The bald area was injected with several doses.　The first case had tried many remedies for nearly a year.　$\frac{1}{4}$ c.c. was injected into the skin of one patch ; in six weeks normal hair was seen upon it. A drawback to the treatment was its painfulness.　Glaubersohn and Posternak [2] described six cases of obstinate alopecia treated with two intradermal injections of $\frac{1}{4}$ to $\frac{1}{2}$ c.c. of sterile milk injected into each patch ; the hair was seen returning in six weeks.　Messieurs H. Gougerot and M. Albeaux-Fernet [3] believed that sympathetic vasoconstriction played the chief rôle in alopecia areata.　They obtained rapid cures with methylacetylcholine injections ; this drug produces immediately a local vascular dilatation which lasts nearly an hour.　Intradermal injections are given twice a week, in doses $\frac{1}{20}$ c.c. of a solution containing 4 mg. to the c.c.　In this country, P. Bauwens has driven histamine into the patch with the galvanic current.　This causes marked dilatation of the blood vessels ; owing to the effect on the general circulation this method should be performed only by an expert.　It had no effect upon one obstinate case on whom I tested the method.　Dosage of the sympathetic with the Grenz rays is sometimes useful.

In all cases of alopecia areata one should *treat the general health* as well as the local patch.　A complete investigation should be made and everything possible done to remove all sources of sepsis and of reflex irritation. In the paragraph on ætiology, emphasis is laid on the rôle played by reflex irritation in the production of alopecia areata.　The administration of thyroid gland is often very effective in cases of alopecia areata.　It is natural to expect benefit from thyroid in the case of women at or near the menopause, and in debility after illness or prolonged strain.　But it is indeed surprising to find how often it is beneficial in the case of apparently healthy subjects.　One of my hospital cases, an apparently normal young man in the late twenties, had almost complete alopecia, without discoverable cause.　He was given thyroid in $\frac{1}{4}$- and up to 1-grain doses twice and thrice daily ; equivalent to $\frac{3}{40}$ to $\frac{3}{10}$ grain of dry extract of thyroid. Ultra-violet light and iodine painting were given twice a week, and sulphur ointment was rubbed in every night.　No blistering or active local reaction occurred, yet he improved rapidly and in less than a year had a fine crop of hair.　No sign of excess of thyroid medication appeared at any time in his case.　Yet in many normal individuals as little as $\frac{1}{2}$ grain of thyroid (fresh gland) daily soon causes headache, irritability and a rapid pulse.

---

[1] *Ann. de Derm. et de Syph.*, 1930, 7$^{me}$ Sér. **1**, 372.
[2] *Urol. and Cutan. Rev.*, 1931, **35**, 362.　　[3] *Bull. Soc. Franç.*, 1936, **43**, 1586.

I was interested to find that in America Bauckus and others found thyroid more effective than other endocrine preparations.[1]

Another typical case was that of a woman aged fifty-four, who came with one large patch of alopecia areata. Whilst it was being treated the disease developed rapidly in adjacent areas. Nothing could arrest their extension ; she was soon almost completely bald. She was a fragile looking woman, with a sallow complexion, who complained of frequent headaches and depression. She was ordered a diet containing plenty of raw fruit, vegetables and salads, marmite and stone-ground flour bread. An aperient with cascara evacuant and belladonna was taken every night and thyroid $\frac{1}{2}$ and then 1 grain ; equivalent to $\frac{3}{20}$ and $\frac{3}{10}$ grain of dry extract. She attended once a week for over a year. On an average of once a week, after having been painted with liquor epispasticus, the scalp was treated with the mercury vapour lamp and high-frequency applications. Strong reactions were obtained, often with blistering, but for a time it seemed as if new hair would never grow in again. Her health altered entirely for the better, the headaches vanished, the complexion became clear. At last her hair returned, thick and dark, with a beautiful gloss and natural curl ; she looked and felt rejuvenated. Nine years later, at the age of sixty-three, this patient still had thick dark hair.

The treatment of universal alopecia and of alopecia of the beard and eyebrows is disappointing.

Good reports have also been published concerning the usefulness of thymus extract.[2] Calcium in various forms has some cures to its credit ; possibly due to the fact that many patients with chronic mild toxæmia require calcium. The beneficial effect of ultra-violet light to the whole body may be due to the resulting better utilization of calcium.

Bengt N. Bengston [3] noted that a woman treated with pituitary gland preparations for Fröhlich's syndrome grew abundant hair during the progress of her cure. Thereupon he studied the effect of pituitary in sixteen cases of alopecia areata. He gave injections of anterior pituitary and whole gland by mouth with some excellent results, but also many failures.

At the end of this book are the formulæ of a few lotions which have been used for years by many physicians for the treatment of alopecia areata and have survived the changes of time.

We turn now to consider the other causes of BALD PATCHES WITHOUT ATROPHY, which were mentioned in the list on p. 118.

---

[1] *New York J. Med.*, 1936, **36**, ii, 1629.

[2] M. L. SPILLMAN, *Bull. Soc. Franç. de derm. et syph.*, 1935, **42**, 64.

[3] *J. Amer. Med. Assoc.*, 1931, **97**, 1355.

II.  SEBORRHŒA OLEOSA is accompanied by hairfall and is dealt with
under Hairfall accompanied by oiliness (see Chapter VIII).  When the
hairfall is severe enough to have caused the formation of bald patches,
these occur usually on the tonsure area and the temporal regions.  They
have not sharply demarcated margins ; the skin of the scalp, for some
years, as the disease progresses, shines through the gradually thinning
hairs on the vertex.

III.  **Senile Baldness.**  There is a natural thinning of the hair, in
both sexes, as age advances, especially visible on the posterior part of the
vertex.  It begins usually between the fiftieth and sixtieth year.  After
a time the openings of the hair follicles are no longer visible, and the
scalp is stretched tight on the skull.  Sometimes, at a late stage, a fine
atrophy can be seen over the region, especially over some of the follicle
mouths.

IV.  PITYRIASIS SIMPLEX CAPITIS.  Small, irregularly shaped bald
areas, the size of a threepenny- or sixpenny-piece, occur with some cases
of pityriasis simplex, usually when it is of rapid onset, spreading, or
associated with coccal infection.  This disease is dealt with under its
characteristic feature, scaling (Chapter XI, p. 159).

V.  IMPETIGO and OTHER PUSTULAR AFFECTIONS are fully described
in the chapter on pustular conditions (p. 216).  These leave bald areas
without atrophy ; the bald area is seen immediately after the crusts
fall ; it is pink at first, and is of brief duration, as hair regrowth starts
at once.  It is only in rare cases that the bald area is very extensive.

VI.  In **Secondary Syphilis** there may occur a form of hairfall so
characteristic that one can diagnose the disease from the appearance of
the head.  In spite of the fact that the description of the " moth-eaten "
look of the scalp in this condition is well known to every medical student,
this form of hairfall was never very common.  Even in the days before
the introduction of arsenical compounds for the early treatment of syphilis,
when every student was familiar with the appearance of secondary and
tertiary syphilitic eruptions, this particular form of baldness was not
frequently seen.  The features special to this form of syphilitic alopecia
are : the rapid onset of a very profuse loss of hair without any history of
the usual causes of heavy loss of hair, such as high fever, operation or
shock (Chapter VI).  The hair falls diffusely from every part of the head,
soon leaving bald areas about the diameter of a pea, all over the scalp,
but especially on the temples and behind the ears.  The hairfall occurs
on the areas affected by the roseolar and papular rash, and therefore it
usually begins about six weeks to three months after the date of infection ;

sometimes it is delayed a little longer. The fall continues heavily for about a month, then decreases ; there is never complete baldness with syphilis. The above described type of syphilitic alopecia is associated with loss of hair in patches elsewhere on the body : the axillæ, genitals, and limbs. These patches are usually overlooked owing to the more obvious loss of hair on the scalp.

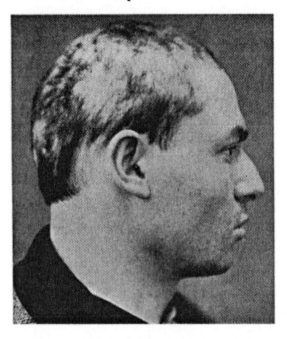

Fig. 30.—Advanced stage of Diffuse Hairfall in Secondary Syphilis.
From J. H. Sequeira's " Diseases of the Skin." J. and A. Churchill Ltd., London.

Another type of alopecia due to syphilis is the so-called *essential alopecia* caused by *neurosyphilis*. With this form, there are no associated cutaneous secondary lesions ; there may even be a negative Wasserman reaction, but the spinal fluid has the increased lymphocyte count characteristic of neurosyphilis. This condition is fully discussed by Wile and Belote,[1] with illustrations of the two types of alopecia.

The *diagnosis* rests on the " moth-eaten " appearance given by the small, irregularly shaped bald areas scattered amongst the remaining hairs, or the other signs of syphilis : mucous patches on the throat and palate, hairs fallen from the eyebrows, enlarged glands in the neck and

[1] U. J. WILE and G. H. BELOTE, *Arch. Derm. and Syph.*, 1926, **13**, 495.

groins, and from the history of the initial lesion, the chancre, about six weeks to three months previously. If the patient is seen when the hair-fall is beginning, traces of the roseolar rash may be seen as it is fading from the head, face and body. Secondary syphilis is distinguished from *alopecia areata* by the absence of the " exclamation hairs " at the margins of the patches. On the other hand, it must be remembered that *alopecia areata* can occur in a syphilitic patient. *Male pattern baldness*, or *seborrhœa oleosa*, being so common in men, may co-exist with many other causes of baldness on the vertex and temples. The distinction between the two conditions can be made by examining the hairs behind the ears ; if these are pulled, they come away profusely when the cause in operation is a general infection, and not when the cause is seborrhœa. To clinch the diagnosis, seek for the other signs of syphilis mentioned above. When *tertiary syphilis* causes baldness, the scalp condition is quite different ; the bald areas are due to the scars left by healed gummata or ulcers (see Chapter XVII).

The *prognosis* is excellent ; the hair grows in again after the anti-syphilitic treatment.

VII. **Baldness over Tumours.** Baldness occurs over TUMOURS, but hairfall is not then the complaint for which advice is sought. The hair usually falls out and leaves a bald region on the skin above the tumour. Thus, the skin over a sebaceous cyst is usually bald. I have seen the whole vertex of a woman quite bald, stretched over secondary malignant swellings. The skin in time becomes smooth and glossy, whilst above the nodules it becomes reddened and shows enlarged blood-vessels. Except in the case of small sebaceous cysts, patients who suffer from these conditions complain of swellings, and not of loss of hair. On the other hand, loss of hair is sometimes the first sign of *cutis verticis gyrata* (p. 266).

Bald patches may be simulated by the presence of NÆVI and MOLES, white or pigmented. The hair is usually entirely absent over verrucose nævi. Over the deep nævi which show no cutaneous vascularity, the hair may be entirely or partly absent ; such tumours are diagnosed by the sensation conveyed to the examining finger ; the swelling yields on compression. When this type of nævus is treated with radium, hair has grown in over the bald region.

VIII. " BALD RINGWORM." This form of ringworm is occasionally seen in a child. There is a clean bald patch, and only after persevering examination is some infected hair found. This variety of ringworm is discussed in the section on ringworm in Chapter XII.

IX.  A rare form of incomplete alopecia is due to **Trichotillomania.**
This condition occurs in nervous subjects, who pull out their hair so
assiduously that they succeed in producing a bald patch.  The bald patch
may be red, indurated and excoriated, or more often the skin is normal,
with most of the hairs absent, those which are left being quite short.
The patch is usually irregular in shape and on it may be seen a few quite
healthy hairs which are short enough to have escaped being pulled out.

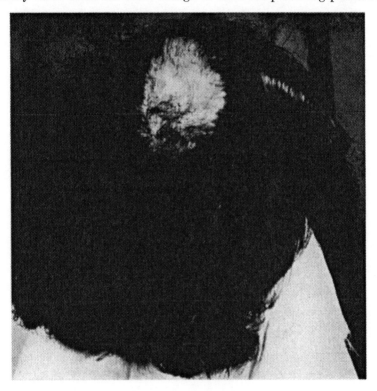

Fig. 31.—Trichotillomania.
(*Photograph kindly lent by Dr. Martin Scott.*)

The hair follicles are visible, and some, with retained hair roots, give the
appearance of being filled with powder.  In some cases the trichotillomania begins with the simple habit of scratching an irritable area on the
scalp (see Chapter X).

I saw a girl aged 11 with extensive baldness over the vertex ; it had
no definite margin ; there were many broken and bent short hairs mixed
with others of varying length.  The child unconsciously plucked at the

scalp all the time of the consultation. As she had suffered two nervous shocks connected with hair and fur, psychotherapy was advised. Two years later, she had a good crop of healthy hair. She volunteered that as she desired to have nice hair she thought how foolish it was to pick at it ; thus she herself broke the bad habit. A similar tic is seen in adults who absentmindedly pull their hair whilst reading. The bald region is usually behind the ear, or on the temples, but this type of patient may pluck the eyebrows, moustache or pubis.

The name **trichokryptomania** is used to describe the condition in which the hairs are not pulled out, but broken off. The condition is seen in neurotic patients ; some have found it in drug addicts.

*Diagnosis.* As a rule this is simple. In a young adult or child who denies having any habit of pulling at the hair, there is occasionally difficulty in deciding the cause of the baldness. Usually it is seen on both sides, in patches near the temples or ears, regions easily reached by the right hand ; the patches have not the rounded outline of alopecia areata, but merge into the surrounding normal hair. A diagnostic feature is the presence of hairs of unequal length and some of these are seen to be freshly growing young hairs which are too short to be plucked. No atrophied " exclamation mark " hairs are present.

*Prognosis and Treatment.* The habit is a very obstinate one and often recurs after apparent cure. The hair should be cut very short, and may be kept shaved in order to make it difficult or impossible for the patient to take hold of it. Collodion or plaster may be applied, or the hands can be covered with gloves day and night, so that every time the patient has the impulse to pull the hair he becomes conscious of his habit and arrests his unthinking movement. An epilation dose with X-ray renders the scalp bald for at least six weeks ; in some this suffices to break the morbid tendency. Psychotherapy is the most promising method of cure when practised by a wise individual accustomed to deal with nervous habits.

X. Monilethrix is described under alterations of the hair shaft in Chapter XVI. At first sight the sufferer appears to be bald. On closer examination, tiny rough cones and scales, with defective short hairs, make one suspect ringworm. Then the microscope reveals the diagnostic feature, the beaded state of the hair shaft.

### Group B. Bald Patches with Atrophy or Scarring

Clinical Investigation. On examination of the bald patches with the naked eye or lens, atrophy or scarring is found. Sometimes the entire patch is scarred over ; sometimes only at the follicles is atrophy discovered. Sometimes the clue to a diagnosis is given by examining the face, ears and other parts of the body, to find out if any eruption is present which is more clearly seen than on the scalp, as in lupus erythematosus, impetigo and lupus vulgaris or other nodular conditions which, as they heal, leave atrophy or cicatrices behind. I have seen a permanently bald area follow a simple but long-neglected pityriasis steatoides.

BALD PATCHES with ATROPHY or SCARRING usually occur with definite margins. In some cases, however, the part involved has extended over a wide area before the physician is consulted. Thus, for example, in causes VII to XI (below) the patients may seek your advice when the whole scalp is almost bald, because years have passed during which they have wandered to various doctors and hospitals. The history of the duration of the bald patch, the rate at which it has spread and its mode of onset gives great assistance in forming a diagnosis. Only a transient baldness occurs after impetigo and other superficial pustular conditions. A degree of erythema complicates the scars of causes I, VII, IX, XI, XV, sometimes of X and the early stages of XIV. Note also the presence or absence of other lesions, such as scales or pus. The differentiating features are described under the various causes, which are named as far as possible in order of frequency of occurrence :

I   Lupus erythematosus.
II   Traumatism.
III   Impetigo, folliculitis and other pustular conditions such as : Kerion ; Boils ; Carbuncles ; Acne varioloformis and Acne keloid ; Acne conglobata ; Chickenpox and smallpox ; After certain drug eruptions.
IV   Alopecia after the menopause.
V   Morphœa and scleroderma.
VI   Herpes zoster.
VII   Favus.
VIII   Pseudo-pelade.
IX   Folliculitis decalvans.
X   Lichen spinulosus and plano-pilaris.
XI   Ulerythema ophryogenes.
XII   Chignon alopecia.
XIII   Lupus vulgaris, sarcoid and other nodular conditions.
XIV   Radiodermatitis dating from many years.
XV   Frontal band alopecia.
XVI   Hyperkeratosis cystica follicularis.
XVII   Congenital defects.

I. **Lupus Erythematosus** is a disease which often causes difficulty in diagnosis when it affects the scalp alone. The discoid form is that most common on the scalp, a dull red patch with marginal adherent scales. As this spreads, with slightly elevated pink or dull red islets, often showing telangiectases and a scaly margin, the centre becomes depressed, atrophic and white. Several patches may coalesce and a large region of the scalp may become atrophied, with permanent destruction of the hair follicles on the involved area. Itching may or may not be present during the early stages. The scales, when present, are adherent, and tender when being removed, often with prolongations dipping into the follicles. In most cases there are lesions elsewhere on the body, especially on the lobe and tip of the ear, on the nose and cheeks, sometimes also on the backs of the fingers. As a rule, when there are many lesions on the skin, there are only a few on the scalp ; and vice versa.

*Ætiology.* The cause remains obscure ; tuberculous or streptococcal infection is usually present. Many causes are listed in dermatological text-books. Women are more often affected than men. The disease occurs at any age, but chiefly between twenty and forty-five. The French School taught that there was usually a tuberculous soil ; in Britain sensitivity to streptococci is more common. H. W. Barber has reported many cases which cleared up after removal of septic tonsils, and the subsequent administration of an autogenous vaccine. I have watched several cases in whom, after a preliminary flare-up following tonsillectomy, the eruption subsided in six to eight weeks.

*Diagnosis.* The diagnosis of lupus erythematosus on the scalp is simple when, as is usual, the eruption occurs elsewhere ; it may be very difficult when there are no lesions on the face, ears or body. *Folliculitis decalvans* shows a smooth atrophy with marginal red points ; the diagnosis rests on the fact that these minute inflammatory areas surround hairs. *Pseudo-pelade* is considered below (VIII). Erythema, telangiectases and adherent scales, tender on removal, dilated follicles with plugs, point to lupus erythematosus. Sabouraud stated that he had sometimes hesitated when confronted with a case of *alopecia* which had been treated with a powerful rubefacient ; the history settles the diagnosis. Occasionally, *favus* presents difficulty. In difficult cases a microscopic section is advisable.

*Prognosis.* The scars are permanent. The prevention of further extension depends upon the response to treatment. The disease in the discoid form is usually chronic and slow ; the disseminated variety, whether sub-acute or acute, is much more serious than the chronic discoid form, and usually terminates fatally.

*Treatment.* When the cause can be traced to a septic focus, it must be dealt with appropriately. Removal of septic foci, such as infected teeth, must be carried out gradually, lest the sudden liberation of organisms into the blood stream sets up the acute disseminated form of the disease. In early cases I have seen quinine and sodium salicylate act like magic. For the obstinate case, bismuth and gold salts have proved to be most valuable. Toxic symptoms may arise (fever, erythematous and lichenoid eruptions) with the administration of gold and bismuth as well as arsenical salts. To obviate these toxic effects, give a diet with adequate Vitamin A, abundance of fruit and green vegetables, high protein and glucose. This regime is based upon the fact that the detoxicating effect of the liver cells requires Vitamins A and C, glycogen and an amino-acid with sulphur content. For the individual case the correct dosage and the suitable preparation demand study ; special manuals should be consulted. For intramuscular injections, bismuth oxychloride 0·2 G once a week for ten weeks is a usual course. In chronic discoid cases quinine can be taken by mouth at the same time. 0·05 to 0·2 G of bismarsen twice a week should be tried. Penicillin has had varying results ; relapse has followed initial improvement. Myocrisin is a good gold preparation : begin with 0·059, and give ten doses of gradually increasing strength up to a total of 1 G. Gold therapy requires careful control by means of frequent tests of the urine and the blood. Leucopenia after a dose is a danger sign ; a fall to 2000 per c.cm. of the white cells has been followed by generalized lupus erythematosus. Exposure to bright sunlight should be avoided. The gold salts are advised for cases of tuberculous origin ; in those of streptococcal origin, iodine has been useful when given in the large doses recommended for arthritis. Sulphonamide therapy [1] has had some striking success ; during its administration the patient must be in bed, and carefully watched lest latent deep-seated foci are stirred into activity. Begin with small doses, such as 0·125 twice daily. The diet is that recommended during metal salt therapy and, in addition, abundant intake of fluids and alkalis. Locally, apply soothing remedies ; calamine lotion or cream, or colloidal bismuth ointment. $CO_2$ snow (20 seconds firm pressure), phenol painting and diathermy fulguration, can destroy chronic patches. The choice of methods depends on the type of lesions on the body.

II.  Baldness due to **traumatism** usually follows an injury, such as a fall on some hard substance which has broken the skin and healed with scar formation. Wounds caused by missiles, such as stones thrown by children at play, or by wounds received in war, from machinery or splinters of glass, account for many scars on the scalp. Permanent

[1] H. W. BARBER, *Brit. J. Derm. and Syph.*, 1941, **53**, 1 and 33.

baldness may follow injury induced by strong chemical irritants, such as were formerly used for ringworm. Extensive scarring may follow the burns due to hot curling-tongs, permanent waving or celluloid ornaments which have accidentally been set on fire. The scars following accidents with strong acids or burns, are usually severe, irregular in form and often extensive. The linear or angular outline of patches due to traumatic alopecia is a diagnostic feature. When the follicles have been destroyed, the hair cannot return.

III. Certain **pustular** conditions are followed by fine atrophy or by scarring, in proportion to the degree of tissue destruction and the proximity of the pustules :

IMPÈTIGO. When many lesions of impetigo have coalesced, and the pustular condition has lasted some time without treatment, it may be followed by large and permanent scars. However, the bald spots following impetigo are usually temporary and of brief duration (see p. 217).

FOLLICULITIS leaves small atrophic areas only when the stage of pus formation has been severe enough to destroy the follicle. In most cases the baldness only lasts several weeks ; in the more serious type, there remains a permanent punctiform scar (p. 220).

BOILS, CARBUNCLES and KERION may leave bald atrophied patches ; but it is extraordinary how severe boils and carbuncles may be, and yet be followed only by temporary baldness (p. 222). The skin may remain devoid of hair for some months, and the follicles be almost invisible, and then the hair may rapidly begin to grow in again.

ACNE VARIOLOFORMIS (Syn., acne necrotica) is a form of folliculitis which leaves small pitted scars of various sizes. The lesions may be widely distributed over the brow, nose and usually the anterior part of the scalp (Fig. 42). The diagnosis is simple, because the folliculitis is continually recurring and the fresh lesions—indolent itchy papules, becoming pustules with an umbilicated centre—are so characteristic. See also pustular conditions (Chapter XIV, p. 225).

**Acne Keloid** (Dermatitis Capillaris Capillitii ; Sycosis nuchæ) affects the nape of the neck and extends upwards for some distance into the adjacent scalp. It is characterized by raised ridges of hard hypertrophic tissue, with keloid-looking scar formation and discrete, deep-seated pustules. The skin is usually oily ; comedones and acne papules are present. The hairs drop out ; but a few are left, scattered sparsely over the affected area. Deep communicating abscesses form, containing a brownish fluid in which are abundant microbacilli without staphylococci.

*Treatment.* Sulphur is of use as for other forms of acne and pustules. For the scar tissue X-ray is given in fractional doses.

The names **Acne conglobata** and **Perifolliculitis capitis abscedens et suffodiens** have been given to describe what is apparently a similar disease which may extend over the whole scalp. It is very rare. The inflammatory condition affects the lower part of the hair follicles, which become enormously dilated, then tunnelled by communicating abscesses (see Fig., p. 226). The pus contains staphylococcus albus and aureus. This inflammatory condition may persist for months, even years. Hard or fluctuating swellings form, usually with little pain. Sometimes spontaneous resolution occurs ; sometimes vegetations, ulceration and hypertrophied scar tissue. Here and there a few hairs are left. It is probable that this condition is analogous to the hidradenitis suppurativa of Verneuil which in men affects the apocrine glands of the axillæ and groins and may also be seen on the neck and scalp. Pyoderma faciale, which is seen in older women, with sudden onset of large so-called acne cysts, without comedones, has been associated in certain cases.

*Treatment.* Tyrothricin 0·1 per cent. solution and intraderm sulphur [1] gave good results in 1949. X-rays can be given in the early stage ; surgery may be required later. For details see footnote below.[2] When abscesses involve much of the body—neck, groins, buttocks, perianal region—and recur for years, Barber [3] uses stilboestrol implantations, 300 mg. Pus and cysts vanish, the seborrhœic pores become smaller, the skin finer. The treatment must not be long continued, as gnæcomastia develops, and sexual changes follow with reduced vigour of mind and body ; but relapse is uncommon.

Scars after CHICKENPOX are minute, hollow cicatrices, smaller than those of SMALLPOX. They are usually few in number, and are distributed over the head. Frequently the patient does not know of their existence ; they are discovered accidentally. It is important not to mistake them for alopecia areata. Scars may be left after BROMIDE and IODIDE ERUPTIONS, which have been pustular and have persisted for some time.

**IV. Alopecia of the Menopause.** Thinning of the hair over the vertex, especially the posterior part, is not unusual after the menopause. On closer examination, in some cases one can see, usually after years

---

[1] *J. Invest. Derm.*, 1945, **6**, 309, and 1946, **7**, 175.

[2] P. A. O'LEARY and R. R. KIERLAND, *Arch. Derm. and Syph.*, 1940, **41**, 451. The following articles should also be consulted : H. A. BRUNSTING, *Arch. Derm. and Syph.*, 1939, **39**, 108 ; L. A. BRUNSTING, *J. Michigan Med. Soc.*, 1943, **42**, 185 ; and H. B. MACEY, *Am. J. Surg.* n.s. 1941, **54**, 643. The last named has good figures of the required surgical procedures.

[3] *Proc. Roy. Soc. Med.*, 1948, **41**, 5, 300.

have passed, an atrophic condition of the follicles. The same atrophy often follows the seborrhœic baldness in men in later life.

*Diagnosis.* Although the age and sex of the patient simplifies the diagnosis, one must not conclude that in every case the thinning of the hair is due to the menopause; other causes must be investigated.

*Treatment.* If this condition is dealt with early and vigorously, arrest is possible and even regrowth in patients of good physique. Ovarian preparations can be tried; and when other indications are present, thyroid and pituitary.

V. When MORPHŒA is present on the scalp it appears as a small patch, which has a smooth surface which feels like wax and has a shiny appearance. Around it there may be a lilac-coloured zone with a few dilated blood-vessels on the surface, or it may be atrophic and depressed. The diagnosis is simple when lesions occur also on the face or body, as is usual.

VI. HERPES ZOSTER. The scars are minute and occur in a group, which lies along the distribution of a nerve. The area of the supraorbital nerve is often involved. See chapter on vesicular eruptions (p. 230).

VII. FAVUS infection of the scalp is followed by baldness with scarring. The areas of erythema, the typical yellow crusts (see p. 198) and the extensive, irregular character of the cicatricial area settle the diagnosis. The finding of the fungus decides the diagnosis from lupus erythematosus and folliculitis decalvans. When the patient is seen after the stage of active infection has passed, the history aids the diagnosis.

Sabouraud pointed out that a certain species of RINGWORM fungus (endothrix violaceum) is also apt to leave fine scars.

VIII. **Pseudo-pelade** (Brocq) is a rare disease which at first sight is often mistaken for a commencing alopecia areata. The onset is insidious; by the time the physician is consulted the disease has already made progress; the scalp shows a number of bald spots of varying size, smooth and atrophied, about half an inch long and somewhat narrower. There may be a degree of tenderness, itching and pinkness of the skin, preceding the development of the baldness. Several patches are usually seen close together, on the vertex, the temporal or the parietal region. The appearance at this stage has been compared to " footsteps in the snow." Sometimes twenty to thirty small patches may be counted. In certain cases these may slowly join, forming after some years a bald area two or three inches long, with intervening tufts of hair marking the borders of the original small patches. In the severe cases, the patches develop more rapidly, coalescing in one or two years to form an atrophic area as large as the palm of the hand. Usually the course of the disease is very much slower.

*Diagnosis.* The skin on the bald patches is white and glossy, differing from that of alopecia areata in that it is atrophic ; no hair follicles are visible on the patches. None of the " exclamation hairs " of alopecia areata are seen on the margins of the patches. Lupus erythematosus never shows so many small patches collected in one region. There are no scales, keratotic plugs nor telangiectases. Brocq first described this disease and pointed out that no evidence of inflammation is seen around the marginal follicles, such

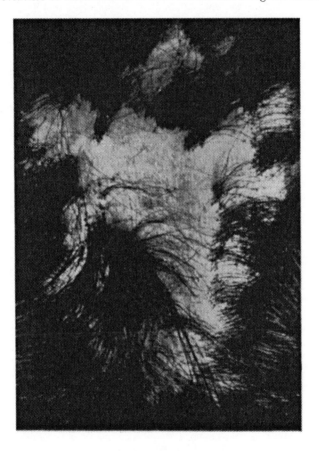

Fig. 32.—Pseudo-pelade.
(*By permission from Roxburgh, " Common Skin Diseases."*)

as occurs in folliculitis decalvans. In the actively spreading cases a certain number of the hairs can be easily pulled out, with the epithelial sheath attached, and such hairs show a minute, almost imperceptible trace of inflammation at the mouth of the follicle ; this redness is rare, and it disappears as soon as the hair falls. The diseased hairs are shown in Fig. 50, p. 239. The shaft is irregular and pigmented, and the root shows evidence of a rapid fall ; it never has the tapered appearance of the root which has had a natural gradual death. No organisms have ever been found on culture. Barber considers that the histology points to a blood-borne toxin, not to a local infection.[1] It has been suggested that it is the atrophic form of Lichen planus.[2]

Forms of cicatricial alopecia are considered at length in *J. Invest. Derm.*, 1947, **8**, 97. Microscopic sections of the various types above described are illustrated in that paper.

The *Cause* remains unknown. Some regard the disease as a sequel to lichen planus. *Prognosis* and *Treatment*, see pages 145 and 146.

IX. **Folliculitis Decalvans** (Quinquaud's disease) has been confused with other forms of baldness with atrophy, especially pseudo-pelade, lupus erythematosus, lichen planus with cicatricial bald regions and the severe type of keratosis pilaris. Folliculitis decalvans starts with a bald patch, usually on the vertex, which has a smooth cicatricial centre and at the margin inflamed follicle mouths, rarely showing any pus. Extensive baldness may develop as adjacent patches coalesce. *Staphylococcus aureus* has been found in cultures made from the affected follicles or the hair roots removed from them. H. W. Barber compares the condition with sycosis of the region of the beard.

X. Bald cicatricial areas on the scalp have been found in association with **lichen planus** and **lichen spinulosus** on the body. The cicatricial area may involve the whole vertex (see Fig. 33). As a rule, only a few or no lichenous lesions are seen on the scalp ; in several of the recorded cases both lesions were present on the trunk and limbs. When the scalp is affected, the bald atrophic patches occur chiefly on the vertex, and there may be found a few horny plugs, sometimes with broken hair stumps in the follicles. In one of Barber's patients a few lichen planus papules were seen on the bald area (see Fig. 34). These rare cases can be diagnosed with certainty only when the eruption affects the body or the mucous membranes. The axillæ and pubis may also be affected : horny follicular papules being followed by atrophy and alopecia. Lichen spinulosus is now (1949) rarely seen on the body. Lichen planus papules on the scalp have also been recorded by French observers. In some patients the lesions became verrucose ; in others, they were followed by smooth atrophic greyish pink patches. Sabouraud believed that a certain number of the latter were in reality a rare form of lupus erythematosus. He also maintained that there are cases of lichen and of pityriasis rubra pilaris which have been erroneously diagnosed as Brocq's pseudo-pelade ; in such cases, the baldness is more extensive and a horny cone is found at the root of the hair which is about to fall. In 1915 E. Graham Little[3] recorded a case of cicatricial baldness which he named folliculitis decalvans. The condition had made slow progress during many years ; then lichen spinulosus appeared on the body. In the same year Wallace Beatty[4] described a similar case which he had watched for ten years before lichen appeared on the scalp and later developed extensively over the body. In his article excellent

---

[1] *Proc. Roy. Soc. Med.*, 1942, **36**, 282.
[2] Q. E. PIERINI, *Revista Argentina de Dermatosifilologia*, 1949, **33**, 45.
[3] *Brit. J. Derm.*, 1915, **27**, 183.　　　　[4] *Ibid.* 331.

illustrations of the clinical and of the histological appearances are published. Reports of apparently identical diseases were described by various Continental observers. Unfortunately these records also employed the label folliculitis decalvans and much confusion arose when the last-named was differentiated from the cicatricial baldness due to lichen. H. Corsi [1] gave a full bibliography and discussed conditions of brittle nails and mucous membrane papules associated with this type of lichenous baldness.

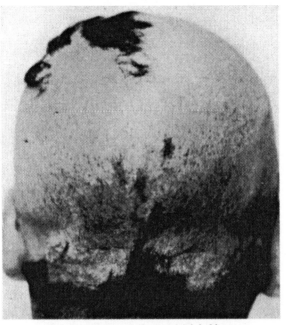

Fig. 33.—Widespread cicatricial baldness.

Patient had severe irritation on the head and body nine months before the hair began to fall. The scalp showed discrete follicular horny papules, with projecting broken off hair stumps and cicatricial baldness. Lichen spinulosus was widespread on the body. Some months previously the scalp had been X-rayed without benefit.

*(Photograph kindly lent by Dr. H. W. Barber.)*

The *prognosis* of the bald areas due to PSEUDO-PELADE and LICHEN is of the gravest, both as regards arrest of the disease and the prospect of regrowth of the hair. The hairfall and scarring usually increase slowly, but with inexorable march, for many years ; with lichen the progress may be rapid.

*Treatment.* Patients suffering from the above diseases usually go from hospital to hospital, and doctor to doctor, seeking cure. Hair cannot return on atrophied areas ; but the march of these diseases can often be arrested by

---

[1] H. Corsi gave a bibliography of these rare conditions in *Brit. Journ. Dermat.*, 1937, **49**, 376.

attention to the general health and to the local condition by adequate, but not by overstimulation of the scalp. Fresh air, nutritious diet, avoidance of emotional strain, tonics, ultra-violet light, all contribute to build up the

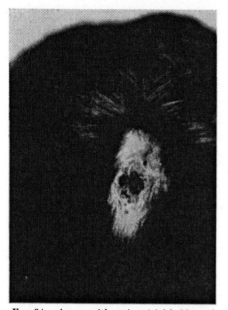

health and thus arrest the progress of pseudo-pelade, folliculitis decalvans and lichen. For pseudo-pelade Sabouraud ordered oil of cade and sulphur applications ; Lee McCarthy has belief in them also. For folliculitis decalvans attack the invading *staphylococcus aureus.* Vaccine given intradermally may be tried; locally, I prefer Ung. Hyd. Ammon. dil. ; others, Ung. Quinolor Co or Penicillin. With the latter remember that the patient may be sensitive to its base, or the organism may not be penicillin sensitive.

XI. **Ulerythema ophryogenes** begins on the eyebrow, whence it may spread to the scalp. In its early stage it resembles keratosis pilaris, with horny papules at the mouths of the hair follicles. The hairs are fine or broken off close to the surface of the skin. No further alteration may occur for years ; in other cases inflammatory changes gradually develop, terminating in atrophy of the follicles and of the intervening skin. Depressed scars are then visible on the affected region.

FIG. 34.—A case with a cicatricial bald patch, shown by H. W. Barber at the Royal Society of Medicine in October, 1931, had raised red patches, the histology of which resembled lichen planus. Over the rest of the scalp were many follicular horny papules, with broken off hair stumps ; on the body were widespread lesions of lichen spinulosus and lichen planus.

(*Photograph kindly lent by Dr. H. W. Barber.*)

After Taenzer in 1889 [1] had described this disease, which he named ulerythema ophryogenes, Brocq [2] independently recorded an apparently similar or allied condition which he named keratosis pilaris. At the outer edge of the eyebrows and usually also on the adjacent temporo-maxillary region the skin shows fine elevations and atrophy of the follicle mouths which at first are invisible except in a good light. At the hair roots redness develops ; gradually the hairs fall and fine cicatrices form. In five of the cases described by Taenzer the disease started in early childhood with horny papules and redness of the eyebrows, with subsequent loss of hair ; then similar lesions extended to the adjacent skin of the brow, cheeks and scalp, leaving marked atrophy at the mouths of the follicles. There is still uncertainty as to the

---

[1] P. TAENZER, *Monats f. prakt Derm.*, 1889, **8**, 197.
[2] BROCQ, *Ann. de Derm. et Syph.*, 1893, 3me Sér. **1**, 97.

pathology of these conditions, but some regard them as a form of the same disease as the ichthyosis follicularis (described by Lesser and others) which is congenital or begins within the first two years of life and occurs in several members of a family. (See Chapter VII, p. 100, and also Keratosis pilaris, Chapter XI, p. 182.)

Treatment is uncertain. The crusts should be removed, and salicylic ointment thoroughly rubbed in. During the war I saw several Service girls with this malady. Large doses of vitamin A were given and the diet supervised so that the vitamins were not destroyed by over-cooking. Improvement was reported, but Army conditions prevented opportunity of following up these patients.

XII. **Lupus Vulgaris** and other nodular conditions. Scars due to lupus vulgaris, syphilitic gummata, sarcoids, leishmaniasis, etc., are recognized by the presence of some unhealed erythematous part of the disease, by lesions on other parts of the body, by microscopic examination of a smear, or by the history of a previous swelling or ulcer. Rarely, if ever, is the scalp alone involved.

SARCOIDS, in particular the *benign nodular* type, may affect the scalp, especially in women. The nodules resemble at first those of lupus vulgaris. They may coalesce to form a plaque which, as it spreads peripherally, may form quite an extensive ringed or circinate eruption. As it heals in the centre, it leaves a depressed and cicatricial bald patch. Several may be present. The *papular form* of sarcoid may appear on the scalp as well as on the body ; the papule may be absorbed, leaving a fine scar, or become pustular and leave a pitted cicatrix. Sarcoids are more fully dealt with under nodules on p. 261.

XIII. **Chignon Alopecia** may be seen in women, Sabouraud said, between the ages of thirty and fifty. At first thinning of the hair is seen on an area about the middle line, towards the posterior region of the vertex. It is a condition in which a slow atrophy of the skin occurs. It used to be attributed to the pressure of heavy coils of hair, pads or combs when their habitual use was fashionable. The disease may form one oval-shaped area, or there may be two parts, one side spreading more than the other. Sometimes the scalp on this region is normal, or shows some scales ; the skin beneath is white and most of the hair follicles have disappeared. Any sparse remaining hairs are like down ; these also gradually disappear. The condition is usually discovered accidentally, when the bald area has attained some size ; it may progress till it is as large as the palm of the hand. Sabouraud tried many forms of treatment without avail. In the early stage it may be mistaken for alopecia of the menopause. The downy hair and the curious shape of the patches, however, are characteristic features of this malady of unknown origin. Sabouraud stated that the disease is not rare ; I have seen several cases since my attention was drawn to this condition some years ago.

XIV. **Radiodermatitis.** Permanent baldness after the use of radium, or after X-ray for ringworm or other disease of the scalp, is not so often seen to-day, when X-ray is administered with the precautions of modern technique. The skin in radiodermatitis is atrophied, wrinkled, showing many telangiectases, and often pigmented patches and a few stray white hairs. The atrophy and its accompaniments may not appear until five, ten, or fifteen years after the X-ray treatment. Nothing can restore the hair in these cases ; the hair papillæ are permanently destroyed. In severe cases, after the lapse of many years, are seen warty growths and ulcers, on which, sooner or later, epithelioma usually develops.

XV. **Frontal Band Alopecia,** which affects chiefly women, was described by Sabouraud [1] (*Alopécie liminaire frontale*) as a low-grade inflammatory process affecting the hair just in front of the ears, and passing in a few weeks like a ribbon across the brow. At first irritable and reddened, the skin becomes cicatricial and bald. A narrow border of healthy hair is usually left intact in front. Often the condition is not seen by the specialist until the patient is elderly and the whole area involved is cicatricial. Cases were reported from Buenos Ayres [2] occurring in young girls : the condition was traced to traumatism, due to curling pins, used very tightly, so that they gave rise to pain and traction on the hair roots. Scaliness and folliculitis followed, and, later, scarring. C. G. Costa and M. A. Junqueira [3] give excellent illustrations of this disease ; the traumatism extended all along the scalp margin. I recently saw an early stage in an elderly woman who had begun to employ hard metal curlers every night ; from ear to ear she had a band of erythema, swelling, and broken off hairs. The condition was cured with soothing applications and the renunciation of her curling appliances.

XVI. **Hyperkeratosis cystica follicularis,** a condition with greatly dilated follicles full of horny plugs, was described in 1929 in Japan ; atrophic alopecia followed. Touraine and Solente [4] had a similar case in 1935 ; they reported histological details and considered that the alopecia was due to folliculitis with keratotic microcysts.

XVII. **Congenital Defects.** Several cases have been reported with a congenital defect which shows as a small area, pin-head to half a crown-sized, usually circular, of depressed cicatricial alopecia. It is often situated on the vertex, or near the sagittal suture, occasionally on the occiput or behind the ears. Kehrer [5] of Vienna collected 32 cases from the literature on the subject, and described one of his own. Anderson and Novy [6] recently reported several cases. The abnormality is congenital and is supposed to be due to amniotic adhesions or to arrested development. Eight per cent. showed congenital defects on other parts of the body. If the patient were an adult and the dermatologist unaware of the condition there would be difficulty in diagnosis. One must review injury at birth, as by forceps, or in later life ; healed angioma ; and congenital depression of the skull. X-ray may aid diagnosis in an obscure case.

[1] *Annales de Dermatologie,* 1931 ; second series ; p. 446.
[2] D. L. BALINA, *Bull. Soc. Franç. de Derm. et Syph.,* 1933, **40,** 1277.
[3] *Arch. Derm. and Syph.,* 1943, **48,** 527.
[4] A. TOURAINE and G. SOLENTE, *Bull. Soc. Franç. de derm. et syph.,* 1935, **42,** 1780. A. TOURAINE, *Bull. Soc. Franç. de derm. et syph.,* 1936, **43,** 363.
[5] KEHRER, *Monatschr. f. Geburtsh. u. Gynak.,* 1910, **31,** 183 ; abstracted in *Surg. Gynec. and Obst.,* 1910, **11,** 108.
[6] N. P. ANDERSON and F. G. NOVY, *Arch. Derm. and Syph.,* 1942, **46,** 257.

# CHAPTER X

## ITCHING OF THE SCALP

**Itching of the scalp,** apart from *urticaria,* is common ; it may be a trivial matter ; it may also be the precursor of serious disease. It may be present even in apparently simple cases of *pityriasis simplex.* It is usually, but not always, present with any *eruption with a red base,* as is seen when generalized eruptions extend to the scalp. Itching is frequent when *pityriasis steatoides* (" seborrhœic dermatitis ") develops in older patients with defective liver function, but is usually absent when this disease affects young people. With *lupus erythematosus* there may be no itching, or it may be severe. In uncomplicated *psoriasis* and in *syphilis* there is a noticeable absence of itching, but irritation develops when there is an accompanying *streptococcal infection.* The patient who has *alopecia areata* can sometimes foretell, by the itching, the position of a patch about to develop. Itching often precedes *acute hairfall,* and may follow overdosage of *microbacillus vaccine.* Itching may precede the initial stage of the formation of pustules, vesicles and bullæ, as in *eczema, kerion, chickenpox, herpes zoster, impetigo* and *dermatitis herpetiformis.* Itching may be the first sign of dermatitis due to an *external irritant* (soap, dyes, various shampoos, " cold perm " or other lotions). Fig. 33 illustrates a case in which extensive cicatricial baldness, with *lichenous* lesions, had been preceded by several months of itching. Itching may be a marked feature in *mycosis fungoides,* before any eruption is visible, but it is rare indeed that this would not first be seen on the body. Itching is felt at a certain stage of the growth of *sebaceous cysts, leukæmia* and other *nodules,* and may precede as well as accompany a patch of *morphæa.* However, in all these examples, itching is not the prominent nor the diagnostic feature. Marked itching accompanies *pediculosis* ; as itching is the symptom for which the patient usually seeks advice, pediculosis of the scalp is described under Cause VI, below. When itching is severe, scratching is constantly indulged in, and if at the same time treatment is neglected, *lichenification* of the scalp may develop in time (p. 150).

Itching is also a prominent feature and is the symptom for which advice is sought, in the following diseases, which are described as far as possible in the order of frequency of occurrence. In the first six causes, there is local evidence of disease of the scalp. In Cause VII, and sometimes in Cause II, no local disease is visible.

149

I   Neurodermatitis.
II  Urticaria.
III Acne necrotica miliaris.
IV  Acne varioloformis.
V   Streptococcal pityriasis.
VI  Pediculosis capitis.
VII Drug habits.

I. *The patient, usually a woman, complains of long-standing and marked itching at the back of the scalp, just above the neck. A scaly patch, often with a red base, is visible.* The disease is NEURODERMATITIS (Lichen Simplex Chronicus).

**Neurodermatitis,** sometimes called **Lichen Simplex Chronicus,** has had several titles since 1907, and may yet acquire a better name in the future.   Severe itching accompanies this common condition, a thickened, red-based, lichenified, scaly patch on the occipital region. The eruption begins at the nape of the neck, at the margin of the hair, and often spreads to the adjoining skin, whilst its upper margin extends upwards under the hair.   Sometimes the patch may grow forward as far as the ears.   Frequently, especially in the older patients, there are also present on the neck lichenified lesions resembling the lichen circumscriptum of Vidal.   In younger patients the patch on the nape may be accompanied by some post-auricular intertrigo.   The patches on the neck are intensely irritating.   Retro-auricular intertrigo may be a super-imposed infection, especially in the younger patients.   The usual oval-shaped patch at the nape conveys to the examining finger a thick, hard sensation, as if part of it lay beneath the skin like a waxen plaque.   On the surface are thin dry scales ; sometimes these are thick, almost psoriatic.   Only rarely is there found a degree of moisture when the scales are rubbed off.   Some hairs may be broken off at the skin level, due to being scratched away, but the disease does not lead to a real hairfall.

The *diagnosis* is simple, because of the characteristic position, the severity of the itching, and the obstinate resistance to the local applications which succeed with pityriasis circinata.   The usual antipruritics can be tried—carbolic, tar, 1 per cent. anethane ointment and anthisan cream, menthol and camphor, but as a rule they give only temporary relief.   A good method is to administer two half-pastille doses of X-ray (with the old gas-filled tube) at a fortnight's interval, filtered half the time through half a millimetre of aluminium.   Follow with two to four doses of iodine ionization, twice a week ;   the patient meanwhile rubs in a mild mer-curial or tar ointment.   The above method cured a few obstinate cases which had long resisted not only various applications but also a course of careful dieting and treatment directed towards improvement of the general health. I am favourably impressed by the effects of crude coal tar ointment, but its use is disagreeable to the patient, owing to its colour and adhesiveness. Sabouraud recommended the treatment which is successful for chronic streptococcal dermatitis : weak iodine (1 or 2 per cent.) in alcohol, followed by massage with 1 to 6 per cent. coal tar ointment. This can be cleaned off with cotton wool soaked in equal parts of acetone, alcohol and distilled water. Insulin, 40 to 80 units, once or twice a day, has benefited some.[1] Corsi reported success with five weekly applications of Thorium X in varnish painted on the region (2000 units to the c.cm.[2]). Some of my worst cases improved most with benedryl and phenergan ; but the benefit was not lasting. Ung. hyd. ammon. is useful when the scales are thick. This malady is largely due to the habit of scratching, almost unconsciously, by day, and on waking in the morning. It provides a form of psychological relief from worry and mental tension. Sometimes the removal of a septic focus relieves the itching and thus breaks the habit of continual rubbing. One obstinate patch I cured by sealing it off with elastoplast. One lady was convinced that all ointments removed the scales, but increased itching ; she preferred to apply siccolam, although it left a dry pink powder. Modern thought advises a psychological line of approach ; but the influence of the physical upon the mental is also marked.

II. Itching of the scalp sometimes occurs as a variety of **urticaria**. This form of urticaria troubles the patient only for a day or two, when there is constipation or other transient disorder of the stomach or intestine. The presence of a few urticarial lesions on the face or neck aids the diagnosis. Urticarial papules may be present on various parts of the body, but may be few or absent. Sometimes the urticarial basis of the itching is not recognized until a temporary gastro-intestinal cause has passed away. If, after a few days' respite, there is a recurrence of the scalp itching, the previous occasion is recalled and the diagnosis becomes clear.

III. **Acne Necrotica Miliaris.** One is not infrequently consulted about a condition of itching of the scalp for which for many years I was unable to find a name. The patient comes because the scalp itches. On examination one finds scattered about the scalp a few tiny oozing points. These lesions are usually much smaller in diameter than a pea ; sometimes a conical crust tops a moist point, about the size of a pin head. It often happens that only two or three of these minute lesions can be

[1] *Arch. Derm. and Syph.*, Chicago, 1941, **43**, 980.    [2] *Lancet*, 1943, **ii**, 346.

found. At other times the brow, part of the cheeks, neck and chest may also be involved.

I have seen this condition recurring at intervals, for many years, in the young and the middle-aged, in men and in women. It improves, but does not vanish under the use of mercurial or sulphur applications, whether in lotion or ointment form. Apparently mild tar and mercurial lotions give the best local effects. I have always found that internal treatment is more valuable than local applications. In men I have seen

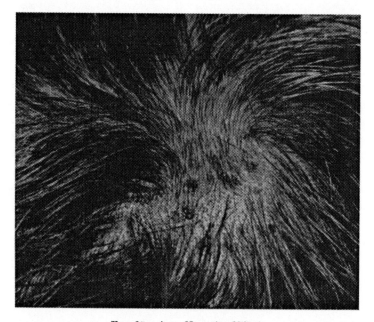

FIG. 35.—Acne Necrotica Miliaris.
(*Photograph kindly lent by Dr. Hamilton Montgomery, from "Diseases of the Skin," Ormsby and Montgomery; Henry Kimpton.*)

the formation of fresh lesions arrested by the prohibition of all forms of alcohol. In other cases treatment on lines of diet, the correction of intestinal toxæmia, the elimination of sweets, and the restriction of farinaceous foods, together with alkalis and laxatives, have given the best results. However, one does not see numerous enough examples of this malady to enable one to draw a definite conclusion as to the cause and the best form of treatment. Sabouraud described this condition and suggested that it was an abortive form of acne necrotica (acne nécrotique miliaire). He found staphylococcus aureus on culturing the crusts. I watched one patient who had attacks, at intervals, for over twenty years ;

true acne necrotica never developed, but on two occasions she had boils on the scalp, due, I believed, to her having scratched the tiny itching vesicles. Hamilton Montgomery [1] reported twenty-five cases who, from the illustrations, suffered from the above described malady (Fig. 35). Itching was the chief complaint ; minute vesicles developed on the itching areas. After about six hours the vesicles broke, oozed serum and crusted over ; a few ulcerated. Histologically, there was found an intradermal vesicle filled with serum ; staphylococci were obtained when ulceration developed. In Montgomery's experience the best form of treatment consisted of an ointment with ammoniated mercury of the strength usually employed for psoriasis of the scalp. In some obstinate types I have found this of much value.

IV. ACNE VARIOLOFORMIS (Syn., Acne necrotica) is described under pustular conditions of the scalp (p. 225). Itching is a prominent feature in the early stages.

V. In STREPTOCOCCAL PITYRIASIS itching may be a marked feature ; but sometimes it is entirely absent (see p. 176).

VI. *The patient complains of itching of the scalp. In the occipital region nits are seen on the hairs, near the scalp. The patient has* PEDICU-LOSIS CAPITIS.

**Pediculosis capitis** is the invasion of the hairy scalp by the pediculus or louse. The patient complains of itching of the scalp ; at times a creeping sensation is felt which leads to scratching. The louse multiplies in those who take little care of the person, therefore it is chiefly found in very young or very old people, especially those living in dirty, unhealthy surroundings. But no class is exempt. It is extraordinary how long a time may elapse in the case of educated wealthy people before the true origin of the scalp irritation is suspected by either the patient or his physician. The degree of irritation complained of depends upon the sensitiveness of the sufferer. In some people the presence of one or two lice on the head causes more misery than an army of lice on the scalp of an insensitive person. In a highly strung individual the health suffers from loss of sleep and the depression caused by the continuous itching. Thirty years ago it was quite common for medical students, nurses and visitors in slum districts to have their heads infected by lice ; the condition remained unsuspected for weeks.

The insects are usually found first on the occipital region of the scalp ;

---

[1] HAMILTON MONTGOMERY, *Arch. Derm. and Syph.*, 1937, **36**, 40. LANE, *ibid.*, 1933, **28**, 10.

thence they spread to the parietal regions. Only in very infected heads do the pediculi take up a habitat beyond the posterior half of the scalp, but in neglected patients the entire scalp may be invaded.

When women wore long hair, and before there was any medical inspection in schools, one often saw such extensive infection that the hair over the whole head appeared to be grey, due to the presence of innumerable ova—the so-called nits. The post-cervical glands of the neck were enlarged, abscesses formed, serum and pus poured from the excoriated scalp, and the sufferer might be seriously ill, with marked anæmia and toxæmia. The medical inspection of schools produced a higher level of cleanliness amongst the general population, and it became rare to see an infected child at a hospital clinic. To maintain this result constant watchfulness was necessary on the part of the nursing staff ;

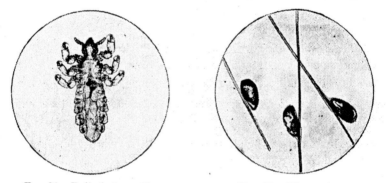

FIG. 36.—Pediculosis capitis.        FIG. 37.—Nits on hair.

during the holiday weeks, the cleanliness of the children tended to relapse. During the war, pediculosis of the scalp became more common in the great industrial towns with the vast army of factory workers, who, in order to retain their waves and curls, refused hygienic care to their heads. Medical officers who inspected the factories reported that among the young women and girls the incidence of lice-infected heads then was greatly increased. When one sees a rash, partly papular, partly impetiginized on the neck at the occipital region, on the cheeks and behind the ears, one can predict with certainty the discovery of lice on the scalp.

*Diagnosis.* The insects may be so few that the physician may long be baffled when searching for the cause of the itching scalp. Careful investigation discovers one or two nits on the hair shafts, close to the scalp, in the occipital region. At first they may be mistaken for scurf, but are distinguished by their firm attachment to the hair shaft (Fig. 37). The presence of tiny papules at the nape of the neck, below the hair margin and behind the ears often provides the clue to diagnosis. The ova are usually laid close to the scalp, so that in long-standing cases the date of infection can be estimated by the distance of the nits from the scalp. Thus, as hairs grow at about the rate of a centimetre a month, the duration of the invasion can be measured by the distance of the nits from the scalp.

*Treatment. Old methods :* to be used when the new drugs are unobtainable, as in emergency. Apply over the whole scalp an ointment containing 2 per cent. ammoniated mercury. Sabouraud said that the insects die even if nothing but simple vaseline is used, because it blocks up the respiratory system of the louse and causes immediate death. He added xylol in the proportions of 50 drops to 50 grammes of white vaseline. The head can be soaped and washed an hour or two after this application has been well rubbed in over the entire scalp. Crusts saturated with the vaseline should be removed on the following day with a fine comb. Other remedies are oil of sassafras, 2 per cent. cresol or lysol (i.e. crude phenol emulsified with soft soap). Some saturated the hair with 1 in 40 carbolic acid, squeezing out the fluid and keeping the head wrapped in a towel for two hours, when ova and lice should be destroyed. For children an efficacious application consists of methylated spirit, 7 parts ; water, 3 parts ; three ounces of this mixture is sufficient to soak the hair. The head is then bound up with a rubber cap for an hour, when insects and ova are killed. *Modern methods :* The above are not in favour when a woman desires to retain her wave setting. Remedies are now employed which leave the hair no more disturbed than with an application of brilliantine. Three effective insecticides are : 25 per cent. technical lauryl thiocyanate in a white oil ; 50 per cent. lethane 384 special, in similar oil ; and derris cream. Of these 2 c.cm. is enough for a child with short hair, and 8 c.cm. for a woman with long thick hair. The hair must be carefully parted and the chosen preparation put on the scalp in several regions, then massaged well in with the fingers. The material remains active for about ten days ; therefore the hair must not be washed for that time. Full details of the composition of these applications are given in the article by Busvine and Buxton.[1] Care must be taken that the ova are destroyed ; the firm outer coating is resistant to alkalis and soap.

Older text-books state that ova are destroyed by soaking the hair in vinegar or acetic acid ; recent writers deny this teaching. I tested the fact on three locks of hair equally and heavily infected with nits. I placed them in three receptacles : one contained strong acetic acid ; another had 33 per cent. acetic acid (equivalent to dilute acetic) ; the third held vinegar. After having lain five minutes in the first two solutions, the nits were readily

[1] *Brit. Med. J.*, 1942, 1, 464.

removed by gentle rubbing along the hair shafts. With the soaking in vinegar the nits were not easily removed from the hairs. Soaking in benzole was not more rapidly effective than in strong acetic acid.

Dead insects and ova can be removed by using a fine comb. Ascabiol [1] is recommended for the removal of nits and the destruction of pediculi ; it is a 25 per cent. emulsion of benzyl benzoate made up with triethanolamine. 10 per cent. D.D.T. powder left on the scalp and the hair for a week destroys lice. It can be used in an emulsified base or a mineral oil. Gammexane L.G. 140 is reported to be even more successful.[2]

VII. Itching of the scalp may be complained of when NO LOCAL DISEASE OF THE SCALP can be seen.

Itching of the scalp I have found occurring as part of the *general pruritus* which sometimes accompanies both functional and organic disease of the liver and gall-bladder, and also in elderly people with so-called senile pruritus.

Here it is necessary to point out that real itching of the scalp must be diagnosed from the *nervous condition* in which a patient develops a habit of absent-mindedly rubbing the head, as if he were suffering from itching. This form of tic can be diagnosed by observing the patient quietly when he is unaware that he is being watched.

Sabouraud described a condition in which the chief symptom is intense irritation of the scalp without visible cause. In nervous women whose sleep is broken by itching, and disturbed by nightmare, he is convinced that the root of the trouble is to be found in secret alcohol or drug-taking. Alcohol, he said, was the drug of women of the hospital class. However, alcohol cannot be mentioned to the patient whose vice is secret drinking ; approaching the subject in his inimitable style, Sabouraud used to advise the sufferer to avoid all fermented drinks : " Of course I do not speak of spirits, which for you is terribly poisonous, nor even of beer or wine." Alcohol should be replaced by an abundant intake of a simple fluid, such as one of the harmless tisanes so widely used in France. In a healthy patient the cocktail habit, which impairs hepatic function, can give rise to pruritus of the scalp and elsewhere.

Another characteristic type we all see frequently—the talkative and argumentative patients who declare they feel and even see insects on the skin. Sabouraud stated dogmatically that these were cocaine or heroin addicts, who misled all their physicians, and that the only means of making certain of the diagnosis was to examine the regions for punctures of the hypodermic needle. Looking back on cases I have met with, I recall one clever medical woman who constantly sought fresh advice and for over a year baffled a score of equally clever physicians. Her malady was eventually tracked down to the cocaine habit. But it is difficult to believe that all these cases belong to the group of drug addicts. Psychiatric treatment is often useful.

[1] ERIC BLACKSTOCK, *Brit. Med. Journ.*, 1944, 1, 115. See also ELIZABETH SCOBBIE, *Brit. Med. J.*, 1945, 1, 409.

[2] J. R. BUSVINE and J. A. REID, Medical Journal of Malaya, 1949, 3, 232.

## CHAPTER XI

## SCALY CONDITIONS OF THE SCALP

As a sequel to all *inflammatory* conditions, the upper layers of the skin are seen flaking off in large, papery, whitish-grey scales ; in these cases there is a definite history of redness preceding and usually also underlying the formation of the scales. A patient may complain of scales, or " *scurf*," which falls from the scalp and makes the hair appear to be covered with dust. On the other hand, scales may be present even when the patient remains unaware of the fact. When the *scalp is neglected*—as frequently occurs with old and lazy people, and young women who fear to dislodge their " waves "—never washed nor cleaned, and inefficiently brushed and combed, it is common to see brownish-yellow scales, because the normal shedding of the upper layers of the epidermis is retained in position by the unbrushed hair. Mistakes may occur even in apparently so simple a matter as diagnosing the presence of scales. Since the introduction of cleansing detergents and frequent washing of short hair, I have been impressed by the increased scaliness which patients have wrongly attributed to dandruff. No pityrosporon is found when these scales are stained. The *ova* of pediculi have often been mistaken for dandruff ; the distinguishing characteristic is that they cannot be gently blown off or brushed off ; they adhere to the hair shaft (see Fig. 37). The heaped-up yellow CRUSTS which follow exudation of serum or of pus are not fully discussed in this chapter.

When a patient has scales which are continually renewed, or which resist ordinary methods of brushing and combing, the following diseases giving rise to SCALES ON THE SCALP should be considered. They are mentioned as far as possible in order of frequency of occurrence :

I Pityriasis simplex and other stages of pityriasis.
II Psoriasis.
III Neurodermatitis (Lichen Simplex Chronicus).
IV Streptococcal pityriasis.
V Scaling due to traumatism.
VI Crusts and scales following exudation.
VII Parasitic infections, ringworm and favus.
VIII Crusts of impetigo and other pustular maladies.
IX Lupus erythematosus.
X " Fausse teigne."
XI Papulo-squamous syphilide.
XII Pityriasis rubra pilaris.
XIII Ichthyosis.

XIV    Dermatitis exfoliativa and other rare generalized eruptions, when
          they involve or extend to the scalp.
XV    Conditions with Keratosis.

*Diseases* with SCALES OR CRUSTS, in which the *microscopic examination*
of the hairs reveals a FUNGUS, are described in Chapter XII.

The doctor may meet with one form of a scaly scalp as soon as a babe
is born.   A layer of sticky material adheres to the head of some infants—the
*vernix caseosa* ; it consists of desquamated scales of epidermis, mixed with
sebaceous secretion.   Microscopic examination shows a mass of exfoliated
horny cells.   Jacquet proved that the sebaceous glands functioned even in
the fœtus.   When the scalp of an infant remains thickly coated with scales,
abnormal intestinal flora are usually found to be present.

I have recently seen a similar condition in two adults who came complaining of hairfall and extensive scaling of the scalp, dating from an acute intestinal
malady (dysentery and colitis).   In these patients microscopic examinations
revealed few or no bottle bacilli.   The scalp condition cleared up without
local antiseptic applications, the lotions employed being merely stimulants
for the hairfall.   Treatment for the general health and intestinal condition
appear to play an important rôle in the cure of the scalp.

CLINICAL INVESTIGATION.   Bearing in mind the facts mentioned in
the introductory paragraph, examine the scales ; in order to detect their
character, the presence of minute exudation or atrophy of the scalp, use
a lens ; a microscopic examination may be required.   Pityriasis simplex
is the most common cause of scales and should be considered first.   Scrape
off any thick scales and find if serous exudation or pus is present on the
underlying surface of the scalp.   Examine behind the ears and other
adjacent regions of the skin beyond the hairy scalp—retroauricular
dermatitis accompanies streptococcal infection, and is persistent ; tiny
papules on face and neck suggest pediculosis.   Note the *age* of the patient ;
then examine the face and the whole body, especially when erythema is
seen below the scales.   Enquire into the *history*.   In a child, fungus
infection is a common cause, *fausse teigne* a rare cause, of scales occurring
in patches.   If there has been redness and exudation, scales and crusts
may be the final, flaking stage of acute streptococcal dermatitis, or the
child may be recovering from impetigo or infantile eczema.   If there is
itching, recent erythema and oozing in some regions, especially behind the
ear, consider chronic streptococcal infection, primary or secondary.   If
the patient is an adult woman with itching on the occipital region, suspect
neurodermatitis.   If the scales are thick and white, on a red base, if
itching is absent or only slight, and there are patches on the body, psoriasis
or squamous syphilide is a probable, pityriasis rubra pilaris a rare cause.
With lupus erythematosus there are usually characteristic red, scaly
patches on the ears and face, and the patient is over twenty-five.   A

history of the use of strong local remedies points to traumatic dermatitis. When causes XII to XIV are present, the patient complains less about the scalp than the scaliness or redness of the body. When the hair is short, and hard cones are seen at the mouth of the follicles, review the various causes of keratosis (pp. 100, 146, and 182).

I. *The patient, who may be of either sex and of any age, complains of scales continually brushed off or falling from the scalp. The most common cause is* PITYRIASIS SIMPLEX CAPITIS.

**Pityriasis Simplex Capitis.** (Syn., pityriasis sicca.) No subject would seem to present a more simple problem than that of pityriasis. Yet no dermatological condition (except seborrhœa oleosa) has afforded more discussion than this apparently superficial condition of scaliness on the scalp.

The commonest malady of the scalp is the state of scaliness, pityriasis simplex, or pityriasis sicca, which is popularly known as dandruff or scurf. In text-books on dermatology of a generation ago the name " seborrhœa sicca " is often met with. The term was first brought into use by Hebra. He taught that an excessive secretion of sebum might either give rise to an increased oiliness of the scalp, or the sebum might undergo a change which led to its becoming deposited on the scalp in the form of somewhat greasy dry scales. To this appearance, which he regarded as a solidified fatty secretion, he gave the name dry seborrhœa, " seborrhœa sicca." Hence this title has been employed until recently, even by dermatologists, although they usually accompany the use of the term with an apology or brief explanation that they do not agree with the meaning implied by such a name. At the present time, therefore, when " seborrhœa sicca " is mentioned, a definite clinical condition is understood, even by those who do not profess to know anything about diseases of the scalp. In the early years of this century the monumental research of Sabouraud in Paris provided the chief massing of facts which disclosed the error of the previous assumption that the grey and the yellow sticky scales so frequently seen on the scalp consisted of a dried-up or solidified secretion of sebum. Although in certain circles, especially where Sabouraud's investigations are unknown, there is a revival of the old conception of solidified sebum, the continued employment of the old terminology is to be deprecated, because it is liable to lead the physician into errors.

*Symptoms and Signs.* With pityriasis capitis there are seen loose dry scales which may affect the vertex or the whole scalp. The scaliness is really a flaking off of the upper layers of the epidermis. The popular name for this condition is dandruff or scurf. The scales are grey, and are usually seen at first in small round patches, especially on the vertex.

These may extend to cover nearly all of the scalp. As they are constantly being shed, they may lie along the hair shafts, and when profuse are seen on the clothing. Occasionally itching is felt when fresh scaly patches occur, but usually the patient complains only of the unsightly scales.

Three clinical stages of pityriasis can be distinguished :

1. *Pityriasis simplex* may remain more or less unchanged throughout the lifetime of a healthy individual. Similar patches of grey scales sometimes occur also on the skin of the face.

2. In other cases the scalp reacts by throwing out a slight serous exudation, which causes the scales to become adherent, not so readily shed, and with a waxy yellow, and later almost a crusted appearance. They are not greasy ; to the finger they convey a sticky, slightly moist sensation. On removing the adherent scales a faint moisture and sometimes even a faint rosiness of the underlying skin is seen with the examining lens. To this condition Sabouraud gave the descriptive name *pityriasis steatoides*. These scaly patches also affect the face, especially the nasolabial folds.

3. Beneath the sticky scales, in some patients, the skin shows more moisture, and below and beyond the scales an eruption, pale red or yellowish red, develops, with a circinate margin. It is especially marked round the edge of the hairy scalp and may spread to the skin of the ears, neck and brow, the *corona seborrhœica* (p. 205). The same eruption may be present on other parts of the body, especially along the mid-line of the front and back of the chest. This characteristic condition Sabouraud named *pityriasis circinata* ; it is an eczematized *pityriasis steatoides* (Fig. 39). This red, scaly eruption had been called by Unna " seborrhœic eczema," and the name *seborrhœic dermatitis* has unfortunately remained. Seborrhœic dermatitis is an eczematized infective dermatitis ; the region becomes eczematized owing to the epidermis becoming sensitized to (as opposed to being merely infected by) the micro-organisms. This causes the formation of vesicles and subsequent oozing of serum. At the present time many leading dermatologists retain the misleading name " seborrhœic dermatitis " because they consider that the eruption develops only where there is a seborrhœic skin, i.e. an altered sebaceous secretion which permits the pityriasis organisms to flourish. This mistaken nomenclature is also discussed in the section on seborrhœa (p. 101) and on ætiology (p. 162).

Although *hairfall* may occur in association with all stages of pityriasis, it is uncertain whether the pityriasis and its associated micro-organisms are the sole cause in operation. On the other hand, many patients have pityriasis sicca, pityriasis steatoides and seborrhœic dermatitis on and off during a whole lifetime and yet have no loss of hair. When there is associated hairfall, it is a good rule to investigate the general health.

*Diagnosis.* The diagnosis of pityriasis is rarely difficult; its early recognition is important, because the prognosis is so good if the correct treatment is carried out. Except in causes I and IV, the scales on the scalp seen in the diseases named in the list on p. 157 do not form the most prominent feature of those diseases; these are dealt with later in this chapter, under their respective headings. Only the chief points and the common causes of error in diagnosis are mentioned here. The introductory paragraph of this chapter should be recalled in this connection.

A scalp affected with dandruff looks untidy and uncared for; the thick grey scales fall on the clothing and body. Mistakes may occur in diagnosing a case of pityriasis sicca when there has been much hard combing, or friction with a stiff brush, or after the use of very drying spirit lotions and many of the modern soapless shampoos (see p. 54). I have frequently seen scaliness when the patient has been over-vigorous in applying remedies for pityriasis. After such causes of *traumatism*, due to external irritants, there are seen loose, fine, branny scales on the scalp and hair shafts. Careful inspection usually renders the diagnosis easy; the apparent scales are seen to be thin layers of epidermis; some are long, and on being pulled, break away from the scalp like a strip of thin skin. The scales of pityriasis are thicker, and usually occur in circular patches on the vertex. However, it must not be forgotten that both conditions may be present together. In elderly people I have seen scaliness associated with *athyroidism*; in young and middle-aged subjects, a generalized scaliness of the scalp is occasionally seen when the *general health* is below par, see p. 158. When the diagnosis is doubtful, the point can be settled by staining and examining the scales under the microscope. With pityriasis sicca, many " bottle bacilli " are seen (Fig. 38). *Psoriasis* may be mistaken for pityriasis steatoides, but the scales are thicker, silvery, and there is usually psoriasis present on the body (p. 173). When psoriasis is complicated with streptococcal infection, the diagnosis from eczematized stages of pityriasis may be difficult (see below).

It is most important not to mistake an early patch of *ringworm* for pityriasis. Ringworm is rare in adults, but common in children under the age of puberty. In the early stage of ringworm the scales resemble those of simple pityriasis, but after careful search broken hairs are detected (see p. 184); a microscopic examination settles the diagnosis. A *chronic streptococcal infection* of the scalp can be mistaken for simple pityriasis or more often for pityriasis steatoides. There is itching of the scalp and on examination one sees fine white scales, and in many cases, dispersed here and there are visible a few small oozing points ; sometimes oozing and a pink hue underlie a small yellow crust. This type of case is aggravated by the applications suitable for simple pityriasis ; this aids the diagnosis (see p. 167). Of recent years staphylococcus aureus has often been found. In *secondary syphilis* the hairfall leads to the formation of bald patches, which produce a characteristic " moth-eaten " appearance to the scalp ; they are numerous ; they may be, but are not necessarily accompanied by pityriasis (see p. 132).

*Ætiology.* Sabouraud's study of the bacteriological flora prevailing on the scalp shed a light on the subject of scaliness and oiliness, and their connection with hairfall, which has had important practical results in prognosis and treatment as well as in diagnosis. Pityriasis is rarely seen under the age of nine or ten ; but it may appear, on and off, during a lifetime. Both sexes are equally affected.

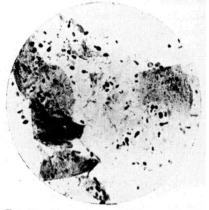

Fig. 38.—Pityrosporon of Malassez (" bottle bacillus ") in a scalp scraping, with scales of epidermis, " dandruff." (Microphotograph × 600.)

1. The invasion of the epidermis by the pityrosporon leads to a multiplication of the cells and consequent scaling of the horny layer. When the scales of *pityriasis simplex* are stained with methylene blue and examined under the microscope, crowds of large flask-like, ovoid and rounded bodies are seen lying between and on the layers of the epidermal cells. For long this organism was known as the pityrosporon of Malassez ; later, Unna described it as the flask or bottle bacillus, because of its resemblance to a flask or bottle (Fig. 38). This name is scientifically inaccurate, but it is pictorially so precise that it will endure long after the more correct term, pityrosporon. Cultures were hard to grow ; it is not decided that the experiments by Mr. Garner in St. John's Hospital for Skin Diseases, London, were true cultures. The " bottle bacillus " is now classed under the group of *Monilia* or yeast organisms. The hyperkeratosis of the mouths of the follicles is now considered to be due to androgen stimulation ; the pityrosporon is found in quantity in the scales which are shed.

2. In *pityriasis steatoides*, the " bottle bacillus " multiplies, and the skin of the scalp reacts by throwing out serum. In this condition a micro-

scopic examination of the scales reveals the presence not only of the bottle bacillus, but also of cocci lying between the scales.   On culture these cocci show a grey growth : Sabouraud refers to this organism as the grey staphylococcus.   The precise staphylococcus has not yet been decided ; it has been named the *micrococcus cutis communis*, and *morococcus* (Unna).

3.  In *pityriasis circinata*, the skin beneath the adherent sticky scales is reddened ;  the same organisms are found as with pityriasis steatoides. This is the stage which arouses dispute.   Many believe that it affects only a seborrhœic soil ;  hence the misleading title, seborrhœic dermatitis.   I prefer Sabouraud's names, pityriasis circinata and eczematized pityriasis steatoides ;  they describe the appearance of the eruption and the causal organism (see case, p. 165, and Fig. 39).

It is advisable here to summarize the modern views and their association with the discoveries of Sabouraud.   Modern dermatology teaches that the pityrosporon of Malassez (or " bottle bacillus "), the staphylococcus albus and the microbacillus are normal flora of the skin, and that it is only when the sebaceous gland secretion is chemically altered and increased that these organisms flourish abundantly.   Certain articles of diet encourage these chemical changes of the sebaceous secretion : cane sugar, excess of farinaceous food, alcohol and certain fats, e.g. bacon.   In the absence of fresh air and exercise this dietetic factor plays a very prominent part.   MacLeod and Dowling carried out a series of important experiments with a pityrosporon (bottle bacillus) culture.   By inoculating the skin with this organism, they produced the typical eruption of Sabouraud's pityriasis circinata on seborrhœic skins ; on normal skins, follicular papules developed, which did not last long.   Hence, it was concluded that the pityrosporon is the chief cause of this dermatitis, and that an increase in the staphylococcus albus is an accompanying feature in the condition. These findings agree with Sabouraud so far as the organisms are concerned, but the claim that " seborrhœic " dermatitis only develops on skin which has an altered or excessive sebaceous secretion is a fresh and important addition to our knowledge, if it proves to be invariably true. H. W. Barber's " seborrhœic state " denotes the type of patient with greasy skin who readily develops dermatitis with erroneous diet.   He found that in many of these patients the urine does not become alkaline till large doses of alkalis have been taken ;  the $pH$ in seborrhœic cases in a series of tests was 4·8 to 5·8, instead of the normal 6·4 to 6·8.   In 1902 Sabouraud noted that in seborrhœic conditions there was a high urinary acidity ;  this fact is discussed under seborrhœa oleosa (p. 106) and also under the treatment of pityriasis circinata (p. 171).

Many years ago I carried out several hundred examinations of scalp

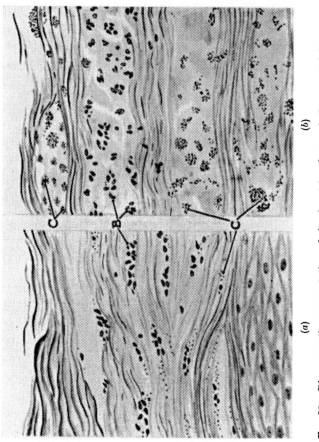

(b)

(a)

(a) Vertical section through scales of pityriasis simplex on scalp. Shows scaling of horny layer; with B many bottle bacilli between and in the scales, and at C a few cocci.

(b) Vertical section through sticky scales of pityriasis steatoides on scalp. Shows C masses of cocci, and B of bottle bacilli in the scales and serous exudation which together form the characteristic moist scales.

Fig. 39.—Diagrammatic representation of the first (a) and second (b) stages of Pityriasis of the Scalp. (After Sabouraud, *Diagnostic et Traitement des Affections du Cuir Chevelu*, Masson et Cie.)

scrapings made from oily, scaly and normal skins, before and after treatment. From these observations I was led to the conclusion that the bottle bacillus is not a normal inhabitant of the skin. It is rare on the scalp unless there is definite dandruff ; then it is usually abundant. After a short course of strong antiseptic treatment, in many patients it was not found on the scalp, even after repeated examination, and the dandruff at the same time had disappeared.

The name seborrhœic dermatitis remains because the prevailing opinion was that it occurs in those with the " seborrhœic diathesis," with tendency to oiliness and acne. There are cases, however, without acne and only slightly greasy skin, who develop pityriasis circinata or steatoides on the scalp and chest when washing is infrequent and warm head-gear and underclothing is worn. The history of a patient whom I have been able to watch for over thirty years is worth recording in this connection. About the age of sixteen to seventeen he had scurf on the vertex, so thick that it was difficult to rub it off with Hebra's soap ; i.e. he had had pityriasis sicca and then pityriasis steatoides. About thirty he began to have " seborrhœic dermatitis " on the front and back of the chest. An ointment containing sulph. præcip. gr. viii with phenol m.ii to the ounce of soft paraffin always quickly cured the active lesions. During twenty years, the eruption in this case appeared on the body whenever a bath had been omitted, even for two days. During the war, 1914–18, when the clothing next the body could not be changed daily, and washing was impossible for several days, the head and chest continually showed recurrence of the eruption. A few applications of the lotion on the scalp and ointment on the body always cleared it up at once. (The lotion consisted of hyd. perchlor. gr.iss ; liq. carb. deterg. m.xx ; phenol. m.iv ; ol. ricini m.v. ; ol. lavand. m.ii ; surgical spirit, aq. dest. āā ad 1 oz.) Scales scraped from the chest lesions showed bottle bacilli and cocci in abundance. The manner of recurrence and ready cure of the eruption favours Sabouraud's contention as to the importance of the pityriasis element. The name pityriasis circinata seems to describe admirably this eruption, its appearance and its ætiology. For in this case the seborrhœic element was always slight. At over fifty, the scalp was healthy, the hair had only the normal thinning of his age ; for years no pityriasis nor a single bottle bacillus had been found on it, except when he left off using the lotion for about ten days.

On the other hand, I often see the other type of case, in whom the " soil " or general metabolism plays the important part. As Sabouraud pointed out, the eruption is specially prone to appear on the scalp of the middle-aged man who takes too little exercise and who eats and drinks too much (" kerose " of Darier, the " seborrhœic state " of H. W. Barber). In such cases, the eruption often resists all local applications until correct diet and exercise are taken.

*Usual Course and Prognosis of Pityriasis.* Pityriasis simplex capitis usually responds to a course of correct treatment, but it tends to relapse, often throughout the life of the individual. It is commonly supposed that everyone in a town community has, or is liable to acquire, the malady popularly described as " scurf " or " dandruff." This is a mistaken belief. Some people never have pityriasis on the scalp ; even after having lived for years in the same house with relatives affected with dandruff they have retained a clean scalp. It is probable that some owe their immunity to their scrupulous refusal to use any brush or comb but their own. On the other hand, in some cases their freedom from scurf may be due to an unknown constitutional cause ; they are immune to the attack of the " bottle bacillus." The course of the malady can be conveniently described under five headings :

1. If pityriasis simplex is neglected, in some persons no bad effect may occur. The hair often becomes dry, brittle and splits (see p. 158). I have even seen grey hairs in quite young men and women affected with pityriasis, but I have never felt certain that this was not in part due to an associated bad condition of the general health. Hairfall can follow pityriasis without the development of any oiliness ; many bottle bacilli, but no microbacilli being found, even on repeated examination. I have gradually been forced to the conclusion that in certain patients the general health plays an all-important part ; the organisms do not return when constipation is corrected and the general health is good. On the other hand, small irregular patches of baldness, about the size of a threepenny bit, appear in certain cases of pityriasis, but the hair returns at once, and regains its gloss, *with local treatment alone.*

2. Another type of case shows quite a different sequel. After one to three years, on combing the scalp, loose dry scales no longer fall ; instead, the scales lie closely adhering to the scalp ; they are massed together with the imperceptible exudation of serum—*pityriasis steatoides.* If the scales are scraped off, there is seen some pinkness of the scalp, with a little serous exudation. The microscopic examination at this stage, as described above, shows staphylococci as well as " bottle bacilli."

3. In young men the most common sequel to pityriasis steatoides is the supervention of *seborrhœa, with hairfall.* This is fully described under hairfall with oiliness, *seborrhœa oleosa* (Chapter VIII).

4. In adolescence, but more often in older and in less healthy subjects there develops a condition in which the yellowish and moist scales lie on a red base with a circinate outline. In some patients an untreated pityriasis steatoides sooner or later always becomes eczematized or impetiginized, with underlying erythema, i.e. *pityriasis circinata,* commonly called seborrhœic dermatitis. If neglected, a permanent bald area may ensue. This eruption usually responds to treatment at the time, but tends to recur at intervals, for years, showing temporary cure, improvement or exacer-

bation. Hairfall rarely accompanies the mild and uncomplicated pityriasis circinata. The rash may appear on a scalp which has been bald for years. The same eruption is often present in other areas, e.g. at the margin of the scalp, especially behind the ears, on the chest, on the back between the shoulder-blades, and on the face, especially on the brow, " *corona seborrhœica,*" and the naso-labial furrows (see case described above, on p. 165). The eyebrows and eyelids may also be affected.

H. W. Barber summarizes the position thus :—

(1) Pityriasis Simplex (" Scurf or Dandruff ") — Pityrosporon infection.

(2) Pityriasis Steatoides (Seborrhœic dermatitis of simple type) — Infection with pityrosporon and cocci (microccoccus cutis communis, Unna's morococcus).

(3) Severer form, often complicated with boils — Superadded infection with Staph. aureus and sometimes with Strept. pyogenes.

(4) Eczematized form of " Seborrhœic Dermatitis " — Here eczematization, independent of superadded bacterial infection, complicates an existing simple " seborrhœic dermatitis." Here diet, emotional upset and metallic intoxication play their part.

Sabouraud and Darier were agreed as to the absurdity of the terms seborrhœic dermatitis and seborrhœide . . . as fallacious as Hebra's " seborrhœa sicca ", which is a contradiction in terms. . . . I would advocate Sabouraud's title, pityriasis steatoides. His descriptions of the transition, clinically and histologically, from simple dry dandruff to pityriasis steatoides . . . should be read in the original. They are a model of clarity.[1]

I am in entire agreement with this summary.

5. Yet another factor may complicate the eruption of pityriasis circinata. This is a *streptococcal* invasion of the affected regions ; it may be acute or chronic. In the acute cases the diagnosis and also the treatment of the case at once become more difficult and the usually favourable outlook is changed. The redness becomes accompanied by a certain amount of swelling and exudation, which remains beneath heavier crusts. Soap and water washing irritates the rash, and makes the exudation more profuse. This condition corresponds to what used to be called " seborrhœic eczema." Streptococcal dermatitis can develop quite independently of the pityriasis ; only when it supervenes on pityriasis does it cause confusion in the diagnosis and treatment as well as the prognosis. The inflammation tends to spread to the skin adjacent to the scalp ; the area becomes swollen and crusted ; and a fissure frequently appears behind the ears. When the post-auricular intertrigo is seen, the physician

[1] " Modern Trends in Dermatology," 1948.

must take precautions to prevent extension of the streptococcal process. The swelling and inflammation may subside completely, leaving an extensive scaling, and the patient may retain only his former condition of the scalp, a simple pityriasis. The condition may continue, rebellious to treatment, for a prolonged period of time. Staphylococcus aureus is often found in the fissures, probably as a later contamination ; but it has become more frequent within recent years. This is discussed under Streptococcal Dermatitis, in the section on Erythematous Lesions (p. 207).

*Treatment of Pityriasis.* Keep the health on a high level ; otherwise the local condition usually relapses as soon as treatment of the scalp is discontinued. Barber thinks that œstrin therapy may be used for women when other symptoms indicate it ; even then it must be given cautiously and never for long. For men he never advises such medication for pityriasis.

Many local methods are successful in dealing with this common disease. When the microbacillus complicates the condition of scaliness, the treatment must be more vigorous ; seborrhœa, see Chapter VIII, p. 109. In the early years of this century, Sabouraud published two large volumes on pityriasis and seborrhœa.[1] I used to follow minutely, and with successful results, the advice given in these two books. This entailed the use of ointments at the beginning of a course of treatment of pityriasis. For severe cases various preparations of mercury and of tar were most effective, and a course of treatment extended over several months. During the first three or four weeks active daily treatment was required ; applications were continued frequently for many months, and resumed at any threat of recurrence. With short hair lotions alone, correctly used, should clean the scalp in a week or a fortnight.

Before using any local application, the hair and scalp should be washed. Suitable ingredients for and methods of washing are discussed in Chapter III. In pre-war days, to wash and dry long, thick hair was so tedious a task that one hesitated to order greasy applications ; their use necessitated frequent washing for the sake of appearance. To save so much trouble patients can wash only the scalp and leave unwashed the long tresses which before 1914 reached to the waist or hips. If only the scalp were washed, drying could be completed in a few minutes ; by this method the use of ointments was rendered less objectionable. Sabouraud advised, in 1922, the same method of localized washing.

[1] " Maladies du Cuir Chevelu." " Les Maladies séborrhéiques," Paris, 1902 ; " Pityriasis et Alopécies Pelliculaires," Paris, 1904. In 1932 he wrote another volume, summarizing the results of his investigations during forty years: " Diagnostic et Traitement des Affections du Cuir Chevelu." Masson et Cie, Paris, 1932.

It is important to employ every method of encouraging the circulation of the scalp. For this purpose nothing surpasses *thorough massage*. After the scurf has gone, all the methods of stimulating hair growth which are recommended in the section on diffuse hairfall (p. 91) can be employed.

Originally I used to give an ointment every night for three weeks, then three times a week for a month ; a lotion was used on the nights the ointment was omitted. To ensure that the selected remedy reached every part of the scalp, the hair had to be divided into many partings and along each a very little ointment was thoroughly rubbed in by the fingers until it disappeared. The results were excellent when the patient had the gift of perseverance. When plenty of time was not devoted to the daily ritual, the cure was indefinitely delayed. After 1918, when women began to wear the hair short, good results were obtained with much less trouble. In some cases ointment was prescribed once or twice a week for a few weeks ; in the average mild case only a pleasant lotion was required.

Innumerable are the combinations of drugs and the forms of spirit which have been recommended for pityriasis. The physician soon finds that he can ring the changes by altering the proportions of the ingredients of a few formulæ, the effect of which he has watched till he understands exactly what to use and how to modify them. The majority of these formulæ are based on sulphur, tar and mercury, or phenol and salicylic acid, with spirit and water, together with an amount of oil or glycerine which has to be varied for the individual case. Only experience can teach the correct proportion of oil and spirit suitable for the individual scalp. A lotion made up with much spirit, without any oil or water, is irritating in pityriasis simplex. For a naturally dry scalp with thick hair more oil can be given without making the coiffure appear sticky. With fine, thin hair and with straight hair, less oil is used than with thick, abundant, coarse or curly hair. Men demand much more oily preparations than women, as they prefer the hair to lie flat and sleeky along the scalp. Drugs useful to combat the organisms of pityriasis can be incorporated in many oils and ointments, such as sesame, olive, almond, castor, arachis and paraffin oil. Recently, the emulsifying bases are being employed because they can be more readily washed out when the hair is thick and long. When deciding on a form of treatment one must remember that much depends upon the character of the patient. If the physician is certain that a lotion will be applied carefully and methodically, he can prescribe more oil than he would for the patient who, he knows, will spread as much of the lotion on the hair as on the skin, and will not take the trouble to rub it well into the scalp.

*Treatment of the various stages* which are described in the section on course and prognosis (p. 165):

1. For diffuse *pityriasis simplex*, an effective prescription consists of hyd. perchlor. gr. ½ to 1½, phenol m.v. to xx. or liq. carbonis deterg. m. 30, made up with ol. amygd. dulc., or glycerine m.v. to xl., in one ounce or one part of spt. Indust. to two of distilled water. Some prefer to add or to substitute a small proportion of salicylic acid. Tar is another useful ingredient; it improves the condition of the scalp and hair; the hair becomes more glossy and appears of better quality. In France, wood tars, oil of cade or of birch were often ordered. Oil of cade has a strong odour, difficult to disguise with any perfume. A process of deodorization is possible, but it impairs the efficiency of the oil of cade. Sabouraud therefore recommended cedar-wood oil, which has a comparatively pleasant odour and is not much inferior in its therapeutic properties. In this country coal-tar preparations are preferred; of these the most popular are liquor carbonis detergens and liquor picis carbonis, usually employed in the proportion of half to one drachm to the ounce. Tar has been recommended for centuries; see frontispiece, which reproduces part of a page in a book dealing with the hair, published as long ago as 1550. Lysol 4 per cent., salicylic acid 2 per cent., and resorcin have their advocates. Resorcin may stain fair hair or hair contaminated with alkali or soap. Oil of cade (m.xxx–lx) to the ounce of adeps benz. often succeeds with excessively thick scales in both pityriasis simplex and steatoides.

2. In cases of *pityriasis steatoides*, sulphur can be used as well as tar. In the rare cases when a few vesicles are seen on the scalp, sulphur is irritating. It is best, in the common form of pityriasis steatoides, to begin with an ointment containing sulphur and a little tar. Or one may give, on alternate days, an ointment containing sulphur and a lotion containing tar. The proportion of sulphur should not be strong, only about 10 to 20 grains to the ounce of vaseline; some add four or five drops of phenol to the ounce. After a fortnight this can be followed by an ointment containing hyd. ox. rub. gr. iv to the ounce of soft paraffin. With long hair, use ointment on alternate nights for six weeks; on the other nights a lotion with tar and spirit, such as: Liq. carb. deterg. m.xx, ol. ricini m.iv–xii, industrial spirit 3 drachms, aq. dest. 1 oz. Then for a month, ointment is used twice and lotion four times a week; then ointment once and the lotion three times a week. When the coiffure looks very untidy, owing to the ointment spreading on to the hair, as mentioned above (see p. 168) the scalp can be washed alone, without

wetting the whole length of the hair shafts. Emulsifying bases are replacing vaseline, being more readily washed out.

3. The treatment of cases in which seborrhœa oleosa supervenes are fully dealt with in Chapter VIII, page 108, et seq.

4. When the scales have an underlying circinate erythema *pityriasis circinata* (*seborrhœic dermatitis*) a weak proportion of sulphur gr. v. to viii to the ounce is effective. It is usually taught that in this condition tar should be avoided or given in very weak dilution. Once I found White's coal-tar ointment (see p. 211), tried in error by a young patient, though unpleasant to use, led to a rapid cure. I have often been astonished at the rapidity with which apparently severe cases on the scalp, even in old people, have responded to a mild mercurial ointment. Again, in cases almost identical in appearance, no good effect may be obtained until attention is concentrated on treatment of the general health. The urine, blood and all the organs of the body must be investigated. Fluids must be restricted, correct diet and exercise instituted, and causes of emotional tension removed. Sometimes the vivid redness yields when full doses of alkalis are given. This is probably explained by the fact that at first most forms of toxæmia are benefited by the use of alkalis. Mild degrees of *B. coli* infection are more prevalent than is commonly supposed, and the use of alkalis, especially citrate of potassium, together with diet and regulation of the bowels, often cures such cases [1] without resort to sulphonamides or antibiotics.

5. In some cases it may be difficult to diagnose whether the dermatitis is pityriasis steatoides complicated by *streptococcal dermatitis*. If the case is rebellious to the above described local treatment the case is probably streptococcal. Washing with soap or detergents is forbidden, and the local applications should be mild. (See Chapter XIII.) Pure spirit is usually irritating.

[1] Alkalis, however, are by no means always successful in pityriasis circinata (seborrhœic dermatitis). Some have suffered from excess of alkaline medication, especially when a sodium salt has been taken. Research on the acid base equilibrium and the mineral content of the blood may shed new light on the medication and the diet suitable for the individual. It is known that in nephrosis, when potassium salts are taken, the œdema decreases ; with sodium salts, the œdema increases. With irritating uterine discharge I have observed that when (with ionization and diathermy) the cause has been cured (invasion with micro-organisms and inflammation of the cervix, uterus or tube) in a certain percentage of patients there returns from time to time a transient discharge which no longer contains any organisms. Such cases in gynæcology seem to have an analogy with the " exudative diathesis " in dermatology ; i.e. the sign does not imply disease of the particular organ (uterus or skin), but some common blood condition.

After the pityriasis has disappeared and the scalp appears clean, in order to *prevent recurrence* it is wise to employ, once or twice a week, for months or years, a lotion containing mercury or tar, made up with oil, spirit and water. Hence this is a suitable place to refer to the various forms of spirit employed in hair lotions.

*Spirit Lotions.* Before 1914 we used to order lotions containing absolute alcohol and rectified spirit. They were attractive in appearance and pleasant to use, and a delicate perfume was usually added. Since 1918 the price of such spirit has become so high that the elegant lotions which were once so freely ordered can no longer find a place in our prescriptions. A bottle which formerly cost half a crown now costs about 18s. 6d. *Absolute alcohol* (99 per cent.) and *alcohol* (90 per cent., also called rectified spirit) are nowadays too expensive for general use in the hair lotions which are dispensed in Britain. When expense is of no account, they are still prescribed, because they smell pleasantly, and can be dispensed with perfume. *Methylated spirit* is ethyl alcohol, with the addition of mineral and wood naphtha ; it cannot at the present time be used on the scalp or skin on account of its disagreeable odour, because it is coloured, and also because it contains pyridin, and mineral naphtha, substances which are irritating to the skin. However, the skilled chemist, accustomed to dispense fine preparations, comes to our aid with industrial spirit. *Surgical spirit* has as a basis industrial spirit ; it has now (1949) four formulæ; the most often used contain:—(1) castor oil, methyl salicylate, ethyl phthalate and Industrial spirit ; (2) castor oil, mineral naphtha, ethyl phthalate, and Industrial spirit. Industrial spirit has nine parts of ethyl alcohol and one part of methyl alcohol. It is frequently used in hair lotions. The chemist supplies it only with a medical prescription ; the physician's full signature is required. The physician must never prescribe Surgical spirit with any other ingredient.

*Bay rum* is still a favourite spirit in hair lotions ; but what is usually called " bay rum " has no standard formula. The compound spirit of bay contains oil of bay, pimento, orange, saponin, quassia and various other ingredients in 90 per cent. alcohol and water. Bay rum is also made up with industrial spirit, and is sometimes employed as a vehicle in the preparation of hair lotions. If a pleasantly smelling preparation is desired, the physician can order ten drops of oil of bay to the ounce of Industrial spirit. Many different brands of Eau de Cologne can be used to convey a pleasant scent to hair lotions. When using tincture of iodine in a hair lotion, prescribe only the acetone-free form of Industrial spirit.

When pityriasis is complicated by seborrhœa oleosa, grease dissolvents are required. See seborrhœa oleosa (p. 109).

II. *The patient complains of thick scaly patches which cannot be washed away. There are usually similar areas present on the elbows and knees. The disease is probably* PSORIASIS.

**Psoriasis** is in the majority of cases easy to diagnose, because the scales are characteristic—thick, hard, dry, silvery ; they lie on firm patches which usually show a dark-red narrow border just visible below and around the area of heaped-up scales. On scratching off the scales, one reaches a layer which bleeds a little. There is no itching and no hairfall in uncomplicated cases.

Psoriasis may occur at any time of life, but the majority of cases are seen after adolescence, and during middle age. In the young and in the old, the scales are not so thick, the red margin is more extensive and less dull red in colour, and the patches tend to be diffused over the scalp. In middle age psoriasis usually shows several large, firm and separate discs, with smaller, equally firm-looking patches between the large ones. Occasionally the whole scalp may be covered with these hard psoriatic discs. This form of psoriasis lasts for a long time ; the patches tend to recur as soon as treatment has succeeded in removing them. Psoriasis does not lead to baldness ; indeed, it is difficult to scrape off the silvery scales, owing to the presence of the hairs growing up through them. If bald areas are seen with psoriasis, they are due to some co-existing disease, such as seborrhœa.

*Ætiology.* Psoriasis is not due to a specific organism as, for example, is typhoid fever. It is familial and often alternates or is associated with rheumatism and arthritis. In the young, throat infection is often found ; in the older patients, some metabolic error such as gout. Many forms of diet have been blamed as causative ; fat, animal protein, excess of fat and carbohydrate. During acute infections psoriasis usually clears up temporarily, but streptococcal processes aggravate it. Streptococcal causes cannot always be found. *B. coli* infection is sometimes causal.[1]

*Diagnosis.* When there are lesions on the elbows and knees, the diagnosis is simple. When only the scalp is involved, the nature of the scales must be carefully investigated. Owing to their powdery, silvery character, the physician rarely makes a mistake in the diagnosis of psoriasis in middle age, except when the disease is complicated by other conditions. The usual slow, chronic course of psoriasis is another distinctive feature. In young people and in the elderly, psoriasis may be mistaken for pityriasis circinata (seborrhœic dermatitis). In pityriasis circinata the scales are more yellowish ; on removing them, there is seen

---

[1] Ætiology is fully discussed by H. W. BARBER, *Brit. Med. Journ.*, 1950, i, 219.

only a slight moisture ; whilst in uncomplicated psoriasis the removal of the scales shows a bleeding layer. On the scalp, pityriasis circinata does not form in large discrete discs, but is more diffuse, and extends to the adjacent skin, chiefly of the forehead, temples, and vertex ; on the body, it affects chiefly the mid-line of the chest. Some twenty years ago it was taught that in certain cases it was impossible to distinguish an acute, widespread psoriasis from " seborrhœic dermatitis." Several authorities indeed maintained that the diseases were identical. The clinical points of distinction in these cases are made out by examining the lesions on the body. In cases of psoriasis one can almost always find on the body some patches with silvery scales, especially on the elbows and knees, and on scratching off the silvery scales one reaches the red easily bleeding layer ; the eruption tends to affect the extensor aspects of the limbs and the nails usually show pitting. Laymon found that sections of psoriasis, seborrhœic dermatitis and neurodermatitis do not aid diagnosis, whereas in active lupus erythematosus and lichen planus the histological features are characteristic.[1] *Pityriasis rubra pilaris* at one stage may be mistaken for psoriasis ; the points of differentiation are given on p. 180. In the *scaly syphilide* the underlying eruption shows a dusky brownish hue and larger scales, tends to leave an atrophic centre as it spreads, shows no bleeding layer when the scales are scraped off, and conveys to the finger a characteristic feeling of induration under the skin. When psoriasis is complicated with a *streptococcal infection*, there may be difficulty in diagnosis. There may be obtainable a history of a lesion resembling a chronic psoriasis, followed by a somewhat sudden development of redness and oozing over the scalp, extending to the adjacent skin ; this flare-up is accompanied by much itching and frequently there is the

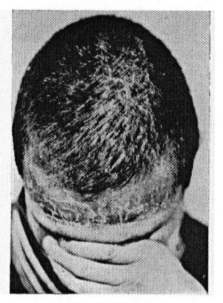

Fig. 40.   Psoriasis.
(*Photograph kindly lent by Dr. Hamilton Montgomery.*)

[1] Scaly dermatoses of the scalp. *Arch. Derm. and Syph.*, 1950, **62**, 181.

post-auricular intertrigo with a fissure which is so characteristic of streptococcal infection.

*Treatment.* Psoriasis of the scalp requires strong remedies, capable of softening the thick adherent scales so that they can be readily removed by washing or rubbing. Chrysarobin and cignolin, which are successfully employed on the body, must not be used on the scalp. Not only would they stain the hair and skin, but they are liable to set up severe dermatitis. Even pyrogallol must be used with caution, and it must not be forgotten that this drug stains fair hair. The remedy favoured by English dermatologists is an ointment containing ammoniated mercury (20 to 30 grains to the ounce); this may be combined with salicylic acid (15 to 25 grains to the ounce). Or salicylic acid can be used alone, 30 to 60 grains to the ounce. In America a higher percentage of ammoniated mercury is employed. Tar is another valuable agent. So much perseverance is necessary that one requires the aid of a nurse to remove the thick scales before the application of fresh ointment. Hard work with soap and soft water may be essential. I found particularly effective Sabouraud's ointment, which combined oil of cade and a mercurial salt (see formulæ on page 304). The general health must be attended to. In the acute spreading cases, rest in bed with alkalis and sodium salicylate is imperative. In one of my patients patches of obstinate psoriasis of the scalp and body gradually subsided, without any local treatment, during a course of intrauterine ionization and pelvic diathermy; as the profuse uterine discharge was thus cured, the skin lesions gradually cleared spontaneously. In some patients, especially when the menstrual periods are scanty, pituitary extract by mouth is well worth trial; I cannot explain its method of action. Arsenic is an old-fashioned remedy again creeping back into favour, especially for chronic types of psoriasis; as malignancy may develop after many years, it must not be given over prolonged periods. Danyz had success with vaccines cultured from the stools; but it was impossible to foretell the type which would respond favourably.

III. NEURODERMATITIS (LICHEN SIMPLEX CHRONICUS) occurs chiefly in women over twenty-five. The occipital region is the usual site of this very irritable and obstinate eruption. There are fine, branny scales above a hard, thickened red base. Neurodermatitis may be mistaken for psoriasis when it has thick scales in its chronic stage, but the presence of itching and the absence of the psoriatic readily bleeding layer beneath the scales enable one to make a diagnosis. As itching is the chief complaint made by the patient, the disease is described on p. 150.

IV. **Streptococcal Pityriasis.** This is the condition described by Sabouraud, in which scales are seen on definite regions of the scalp, due to a chronic streptococcal infection of the skin. The scales are white, fine, dry ; the underlying scalp may be normal or pink. Itching may or may not be present. Examination with a lens sometimes reveals slight exudation in some parts, between the scales. Compare here the section on Fausse Teigne (p. 179). The scales may develop, with itching, on the scalp of an adult who has never suffered from dandruff. The condition is in fact the same as the dry pityriasis patches, " *dartres volantes* " (due to streptococci), which are so often seen on the faces of some people during the windy cold months of spring.[1]

*Diagnosis.* Dry scaliness is the final stage of *acute streptococcal dermatitis* (p. 207) ; the inflamed skin flakes off, and the crusts of dried serum break up ; the history of acute dermatitis in such cases renders the diagnosis simple. When streptococcal pityriasis has been chronic from the beginning it is usually mistaken for ordinary *pityriasis simplex*. The limited areas on which the scales are found and, in some cases, the presence of post-auricular fissure simplify what may be a difficult diagnosis. Microscopic examination of the thick, grey scales in pityriasis simplex shows many " bottle bacilli " ; in the thin, white scales of strepto-coccal pityriasis these are rare or absent. The examination can be carried out in a few minutes, with a methylene blue stain. A streptococcal scaling condition is irritated by soap, detergents and by vigorous treat-ment of pityriasis simplex ; when a microscopical examination has been omitted, this may be the first fact which leads to a correct diagnosis.

*Treatment.* The general health in these cases is usually at fault ; such patients require the tonic air of mountains or the sea. Often a septic focus is present and must be dealt with ; see remarks on Fausse Teigne, p. 179. The strong lotions so useful in pityriasis simplex may cause an angry reaction. Even washing with soap and water may set up oozing of serum and the formation of crusts. When the skin has become thus sensitized, use soothing applications with zinc and oil, and Burow's solution. Tar is the best application in chronic cases ; Sabouraud used coal tar, in inverse proportion to the amount of underlying redness.

V. Scales due to **traumatism** or other **external causes** may often be mistaken for pityriasis, unless one is aware of the existence of this

---

[1] This description has shed light on cases suffering from scurf with considerable itching. In my pre-1914 notes I find references to such patients, with the remark : " much itching, no bottle bacilli, only cocci found in the scales." This form of pityriasis accounts for the recurrence in medical literature of claims that dandruff is due to streptococci.

cause of scales, and is on the alert not to be deceived. Excessive and vigorous combing may cause scaling of the scalp. A common cause of scales is the over-frequent use of strong, stimulating lotions ; this is especially true when the lotions contain too little or no oil or glycerine, and a high percentage of spirit. After the use of these lotions, for some days or weeks, large, fine, translucent scales may be seen ; on pulling these gently from the scalp one finds that they are thin strips of epidermis. A similar condition may be seen after frequent washing with soft soap and with the modern detergents which are so commonly employed for washing the hair. After the inflammation caused by the use of blistering fluids, iodine, strong acids or certain dyes has subsided, scales are left which can easily be recognized when their origin is known or suspected. Strong therapeutic remedies, such as sulphur, chrysophanic or salicylic acid, give rise to scaling after the local reaction has passed off. The list of such causes could be multiplied indefinitely ; instances will occur to the mind of every reader. Another form of traumatic scaling occurs with the FRONTAL BAND of ALOPECIA, which later develops a cicatricial condition. It was first described by Sabouraud, who observed it both in young and in elderly women. It may begin in girlhood ; some cases were caused by undue traction of the hair by tight curlers. See p. 148.

*Treatment* consists in leaving off the use of the irritating agent, and in applying a lubricant such as castor, almond or olive oil. Washing, especially with detergents, should be avoided for a time. If the traumatic cause is not discontinued, the skin may become invaded by micro-organisms, and folliculitis or streptococcal dermatitis follow.

VI. Crusts of dried serum occur after the first stage of ACUTE STREPTO-COCCAL and TRAUMATIC DERMATITIS and with ECZEMA. There is always serum and an underlying inflammatory condition, especially of the skin adjacent to the scalp ; therefore these diseases are described in erythe-matous conditions with exudation (p. 207). The crusts may be heavy and the chief complaint of the patient, who may omit to mention the preceding acute inflammation.

VII. PARASITIC INFECTION. In both ringworm and favus the patient may be brought to the physician on account of scaly patches. Ringworm occurs almost always in children under puberty ; its early stage may easily be mistaken for pityriasis sicca. Broken hairs amongst the scales, and the presence of fungus seen on microscopic examination, form the diagnostic features of ringworm. In favus, the scales lie in thick cup-shaped masses ; the microscopic examination clinches the diagnosis. Both diseases are described in the following chapter.

VIII. The scales of IMPETIGO rarely cause difficulty in diagnosis, except when the condition is clearing off, and there are left only scales from the drying up of the moist lesions. In the earlier, moist stage, the scales are really yellowish crusts. D'Alibert's name is connected with the form of impetigo which has a thick crust. The so-called crusts may resemble a thick layer of grey scales ; the patient is usually sent to the out-patient departments with a diagnosis of " persistent pityriasis, which will not respond to treatment." The adherent scales may be hard to remove, so firm that the physician may at first regard the condition as

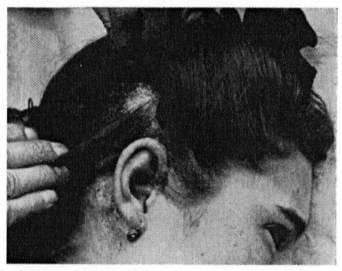

FIG. 41.—Streptococcal infection of the scalp, showing the heaped-up layer of scales (resembling *Fausse Teigne Amiantacée*), and the frequently associated postauricular dermatitis.

(Kindly lent by Dr. R. Sabouraud, from *Diagnostic et Traitement des Affections du Cuir Chevelu*, Masson et Cie. Paris, 1932.)

one of Fausse Teigne (see p. 179). After removing the thick layer one arrives at the diagnostic feature, the moist surface exuding serum, often also pus. Streptococci are found in abundance, usually hæmolytic. The condition may occur over a small or an extensive area of the scalp, and retro-auricular dermatitis is also present. (Fig. 41.) I have seen this disease in adults, but it affects children more frequently. CRUSTS from OTHER PUSTULAR CONDITIONS, such as lesions due to pediculosis and folliculitis (Bockhardt's impetigo), have identifying features, and the history usually simplifies the diagnosis. Impetigo and its treatment are discussed on p. 216.

IX. LUPUS ERYTHEMATOSUS often affects the scalp. As its characteristic lesion is erythematous rather than scaly, and an atrophic area develops as it progresses, the disease is described in the section of bald patches with atrophy (p. 137). Scales, indeed, may be entirely absent when the disease occurs on the scalp. Lupus erythematosus is readily diagnosed when other lesions are present, as is usual, on the nose, cheeks, ears and backs of the fingers.

X. **Fausse Teigne Amiantacée** is seen more often in children than in adults. Thick scales are heaped up in layers, some sticking firmly to the scalp, some adhering to and appearing as if climbing up the shafts of the hairs. Sabouraud considered it to be a form of eczema, beginning with a moist exudation which soon became crusted. The scales are white above, more yellow below. The dry crust of scales resembles asbestos, being silvery grey and white, crumbling on the top. Often the disease is seen only on the localised patch, but in another form it is widespread. Opinions as to its ætiology are very varied. No organisms are to be found in most cases ; this distinguishes it from the crusted impetigo with which so many writers have confused it (see Fig. 41). H. W. Barber considers that there are several types : (i) the common form usually associated with retro-auricular intertrigo. In this variety Sabouraud succeeded in obtaining streptococci, but after many attempts Barber failed to confirm this, and regards the condition as a streptococcide, the streptococcic toxin being absorbed, possibly by the lymphatics, from the adjacent focus behind the ear. (ii) Another type occurs without any local streptococcal skin infection, but is associated with a streptococcal toxin with its focus in the nose, teeth, tonsils, antrum or elsewhere ; (iii) an eczematized tuberculide, associated with other tuberculides, such as lichen scrofulosorum.

Success in *treatment* depends upon the correct application of the remedies. The crust must be rubbed off the scalp with some blunt instrument, then removed gently by combing down the hair. Ointment is then applied to the scalp over the area to which the crust adhered. In cases with very thick scales it may be necessary at first to loosen these with sulphur and salicyclic acid, 10 per cent. of each. Montgomery recommends ung. hyd. ammon and 5 per cent. sulphur ointment. As in the treatment of chronic streptococcal scaly conditions, the remedies must be continued long after the condition seems to be cured ; otherwise it will relapse. I like oil of cade ℥x in an ounce of almond oil. Sabouraud recommended at first coal tar 1 in 30, and later oil of cade, 1 in 3 parts of vasolanoline, cleaned off in the morning with alcohol 90 per cent. 30 parts, acetone anhyd. 30 parts, distilled water 60 parts.

XI. The **Squamous Syphilide.** Since the introduction of methods of treatment with arsenical compounds, secondary and tertiary lesions are less frequently seen nowadays. Some twenty years ago they were very common. The scalp is a frequent site for the early eruption of secondary syphilis (see pp. 86 and 132). A little later, papules tend to appear on the forehead at the edge of the scalp—the *corona veneris.* In the secondary stage of syphilis the papules may be so covered with scales that they have been described as psoriasiform syphilides. The papules may be small, pea-sized, appearing in rings or in segments of circles. In colour they are of more dull violet than the vivid red of psoriasis. To the examining finger they convey a characteristic feeling of hard *induration* under the skin. The scales may be plentiful, but are more grey than those of psoriasis. Other lesions are usually present on the body and these vary in appearance, owing to the polymorphic nature of the eruption ; this is a diagnostic feature. Some are papular without having much scaling. In the later or more severe type of syphilis (usually called tertiary) the lesions are larger and flatter ; many have abundant scales. They appear in circinate patches, or in segments of circles, healing in the centre and leaving a depressed centre ; they do not appear in large numbers over the whole body, but tend to be concentrated in one large group on certain areas. A common position is the forehead or other region at the margin of, and spreading on to the scalp. In still more severe cases, the scales are really crusts above an area of serpiginous ulceration ; therefore this form is described in the section on erythematous eruptions (p. 205). In both forms, the serum reaction and the preference of diffusely spread body lesions for the flexor surfaces of the limbs aid the diagnosis from psoriasis. The lesions disappear in two or three weeks with antisyphilitic remedies.

XII. **Pityriasis Rubra Pilaris** is an uncommon disease, which may first be seen on the scalp as fine branny scales on the skin between the hairs. On the scalp no horny cones are seen, but scales which are profuse, small, white and dry. At later stages thick crusts adhere to the hairs, but are easily removed from the skin, which is then seen to be smooth and sometimes red. The early lesion on the skin of the body is a red, acuminate papule, with a horny scale, due to hyperkeratosis at the mouth of the hair follicle. In the early stage of the disease the papules are seen on typical positions— the backs of the proximal phalanges of the fingers and the extensor aspect of the forearms. From time to time the disease has exacerbations, with erythema, appearing somewhat suddenly. Or the malady may proceed more slowly, and the papules coalesce, forming erythematous patches, with thick scales, and the condition then may be mistaken for psoriasis. These patches may gradually extend over the whole body. A generalized erythrodermia may follow, and this may recede and disappear, except from certain regions, such as the face, palms and soles, which usually remain red, with thick scales. With the tightly stretched condition of the erythematous face, ectropion is common. Except when the disease affects seborrhœic patients, no hairfall occurs until the onset of erythrodermia. The disease lasts for years ; the general health may not be affected except during the periods of erythematous exacerbation.

*Ætiology.* The cause is unknown. Some maintain that it is due to vitamin A deficiency, but this has not been confirmed by other observers.

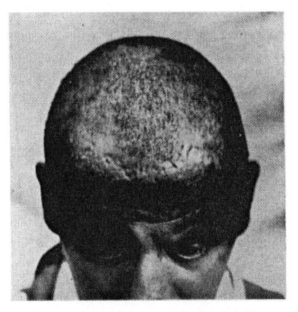

Fig. 42.—Case shows acuminate horny papules of pityriasis rubra pilaris and also old scars of acne varioloformis (acne necrotica).

(*Photograph kindly lent by Dr. H. W. Barber.*)

*Treatment* is symptomatic, and far from hopeful, although eventually, after many relapses, many become cured. In the early stages, thyroid has appeared to arrest the progress of the disease for a time. Ultra-violet rays have aided some patients. Some cases have responded to gold injections and to shock therapy. Reports of cure and of failure are published concerning treatment with large doses of vitamin A.

XIII. **Ichthyosis.** When first seen by a dermatologist who is consulted about the scalp, the patient is usually a child of two or three years, with dry, lustreless and scanty hairs, especially on the top of the head. Over the vertex are seen thick scales, grey to dull brown in hue, adhering to the scalp in their centres and with raised, rough, free edges, often with quadilateral cracks between the masses of scales.

*Diagnosis.* This is aided by the history of normal hair at birth, with scales developing a month or two later, and gradual loss of hair as the scaliness became more marked. No history of any acute lesion precedes the formation of the scales. From these facts a correct diagnosis may be arrived at even before the body is examined. A dry, scaly condition of the body, dating from early infancy, is characteristic. Conditions which may be mistaken for ichthyosis are keratosis pilaris (see below), and ichthyosis follicularis, a congenital, usually familial malady (p. 100).

*Prognosis.* The outlook depends upon perseverance with local treatment ; if it is not carried out systematically the hair in time ceases to grow and the scalp develops an almost cicatricial condition.

The *treatment* is similar to that of ichthyosis of the body—in mild cases, resorcin 2 to 3 per cent., and in severe cases 5 to 15 per cent., in glycerine of starch. Salicylic acid in vaseline, lanoline or oil is also valuable. Thyroid, natural and artificial sunlight are very beneficial. Large doses of vitamin A are now advised.

XIV.    Rare **generalized diseases,** in which scaliness is a marked feature, often involve the scalp. The following merit mention :

In DERMATITIS EXFOLIATIVA, the desquamative process which affects the whole body involves also the scalp. The skin is red, dry and covered with large papery scales, falling freely from all over the body. The hair and nails are affected. The disease may be slow or rapid in course ; it may be primary or may follow other maladies (see Erythematous Eruptions, p. 206). The diagnosis of the condition of the scalp presents no difficulty because it is only an extension of the widespread disease.

When DERMATITIS HERPETIFORMIS affects the scalp, the bullæ, as they dry, leave large flaky scales. Here, itching during and before the formation of the bullæ may be very marked. PEMPHIGUS (simplex and foliaceus) is comparatively rare on the scalp. Both these conditions are unlikely to affect the scalp alone, and are diagnosed by their presence on the body and on the mucous membranes.

Bullæ due to other causes (e.g. bullous impetigo) may also invade the scalp and leave large flaky scales. (See Bullous Eruptions, p. 233.)

XV.    KERATOSIS, which may be mistaken for scales, affects the scalp in the following conditions :

In **Darier's Disease** (keratosis follicularis), a very rare condition, the scalp is involved. The lesions are usually bilateral and symmetrical. There is no loss of hair. The disease may begin on the scalp and face with grey, firmly adherent scales topping minute papules at the mouths of the follicles and sweat ducts. These coalesce into extensive patches of sticky brown crusts.

The *diagnosis* is difficult at first. On removing the adherent crusts the underlying papules show hollowed depressions. As the disease progresses, secondary staphylococcal infection may occur, with pus formation. Malodorous vegetations may develop, especially in the flexures of the joints and the folds of the body.

**Keratosis pilaris,** though common on the extensor aspects of the upper arms and sides of the thighs, is rare on the scalp. Keratosis pilaris is one of the dermatological names about which considerable misunderstanding can arise. The name, as commonly used, denotes a condition in which horny papules occur at the mouth of the hair follicles on the extensor aspect of the upper arms and the sides of the thighs, especially when the limbs show the blue colour so often present with thyroid and pituitary deficiency. Phrynoderma is the same malady. To the examining finger a rough grater-like sensation is conveyed, due to the heaped-up horny material which forms a cone at the mouths of the follicles. Stannus [1] reported a condition of follicular keratosis seen in many children in countries with malnutrition during war. It was usually associated with hyperkeratosis of the elbows, knees and ankle joints where it resembled ichthyosis. Other symptoms of Vitamin A deficiency such as night blindness, xerophthalmia and response to treatment with Vitamin A, were also present. On the scalp some of the hair growth is so strong that it carries up pieces of the horny matter along its shaft ; this has been mistaken for the nits of pediculi. When keratosis affects the scalp, it is usually the first stage of other diseases : MONILETHRIX (Fig. 52), LICHEN SPINULOSUS (p. 144), ICHTHYOSIS FOLLICULARIS (p. 100) or ULERYTHEMA OPHRYOGENES (pp. 97 and 146) ; Sabouraud said that it also occurred in rare forms of LUPUS ERYTHEMATOSUS. In those diseases, areas of baldness develop after some time ; and as the baldness is usually the symptom of which the patient complains, the diseases are described in the section dealing with that symptom. In ulerythema ophryogenes the eyebrow is involved ; this forms a diagnostic feature.

The type of RINGWORM (p. 185) which sometimes causes lesions resembling keratosis pilaris must not be forgotten, especially as it may be seen in young adults.

The *treatment* of keratosis is symptomatic. Keratolytics and X-ray are both useful. It is now believed that Keratosis pilaris is associated with deficiency of Vitamin A ; it is unlikely that this alone can account for the condition.

---

[1] *Brit. Journ. Derm.*, 1945, **37**, 208.

# CHAPTER XII

# SCALY CONDITIONS WITH FUNGI IN THE HAIR

*The patient, usually a child, is brought with a patch on the scalp covered with scales and broken-off short hairs. The most common cause is* RING-WORM.

**Ringworm** used to be the scourge of the schools. In 1901 twenty thousand London Elementary School children were affected ; in 1938 only 103 cases were reported. This reduction was due partly to improved methods of control and partly to the more effective treatment which became possible after Sabouraud and Noiré discovered in 1905 a safe measurement of X-ray dosage for epilation of the scalp. During the second World War the incidence of ringworm again increased and in some countries reached serious epidemic proportions. Since the end of the war the numbers have fallen, but the disease is still far from uncommon.

*Symptoms.* The many species of fungi which can cause scalp ringworm give rise to a number of different clinical appearances. (1) The type met with most frequently in childhood is caused by the *Microsporon audouini*, which is of human origin. This infection usually begins as a pink patch but is rarely seen by the physician till a later stage, usually after a few days, when the infection appears as a circular area, covered with grey scales and short broken hairs, about 3 millimetres long, showing above the scales. The patch spreads rapidly, almost doubling its size in two days, and may coalesce with adjacent diseased areas. The whole scalp may become involved. The infected hairs may be almost buried under the heaped-up scales ; they are brittle, without lustre, and frayed at the ends ; they break on being pulled. The patches are usually first seen on the vertex or the occipital region, but any part of the head may be involved. As a rule no sensation is complained of ; in a few cases there is a mild degree of itching. Except in infants and young children little or no inflammatory reaction occurs in most infections with this type of fungus. The glabrous skin may also be infected ; on the face, neck and eyelids, red discoid patches may be seen.

(2) Another type of ringworm is due to *Microsporon canis*, which is of animal origin and is usually associated with a degree of inflammatory response. Several patches are usually found, with broken hairs about 2 or 3 millimetres above the surface. In the middle or at the margin of

the infected region there may be tiny vesicles, scales or crusts.  With
this fungus there are frequently patches on the glabrous skin, pink or
red, circinate and discoid.  This type of infection tends to spontaneous
cure, but re-infection may be constantly recurring from pet animals,
especially kittens and puppies.

(3) *Black Dot Ringworm* is caused by a fungus of human origin, an
*endothrix trichophyton*, most frequently *T. sulphureum* or *T. tonsurans*.
Black Dot is the clinically descriptive name given to a form of ringworm
in which the infected areas have few or no scales, but black dots are
seen at the mouths of the follicles, where the hairs have broken off below
or at the level of the scalp.  Elevated black spots may also be seen, where
the hair stumps have bent over when failing to penetrate the upper layers
of the skin.  Several patches are usually present.  Black dot ringworm
is persistent and may lead to loss of hair with or without atrophy.  Bald
ringworm is a clinical variant due to this infection.  The patient usually
comes with a diagnosis of alopecia areata, but no exclamation hairs are
found at the margin of the patch, only hairs broken off at skin level.
Scattered over the bald region may be a few long hairs.

(4) *Pustular ringworm.*  Any kind of ringworm may become infected
with pyogenic organisms, but the typical pustular form is usually due
to infection with a trichophyton, especially an ectothrix trichophyton ;
occasionally it is caused by a microsporon.  The markedly pustular form
of ringworm, Kerion, has a characteristic raised, red, " boggy " nodule,
pierced with holes, through which oozes a sticky serum or serum and pus.
Kerion is usually restricted to one area of the scalp, but occasionally
may be multiple (see Fig. 47, p. 221).

*General symptoms.*  (*Trichophytides: microsporides.*)  It has long been
known that general symptoms sometimes accompany severe pustular
forms of ringworm, such as kerion.  General symptoms may also occur,
apart from any pustular condition, with both ringworm and favus infection of the hair of the scalp or beard.  Fever, glandular swellings, splenic
enlargement and leucocytosis sometimes occur.  Many forms of cutaneous
reaction are seen.  The most common is a lichenoid eruption, affecting
chiefly the trunk and limbs.  The papules are small, pale or red, often
acuminate, sometimes flat, less often capped with scales, vesicles or
pustules, or with spines like those of lichen spinulosus.  In other cases
the eruption may be eczematous, scarlatiniform, macular, papular or
urticarial.  The rash usually comes on suddenly, about three to eight
weeks after the original local infection.  J. M. H. MacLeod, with a wide
experience of ringworm, says that the trichophytides appear with three

types of ringworm—with kerion ; after X-ray treatment with the fall of hair whilst some infected hairs remain on the scalp ; and with irritating local treatment. Bloch stated that they followed local treatment, X-ray and trichophytin ; i.e. after measures calculated to bring about a sudden influx of living parasites into the blood stream. Much research has been carried out on the nature of microsporides. The fungus has been found in the blood stream, the lymphatic glands and the skin lesions. Microsporides occur when dissemination of the fungus or its products takes place in individuals who have become allergically sensitized.[1]

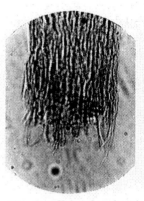

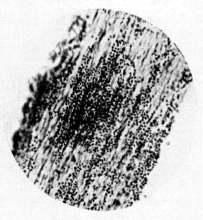

Fig. 43.—Hair infected with small-spored ringworm. Shows free end of hair eroded, owing to invasion of hair shaft by the fungus. (Mag. × 300.)

Fig. 44.—Commonly seen small-spored ringworm, stained by Gram's method. The hair is surrounded with a mosaic of small spores ; the cuticle is invaded and destroyed ; a few fine mycelial threads are visible in the substance of the hair. Microphotograph, Mag. × 425.

*Ætiology.* Ringworm is a highly contagious disease due to the invasion of the scalp hair by a fungus. Only a limited number of fungi are able to invade the hair and even fewer are of common occurrence in this country. The nomenclature and the classification of the ringworm fungi has been revised recently, but a full discussion of this subject would be out of place in this book. For detailed information the reader is referred to the still valuable volume by Sabouraud in 1910 [2] and to the publications

[1] The literature on the subject is extensive. A few of the chief publications are :
    BRUNO BLOCH, " Les Trichophytides." *Ann Derm. et Syph*, 1921, **2**, 1 and 55.
    SULZBERGER and WISE. *Arch. Derm. and Syph.*, 1937, **36**, 548.
    BECK. *New York Journ. Med.*, 1936, **36**, ii, 1237.
[2] " Les Teignes," Masson et Cie., Paris, 1910.

of Emmons [1] and J. T. Duncan.[2] The nomenclature used here follows the recommendations of the Medical Research Council Memorandum.

Two groups of dermatophytes invade the scalp : the microsporon and the trichophyton. The important species of microsporon are *M. audouini*, which is a human parasite (i.e. man is the natural host), and *M. canis*, which is an animal parasite. Duncan found three fairly constant varieties of *M. canis*, differentiated by culture—(1) *M. felineum*, with much orange yellow pigment; (2) *M. lanosum*, unpigmented ; and (3) an intermediate primrose yellow variety. He found that in London to-day *M. audouini* and *M. canis* were equally frequent. In parts of Devonshire all cases were due to *M. canis* (pigmented) ; in Portsmouth all were infected with *M. canis* (non-pigmented). In other parts of the country there is wide variation in the numbers of the two species. Occasional infections are due to *M. gypseum*, also an animal parasite. *M. ferrugineum*, a human parasite, causes widespread epidemics in Eastern Europe but is not yet known to have reached this country.

*Diagnosis.* Microsporon ringworm occurs almost exclusively in childhood, the maximum incidence being between the ages of five and seven, boys being more affected than girls. Large epidemics are usually due to the human types, the animal types giving rise to small outbreaks or to sporadic cases. The differentiation of human from animal infections is important both from the point of view of epidemiological control and of treatment.

(A) *Human Species.* (i) As the infection is readily passed from child to child, other members of the household below the age of puberty are frequently infected. Case to case spread in schools and institutions is perhaps less common but is relatively frequent and is of great importance. The fungus is transmitted by shared hats, caps, towels, pillows, brushes and combs. (ii) That barbers' and hairdressers' shops are occasionally the source of infection is suggested by the frequent occurrence of the first lesion in the clipper area in boys and the region of the parting in girls. (iii) Bus and cinema seats. There is some evidence that *M. audouini* can survive as long as a year in fallen hairs. (iv) *M. audouini* with minimal infection and no loss of hair may remain unsuspected, therefore not diagnosed, for years ; such cases are reservoirs of infection.

(B) *Animal Species.* (i) Transmission from one child to another is limited ; probably not more than four transmissions occur without renewal from an animal reservoir. (ii) Animal to human transmission.

[1] *Arch. Derm. and Syph.*, 1934, **130**, 337.
[2] " Modern Trends in Dermatology," 1948.

The initial human infection is often severe, with extensive skin lesions. The infection becomes milder as it passes from one person to another and finally dies out. A veterinary surgeon may easily miss the presence of ringworm, because a mild degree of infection can be detected only by inspection under Wood's light. In kittens the muzzle and whiskers must be carefully examined.

Certain clinical features enable one often to decide whether the infection is of human or animal origin. The following table, modified from Henrici,[1] is useful for this purpose.

| *M. audouini.* | *M. canis.* |
| --- | --- |
| Perfect hostparasite equilibrium, therefore non-inflammatory. | Unstable hostparasite equilibrium, therefore inflammatory, sometimes pustulation. |
| Occasional ring or discoid lesions, scaly and very mildly inflammatory on face and neck. | Frequently multiple small lesions of smooth skin, circinate, bright red, sometimes with vesicular border. |
| Skin rarely affected in absence of scalp infection. | Skin infection common with normal scalp. |
| Untreated, may persist until puberty. | Untreated, seldom lasts more than a year. |
| Microsporides rare. | Microsporides more common. |

TRICHOPHYTON infections are less often met with. They fall under two main groups : (A) Endothrix and (B) Ectothrix.

(A) The most important Endothrix species are *T. sulphureum, T. tonsurans, T. sabouraudi* and *T. violaceum*. The endothrix trichophytons are essentially human parasites, and produce a persistent infection without much inflammatory reaction. Infected hairs break off at skin level, leaving smooth bald patches on which the broken and diseased hairs appear as black dots. Occasionally these broken hairs are present only at the margin of the patches—the so-called " Bald ringworm." *T. sulphureum* is the species usually met with in Britain. *T. violaceum* is frequently seen in Southern and Eastern Europe ; it causes a particularly persistent and refractory infection. Endothrix trichophyton infections, unlike microsporon infections, show no tendency to spontaneous cure at puberty.

(B) *Ectothrix* and *Endoectothrix* infections are frequently of animal origin. The principal species are *T. flavum* (endoectothrix), *T. mentagrophytes, T. discoides*, which are ectothrix fungi.

---

[1] Molds, Yeasts and Actinomycetes, 2nd edition, New York and London, 1945.

Infections with the endoectothrix fungi are rare in Britain. The various related ectothrix species, for which the term *T. mentagrophytes* is now employed, give rise to lesions which begin as slightly raised areas of erythema with adherent scales and thin yellowish crusts. Some of the infected hairs are broken ; others are of normal length, and have a powdery greyish appearance. In about ten days perifollicular pustules develop, and a kerion may form. Infections with *T. discoides* are highly inflammatory, with early formation of a deep kerion. The hairs are not so brittle as with endothrix fungi ; therefore they are more easily pulled out.

Trichophyton infections may invade the beard and glabrous skin, showing patches or rings, erythematous or with vesicles or pustules. Large vesicular and pustular rings are often seen in the country, especially on the hands of those whose occupation lies with cattle and horses.

All the above mentioned species of ringworm are differentiated readily by their appearance on culture. In every case of ringworm a culture should be made, because on that report depends the correct choice of treatment.

*Clinical Diagnosis of Ringworm.* In microsporon ringworm the scales and broken hairs are characteristic. When a patch is rapidly rubbed over with a few drops of chloroform on wool the infected hairs stand out, looking as if covered with hoar frost. The presence of microsporon ringworm is quickly decided by the Fluorescence test. The scalp is examined in a dark room under Wood's light, i.e. ultra-violet rays passed through a glass filter containing nickel oxide. Under this lamp certain infected hairs show fluorescence. The endothrix trichophytons and indeed the majority of trichophyton infections, show no fluorescence ; a few species are said by some authorities to show a dull greyish hue. Hairs infected with microsporon fungi appear as if dotted thickly over with greenish blue beads. It is essential to examine by this method after X-ray epilation, so as to make sure that no infected hairs remain. Before this test the suspected patches on the scalp should be washed with soap and water in order to remove any " hair tonic " or " pomade " which may have been applied ; such often contain quinine, vaseline, or mineral oils, which can cause a blue fluorescence and therefore lead to a mistaken diagnosis. Thus a physiotherapist, new to the X-ray department, reported to me that a child had extensive ringworm, but on examining the scalp I found that the shining white fluorescence of pityriasis scales had been mistaken by the novice. In the event of an epidemic, children entering a new school should first be submitted to the fluorescence test. With Wood's light one can also diagnose the presence of infection in the coats of animals. When the source of infection is doubtful the fungus may be detected in the fur of apparently normal pets; Davidson and Gregory [1] found that kittens which looked normal were sometimes infected with ringworm.

For a *microscopical* examination it is important to select only infected hairs. Such hairs are loose, broken off short, or break when gently pulled with forceps. With " black dot " ringworm it may be necessary to dig out the buried stumps with a comedo extractor or pick with a needle. The suspected hair is placed on a glass slide with a few drops of liquor potassæ ; a cover slip is applied over it. In about ten minutes examine first with the low, then with the high power lens; the fungus is readily seen. For permanent preservation the specimen can be stained with gentian violet and mounted. The *microsporon* ringworm forms a close sheath or mosaic of spores which passes down from just above the mouth of the follicle to the hair bulb.

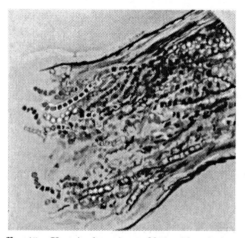

FIG. 45.—Unstained specimen of hair with endothrix infection. Note ladder-like square-ended spores lying in length of hair, and cuticle not invaded. Mag. × about 450.

(After Sabouraud, *Diagnostic et Traitement des Affections du Cuir Chevelu*, Masson et Cie.)

Within the hair shaft are branching threads of mycelium running in a longitudinal direction in the horny part of the hair. They stop short at the soft bulb ; this terminal appearance is known as " Adamson's fringe " (Fig. 43). The hair cuticle is destroyed. The conventional division of the tricophytons into ectothrix and endothrix groups has been referred to. The distinction is not entirely reliable but is useful, as the predominantly endothrix species are of human origin and the ectothrix species are of animal origin. In the endothrix variety the microscope reveals the spores invading the hair shaft ; in the ectothrix type, the fungus surrounds the hair shaft. Sometimes the spores both surround and invade the hair ; the ectoendo-

[1] *Journ. Canad. Med. Assoc.*, 1933, **29**, 242.

thrix fungus. Microscopic examination shows the hair-shaft filled with long mycelia with almost square "ladder-like" divisions into spores (Fig. 45). They resist the action of potassium hydrate solutions.

Diseases which have been wrongly diagnosed as ringworm may be briefly mentioned : seborrhœic dermatitis, pyoderma, monilethrix, trichotillomania and tinea amiantacea. The microscopical examination of the hair and culture growth at once distinguish these because no fungus is found. Much, however, depends upon the skill of the physician in selecting the hairs to be examined.

*Treatment.* The head must be covered with a washable cap, so that no infected hairs or scales can be conveyed to other children, and the child must be excluded from school until the treatment is completed. An antiparasitic ointment must be used regularly, until the hair falls out, or until a cure has been achieved.

*Choice of Treatment.* The choice of treatment will depend on the age of the patient, the nature and extent of the infection, whether it is of animal or human origin, whether the mother or guardian is likely to co-operate fully in a somewhat exacting routine, and finally on the facilities available. Local applications are preferred if the infection is of animal origin, is inflammatory and is of limited extent. These will also be employed if the patient is too young (under one year) for X-ray epilation, when X-ray epilation is not accepted by the parents, and of course when skilled epilation is not available. Occasionally it may be justifiable to withhold epilation in a child approaching puberty, in the expectation that spontaneous cure will occur.

Although the recent progress in the use of penetrating bases has considerably increased the efficacy of local applications, X-ray epilation remains the treatment of choice for the majority of children with *microsporon audouini* infections, for *M. canis* infections which are relatively non-inflammatory or unusually extensive, or when it seems improbable that the child's parents will co-operate fully and the most rapid possible cure is essential. With efficient epilation a cure should be obtained in an average of 40 days, and with no other method of treatment at present available can so rapid a cure be guaranteed. Thallium acetate should be employed only in exceptional circumstances and then only under the direct supervision of a dermatologist experienced in its use.

As spontaneous cure often follows an inflammatory reaction such as occurs with animal ringworm infection, the older methods of treatment aimed at bringing about inflammation in the hair follicles ; some of the time-honoured remedies employed should here be mentioned. Aldersmith produced folliculitis deliberately, by painting on croton oil after cutting the hair short and protecting the healthy skin around the diseased part. The oil was left on for four hours ; then a linseed poultice was applied, removed next day, reapplied and changed every four to six hours. This was continued until folliculitis developed ; then the loose hairs were epilated. Whitfield used croton oil with a number 16 sewing needle, bent to an angle of forty-five degrees. The eye was dipped in the oil and passed down into the follicle ; the hair was pulled out in a few minutes. A popular formula known as Coster's paint (iodine one to two drachms, in an ounce of oil of wood tar) was applied daily with a stiff brush. In a few days a crust formed and was removed ; then the paint was reapplied after washing the area with soap and water. Another method was painting over with strong iodine, then covering with collodion or strapping which hermetically sealed the part, preventing the entrance of air required for the existence of the fungus. Jackson used, twice daily, crystals of iodine, a drachm to the ounce of goose grease, which he claimed penetrated better than other excipients.

When epilation is necessary the most rapid results are obtained by X-ray or thallium. Manual epilation can be used when these are unobtainable and when the lesion is limited. For limited lesions I was pleased during World Wars I and II with Dr. Winkelried Williams' method ; picric acid 7 gr., camphor ½ oz. and Spt. Indust. The camphor must be thoroughly dissolved in the spirit : and the lotion must be well shaken up before use, so that no camphor remains at the foot of the bottle. The hair must be cut short on and around the diseased patch ; the lotion is painted on with an ordinary camel-hair brush, morning and evening. As the lotion evaporates, a yellow powder accumulates on the head. This powder must be washed away lightly at least twice a week, so as to ensure that the fresh application reaches the scalp. The hair should be cut short, by clipping or shaving, two or three times a week ; otherwise the lotion cannot penetrate to the follicles, but accumulates on the hairs. If these details are carefully observed, the hair loosens in three or four weeks, and can readily be pulled out by epilation forceps. Epilation must be performed carefully : otherwise the hair is broken off above the scalp, and the disease remains in the follicles.

Rothman and others found that tinea within the hair is not curable without preceding epilation because no fungicidal preparation penetrates deep enough into the follicle.[1] This brings us to a consideration of the newer fungicides and the rationale of their use. Even for the non-inflammatory infections these may be tried when the disease is limited

[1] *J. Invest. Derm.*, 1947, **8**, 81.

to one small area. At puberty the sebaceous glands of the scalp begin to secrete a sebum which has a fungistatic action on *M. audouini*. From that fact it seemed possible that endocrine therapy would hasten cure before puberty ; for results, see p. 197. In the hair are ether-extractable substances which inhibit the growth of *M. audouini* in culture media. In adults this extract is five times as effective as in childhood ; thus is explained the rarity of this infection in an adult. Higher concentration however is necessary to inhibit the growth of certain forms of animal infection, *M. canis* and certain trichophytons ; hence adults are not immune to infections by those fungi. Adult hair fat has normal aliphatic monobasic acids with odd numbers of carbon atoms, including pelargonic acid. The adult type of hair fat does not kill the fungus which is *in the hair*, but it prevents infection of the new hair growing up to replace the falling one.[1]

Peck and Rosenfeld found that undecylenic acid in sweat was fungicidal.[2] Later work [3] decided that this acid in itself was fungicidal. A good formula is zinc undecylenic acid 5 per cent. in a vanishing emulsion base of $pH$ 6·5. The sole advantage of this preparation is that it is non-irritating ; its fungicidal property is not better than that of sulphur and salicylic acid. Except for monilial infections, gentian violet and hyd. ammon. chlor. are not fungicidal. Fungistatic and fungicidal remedies which are under trial include phenyl-mercuric compounds, and salts of the long-chained fatty acids, especially undecylenic and propionic acids. Antibiotics are being examined as well as chemical fungicides. Research is now being directed to discovering a suitable vehicle to enable the new fungicides to penetrate deeply into the follicles. R. T. Brain and others give a summary of these bases and their results with certain infections.[4] As some of the emulsion bases, such as carbowax, cause sensitization, the subject is still under consideration. Many dermatologists agree that success depends largely on the thoroughness with which treatment is carried out. When properly applied, the old remedies, such as mercury and iodine in goose grease, are quite as effective as the newer applications.

*Epilation* by X-ray and by thallium salts. When skilfully administered X-ray and thallium salts reduce to 28 to 40 days the duration of the disease and the possibility of infecting others. Only those who remember the long course of the disease before X-ray was available and how children could not attend school for years, can realize the gain

---

[1] ROTHMAN and SMILJANIC, *Science*, 1946, **104**, 201.
[2] *J. Invest. Derm.*, 1938, **1**, 265.
[3] SHAPIRO and ROTHMAN, *Arch. Derm. and Syph.*, 1945, **52**, 166.
[4] *Brit. Med. J.*, 1948, **1**, 723. See also "Modern Trends in Dermatology," 1948, p. 357.

to the community. Before the work of Sabouraud and Noiré with X-ray, the dosage was unsafe. Early in 1905 their method of measuring an " erythema dose " was published, and X-ray treatment was revolutionized. The safe dose was gauged by a pastille of barium platinocyanide, which changes colour when exposed to X-ray. Gas-filled X-ray tubes were used and the older dermatologists still prefer them. The pastille changed from light green to fawn and brown; booklets were supplied which showed when the correct, " safe " stage had been reached. If the pastille had darkened too much, there had been overexposure and the scalp developed a reaction with more or less severe damage. After a correct dose the hair fell out in 10 to 20 days.

The difficulty of matching the tint of the pastille, and the modification of X-ray tubes and apparatus led to other methods of calculation of the safe dose. Details of dosage differ with individual apparatus and radiologists; X-ray manuals must be consulted and practical lessons studied. X-ray epilation is a difficult procedure; outside the large towns few experts are available. The average modern dose is 400 roentgens to each area with a five inch diameter. The scalp is mapped out into five regions, the Kienbock-Adamson method. Some radiologists use four areas.[1] Owing to the danger of " scattered " rays, no metallic application should have been used for some time before the X-ray exposure.[2]

The hair begins to fall about 10 days after exposure, and continues to be shed during three weeks. Careful scrutiny is necessary lest any diseased hairs remain. These can be epilated, very carefully, so that no diseased roots remain in the follicle. During the weeks of hairfall a fungicide must be rubbed in, and a cap must be continuously worn. If all goes well the hair begins to return after 14 weeks and grows rapidly. Sometimes straight hair may grow in curly, but usually reverts to its original form.

X-ray treatment is not usually recommended for children under three or four years of age, owing to the difficulty of ensuring immobility. However, this trouble was surmounted by J. M. H. MacLeod who, with Shanks, had many thousand cases of ringworm to deal with in the Goldie Leigh Hospital, connected with the London County Council. The child is bound down to a couch by webbing straps, and the head is restrained by a closely-fitting calico cap which is attached to the couch by tapes.[3]

*Thallium acetate* is given by the mouth : the correct dose leads to

[1] SHANKS, " Four Area Method in X-ray Epilation of the Scalp," *Brit. Journ. Derm. and Syph.*, 1938, **50**, 440.

[2] " Modern Trends in Dermatology," 1948.

[3] See an illustrated article, with full particulars, *Brit. Journ. Derm. and Syph.*, 1931, **43**, 477.

hairfall, which begins just after a week and continues till all the hair has fallen in about 18 days. After a month the hair begins to grow in again; and there should be a strong growth in about three months' time. It appears that the drug does not act directly upon the hair roots, but through the sympathetic trophic nerves, so that those areas escape which are not controlled by the sympathetic, i.e. the eyebrows, eyelashes and the fringe on the brow. The measurement of the dose is based on the body weight; 8 milligrams of the drug are given for each kilogram of body weight. Tables are published stating the correct amount of thallium acetate per pound and per kilogram of body weight. One cannot exaggerate the importance of precision in noting the weight of the patient and adjusting the dosage in accordance with it. Doses slightly too large cause pains in the muscles and joints, particularly the knee-joints. Albuminuria and fits are amongst the general symptoms caused by over-dosage. The drug is more dangerous if given after puberty. To overcome the disadvantages of this drug Buschke and Lange advised the administration of thallium acetate with the application of X-ray, by using half the usual dose of both agents. The Ministry of Education prohibited the use of the drug for ringworm in school children. Fatal cases have been recorded from mistakes in the measurements of the dose. Poisonous doses cause acute abdominal pain, glossitis and vomiting of the cerebral type; symptoms also occur in the heart and lungs, in the kidneys and the nervous system—persisting somnolence, frontal headaches, muscle clonus, signs of involvement of the cranial nerves. In some of the fatal cases no hairfall occurred.[1]

As mentioned above, during the time which elapses between the administration of thallium acetate or X-ray and the final resulting complete loss of hair, the falling hairs must be prevented from infecting others. A cap must be worn and a mercurial (e.g. hyd. ammon. chlor. gr. 20 in 1 oz. or hyd. ox. flav. gr. 10 in 1 oz.) or other fungicidal or fungistatic ointment applied daily over the scalp, especially on the diseased patches. Adhesive plaster may be applied during the last stages to ensure that the hairs are pulled out gently. Rough traction causes the brittle shaft to break off and the diseased root is left in the follicle.

*Causes of Failure.* Sometimes all the hairs do not fall out; when they are loose they must be gently extracted or they will grow firm again, retaining the infected roots. This is not infrequent after thallium acetate. Regrowth may occur too soon after thallium and thus reinfection takes place from retained stumps. It also occurs after faulty X-ray

[1] An account of the literature of this subject is given in the *Brit. Med. J.*, 1934, **1**, 25.

technique.  Not infrequently the after-treatment is careless, and the child becomes reinfected just at the time when the new hairs are returning. X-ray treatment cannot be given a second time with safety until after the lapse of several months.  In cases of early reinfection or incomplete defluvium, we have to fall back on the methods which were employed before the introduction of X-ray and thallium acetate.

When it is not possible to have the X-ray administered by an expert we are obliged to use the local applications of former days.  Provided these are perseveringly applied, they should bring about a cure in a few months.  Partly owing to laziness in applying the remedies and partly owing to reinfection, cure may be delayed for months or years. In 1912 I was very pleased with the rapid results obtained by a method first advocated by Dr. Winkelried Williams.  I published a number of cases successfully treated by his lotion, which contains picric acid 7 gr., camphor ½ oz. and Spirit Indust. ½ oz.[1]  The camphor must be thoroughly dissolved in the spirit ; and the lotion must be well shaken up before use, so that no camphor remains at the foot of the bottle.  The hair must be cut around the diseased patch in the usual way, and the lotion is painted on with an ordinary camel-hair brush, morning and evening. As the lotion evaporates, a yellow powder accumulates on the head. This powder must be washed away lightly at least twice a week, so as to ensure that the fresh application reaches the scalp.  It is important that the hair should be cut short, by clipping or shaving, two or three times a week ; otherwise the lotion cannot penetrate to the scalp, but accumulates on the hairs.  If all these details are carefully observed, the hair becomes loosened in about three or four weeks, and can readily be pulled out by epilation forceps.  Epilation must be performed carefully, with the forceps applied as closely to the root of the hair as possible ; otherwise the hair is broken off above the scalp, and the disease remains in the follicle.

Spontaneous cure often follows an inflammatory reaction, such as occurs with animal ringworm infection.  Hence some of the time-honoured remedies aimed at bringing about inflammation in the hair follicles. Croton oil, ½ or 1 drachm to the ounce of sulphur ointment, was a favourite remedy ; pus formed and the hair fell out or could readily be extracted. Aldersmith's method was often used ; he applied twice daily :

| | | | | | | |
|---|---|---|---|---|---|---|
| Sulph. Praecip. | . | . | . | . | . | 6 to 12 parts. |
| Hydrarg. Ammon. | . | . | . | . | 1 ,, 2 ,, |
| Ac. Salicyl. | . | . | . | . | . | 1·3 ,, 4 ,, |
| Ol. Amygd. dulc. | . | . | . | . | . | 8 ,, |
| Adeps Lanae | . | . | . | . | . | 32 ,, |

Aldersmith also produced folliculitis deliberately, by painting on croton oil after cutting the hair short and protecting the healthy part around the diseased patch. The oil was left on for four hours, then a linseed poultice was applied, removed the next day, reapplied and changed every four to six hours. This was continued until folliculitis developed ; then the loose hairs were epilated. Whitfield used croton oil with a number 16 sewing-needle, bent to an angle of forty-five degrees. The eye was dipped in the oil and passed down into the follicle ; the hair was pulled out in a few minutes. Electrolysis can be used when there are only a few infected hairs.

Mercury was formerly much employed in various ways, e.g. the oleate of mercury ointment, a solution of the bichloride, two grains dissolved in alcohol and mixed with half an ounce of kerosene and olive oil. Iodine was another favourite. A popular form, known as Coster's paint, consisted of iodine 1 to 2 drachms to the ounce of oil of wood tar. It was applied with a stiff brush daily ; after a few days a black crust formed, which was removed, the part washed with soap and water, and the paint again applied. Cure was often obtained after a few applications. Another plan was to paint over with strong iodine and cover with collodion or strapping which hermetically sealed the part, and prevented the entrance of the air necessary for the existence of the fungus. Jackson found great success with the application, twice daily, of crystals of iodine, a drachm to the ounce of goose grease ; he claimed that the goose grease penetrated better than other excipients. Other remedies were glacial acetic acid, formalin, naphthol and oleate of copper.

Injections of ringworm fungus have been tried : the best results were obtained in cases which had a degree of inflammatory reaction in the follicles.[1] As ringworm tends to die out at puberty, it seemed reasonable to deduce that endocrine therapy should be beneficial, even curative. Poth and Kaliski [2] gave theelin and diethylstilboestrol, 1 mg. thrice daily, and also tried 5,000 International Units in a daily capsule ; and locally, 1 gm. (5,000 I.U.) in ointment. The results were disappointing.

*The patient has scaly patches, yellow, cup-shaped dry crusts with mouse-like odour, and bald patches with atrophy. The disease is* FAVUS.

**Favus,** the infection of the hair and the scalp by a fungus, the *Achorion schönleinii,* is characterized by sulphur-yellow crusts, thick layers of

---

[1] L. M. SMITH, *South M.J.,* 1935, **28,** 610, and *Year Book Derm. and Syph.,* Chicago, 1937, pages 7 to 26.
[2] D. O. POTH and S. A. KALISKI, *Arch. Derm. and Syph.,* 1942, **45,** 121.

grey scales, and pink bald patches which in time become white and cicatricial. The disease affects chiefly the scalp but may also appear on the skin of the body and on the nails.

On the scalp favus starts with one or more pink areas, or sometimes with tiny yellow scales, or even with vesicles. By the time the physician sees the case this stage is usually past and there are found many of the typical scutula or yellow crusts, slightly hollowed, like a shallow cup, and perforated by a few hairs. Thick grey scales are also present in quantity ; the hair is dry and dull, and as it falls out, it leaves in its place bald patches of irregular shape and size. The crusts begin near the hair follicles, often as intradermic beads of pus. The typical saucer shape of the crust or scutulum is seen quite early. At first the size of a pin head, the scutulum grows to the diameter of a pea. The scalp beneath it is depressed and moist, or red and atrophied. In long-standing cases few of these crusts may be seen, for the coalescence and subsequent breaking down of the saucer-shaped crusts leads to the formation of mortar-like masses of friable grey scales, composed of infected epithelial scales and fungus. The hairs go on growing for a time after the crusts form, but as the fungus eventually invades them, they lose all lustre, become brittle and fall out. The bald patches are of irregular outline, vividly red at first, white and atrophied in the course of time. Suppuration sometimes accompanies the infection.

*Ætiology.* Favus is contagious, but less so than ringworm. Favus attacks chiefly children between the ages of six to fifteen, especially boys, but is also seen in adults. It is rare in infants. It used to be common amongst the poor of Eastern Europe, e.g. Poles, Russians and Hungarians. Some forty years ago it was frequently met with in Scotland, but was rare in England and America. It spreads by means of caps, combs and brushes ; some say an abrasion is necessary before the fungus can take hold. It affects mice, cats, rabbits and fowls. The fungus infecting the human scalp is *T. schönleinii*. The favus which attacks animals may belong to several other species of trichophyton. The only species of importance is *T. quinckeanum*, which infects mice.

After the infected hair has been soaked in liquor potassæ, it is examined under the microscope. Under the low-power lens a large number of tiny air bubbles can be seen on the hair surface ; this is a feature so characteristic that Sabouraud considered it was practically diagnostic. The hair is infected along its whole shaft, except at the root. The mycelia run along like thin threads, not so numerous as ringworm mycelia (see Fig. 46). The spores are of various shapes, round or oval. At first the infection is outside the cuticle, but later the fungus penetrates the hair and the mycelia grow down towards the root. The hair infected with favus is not so brittle as that infected with ringworm.

*Diagnosis.* The mouse-like odour which emanates from the infected scalp is unmistakable. The yellow cupped crusts, the dead appearance of the hair, the irregular red bald patches and the mousy odour form the four diagnostic features of this disease. There is rarely any difficulty in distinguishing this infection from ringworm. Ringworm infection does not lead to cicatricial bald patches. In both diseases the hairs lose their lustre, become brittle and break off, but in favus the hairs do not show the broken stumps, close to the scalp, so characteristic of ringworm, and the yellow colour and mousy odour of the favus hollow crusts is distinctive. When one tries to epilate the hair it breaks off when infected with ring-worm, whereas with favus the root comes out. Sometimes in old cases, and those with many cicatricial areas, it is necessary to eliminate the diagnosis of *lupus erythematosus* and of *folliculitis decalvans.* In lupus

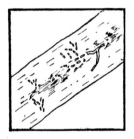

FIG. 46.—Favus Fungus. (Mag. × 450.)

(*Drawn by Dr. I. Muende*).

erythematosus the scar is red, becoming white, and there may be a few scales, but there is no mousy odour, no yellow crusting, nor are the hairs lustreless. In folliculitis decalvans there is difficulty in diagnosis only when the crusts and scales of favus are absent. The scar of folliculitis decalvans is irregular and white. A red spot surrounds the hairs at the margin of the bald patches in folliculitis decalvans, but the hairs are not broken and lustreless as in favus. However, whenever there is any possibility of an error in diagnosis, the microscopic examination of the scales and hairs settles the point. In favus the fungus is seen, with spores larger than those of ringworm, and the hairs showing more mycelia than spores.

*Prognosis and Treatment.* Favus of the scalp is not easy to cure, although favus affecting the skin of the body is as readily responsive as is the ringworm fungus to anti-parasitic remedies. Epilation is necessary, and this is best carried out by X-ray. To ensure that the X-ray does reaches the scalp it is necessary to remove the thick crusts and masses of scales. In order to do this successfully the scalp must be soaked in olive or almond oil for one or even two days ; then washed with soap and soft water and thoroughly cleansed of all debris. When the hairfall begins, scrupulous care must be taken to destroy the loosened hairs. Sulphur ointment or other strong anti-parasitic remedy should be rubbed in daily and a cap worn during the whole period of hairfall. When epilation appears to be complete, every inch of the scalp should be scrutinized, lest a single diseased hair remains.  In any case of doubt, rub in strong remedies, such as hydrarg. perchlor. ½ per cent. in alcohol, sulphur 20 per cent., mercury or camphor oleate, etc.  Jackson considered that crystals of iodine 1 in 8 of goose grease formed the best of all the parasitic ointments he had used for both favus and ringworm. Epilation of all hairs remaining must be most cautiously performed. Owing to the fact that hair infected with favus is less brittle than in ringworm infections, epilation is a comparatively simple operation. Indeed, before the introduction of a safe means of measuring the X-ray dose, manual epilation was the chief method of treating favus.

**Staining** *Hairs* INFECTED WITH FUNGUS.

To obtain good specimens, it is necessary to *epilate the hair*, bringing away the bulb with steady traction.  Do not draw it away with a jerk or the hair breaks off above the bulb.  Soak for several minutes in ether in a watch glass, then wash in 10 per cent. spirit.  Transfer the hairs to a clean slide, and let dry ;  then drop on the stain.

J. M. H. MacLeod gives the following directions for the anilin gentian violet stain :  " Shake up 5 parts of anilin oil in a hundred of distilled water, and filter.  Add to the filtrate sufficient of a saturated alcoholic solution of gentian violet to make the mixture opalescent.  Prepare freshly each time. As this solution rapidly evaporates, add fresh drops from time to time.  In the case of the microsporon, ten minutes is sufficient for staining ;  but with endothrix an hour may be necessary, and the slide should be heated now and then over a flame to soften the keratin and increase the power of penetration of the stain.  Decolourize for five minutes in Gram's iodine solution, poured on without washing the hairs.  The iodine solution is then poured off the slide, and the hairs are further differentiated in anilin oil.  This is the most difficult part of the process, and on it depends the success of the specimen. It should be watched from time to time under a low power.  The time taken varies from a few minutes for the microsporon to several hours in the case of the endothrix.  The action of the anilin oil may be greatly accelerated by the addition of a few drops of nitric acid to a watch glass of anilin oil. Clear in xylol and mount in Canada balsam."

If it is desired to make a rapid examination, as during a clinic, place the suspected hairs or skin scrapings on a clean slide with a few drops of liquor potassæ ;  warm gently for a few minutes, taking care not to let the specimen be boiled.  If it is wished to preserve the specimen for a day or two, run in equal parts of glycerine and water ;  leave for some twelve hours, then press gently with blotting paper and seal.  For preserving the specimen, place it in this solution—lactic acid, 20 gm. ;  phenol crystals, 20 gm. ;  glycerine, 40 gm. ;  distilled water, 20 gm.  If staining is required, add to the above Cotton blue, 0·05 gm.

The Cotton blue lacto-phenol method of staining is useful for identifying the fine spores and mycelia in a thin skin scraping, as from pityriasis versicolor, also for staining spores and other features obtained from cultures.

Permanent specimens can be made by staining with the above, then sealing with Waller's cement (equal parts of purified beeswax and gum dammar).

# CHAPTER XIII

## ERYTHEMATOUS ERUPTIONS

When a patient complains of redness or a rash on the scalp, erythema may be the sole or the outstanding feature, or it may be accompanied by scaling, or by some degree of exudation, with a sensation of tension, burning or itching.

CLINICAL INVESTIGATION. Erythema may be noticed by the physician, but is unlikely to be the cause of complaint on the part of the patient or relatives, in the following conditions :

A mild degree of erythema occurs after the *crusts of impetigo* and of other pustules have dropped off ; this lasts a few days and is followed by pallor and transient baldness.

A pink flush often accompanies the itching of *urticaria*, and precedes the development of the scales in *ringworm and favus*, and sometimes actively spreading patches of *alopecia areata*.

Erythema is definitely present, underlying and extending beyond the scaly margin of many eruptions in which the *formation of scales* is the distinctive feature : as, for example, *psoriasis, neurodermatitis* and *seborrhœic dermatitis* (pityriasis circinata or eczematized pityriasis steatoides of Sabouraud). Erythematous patches precede the papules, vesicles and bullæ of *dermatitis herpetiformis*, but these are not easily seen on the scalp.

An erythematous zone surrounds many of the *pustular* conditions, especially deep-seated pustules with an indurated base. *Anthrax* is a rare disease in which a ring of vesicles may be surrounded by a zone of inflammation with œdema (see page 232). The patient usually seeks advice before this stage. An actively inflamed red patch may lead to a diagnosis of *Trichophyton* infection on the scalp of a child, as on the beard of an adult. Erythema is always present with *ulceration*, and over rapidly enlarging *cysts, nodules* or *tumours*. A minute red zone is visible, encircling the hair before the development of pus in various forms of *folliculitis*. This zone of redness round a hair may provide diagnostic aid in the rare cases of baldness with atrophy, due to *folliculitis decalvans*.

The flat *capillary nævus* must not be mistaken for a patch of erythema. Many infants are born with this type of nævus, which may spontaneously vanish or may persist throughout life (p. 268).

When erythema forms the *predominating or the diagnostic* feature of an eruption, one of the following conditions may be suspected :

GROUP A. ERYTHEMA with raised surface and defined margin, preceded and accompanied by FEVER—ERYSIPELAS.

GROUP B. ERYTHEMA accompanied or soon followed by SCALING :

I Seborrhœic dermatitis (eczematized pityriasis steatoides).
II Certain cases of ringworm.
III Lupus erythematosus.
IV Early stage of herpes zoster.
V Syphilis.
VI Pityriasis rubra pilaris.
VII Part of a generalized erythrodermia.

GROUP C. ERYTHEMA accompanied by EXUDATION.

VIII Subacute and acute streptococcal dermatitis.
IX Infantile eczema.
X Dermatitis due to traumatism.

In these diseases there is early exudation of serum, with, in eczema, preliminary vesicles. At a later stage, there are crusts, and sometimes pus. If the patient is seen at a still later stage, there are dry scales, due to exfoliation of the inflamed skin. Dermatitis due to traumatism may have a profuse exudation, with yellow crusts, and the erythema may be visible only on the skin adjacent to the scalp.

GROUP D. ERYTHEMA not NECESSARILY accompanied by EXUDATION IN THE EARLY STAGE.

X Dermatitis due to traumatism.
XI Dermatitis due to dyes.

In the early stage of these conditions there is swelling and itching as well as discomfort. The presence of œdema, or of vesicles, bullæ and exudation, depends upon the severity of the process.

GROUP E. Certain NODULAR CONDITIONS, in their early stage, are regarded by the patient as a red rash. (See Chapter XVII.)

GROUP A. **Erysipelas** is an acute contagious disease, due to a streptococcus which enters by a minute abrasion. After a brief incubation period of three to six days, fever sets in, usually suddenly, with back pains and vomiting. The rash follows in about a day, as a small red patch, near a tiny wound, often invisible to the eye. The erythema is raised and tense, with a characteristic defined margin which extends day by day. The face is frequently attacked, and thence the eruption extends to the scalp. The constitutional disturbance and the raised, defined margin make the diagnosis usually simple. Immunity is not gained by one attack. *Recurring erysipelas* is common in elderly people, and in connection with sinusitis and local fissure ; chronic œdema with lymphatic blockage often results. Hairfall occurs over the inflamed area in about two weeks ; later is seen the diffuse loss of hair which always follows high fever (p. 85).

*Treatment.* Penicillin and the sulphanilamide group of drugs have revolutionized the treatment of erysipelas. When the organism is penicillin sensitive 1 to 2,000,000 units may be injected every eight hours, or 30,000 every three hours for five to seven days, or given in oil with a local anæsthetic ; or 1 G. sulphadiazine can be taken every four hours until recovery, and then thrice daily for a fortnight. Local applications are rendered unnecessary. In the past many forms of treatment had their quota of success : X-ray, ultra-violet light, anti-streptococcus serum, and 10 per cent. ichthyol in glycerine painted on the area.

*Recurrent erysipelas.* Seek for the site of entry of the infecting organism. Recurrence may be prevented by a prolonged course of autogenous vaccine, preferably administered intradermally.

GROUP B. *Erythematous eruptions preceded, accompanied, or soon followed by some degree of scaling.*

I. **Seborrhœic Dermatitis** (pityriasis circinata or eczematized pityriasis steatoides of Sabouraud) has usually a clear history of scaliness of the scalp (p. 160) having preceded the erythema. When erythema develops, it shows a pale red rim with festooned margin, and here and there are superimposed yellow-grey scales, large or small. Owing to the underlying serous oozing, the scales convey a sticky or greasy sensation to the touch. There is no induration. The rash is commonly seen extending widely along the margin of the scalp and forehead (the *corona seborrhœica*), backwards along the vertex, and often passing down behind and on the skin of the ears. Usually there are also patches on the face, along the naso-labial folds, the middle of the front and the back of the chest, where the sebaceous glands are most active. In the middle-aged especially, the rash may be widespread ; the outlying regions of follicular, soft papules aid the diagnosis in these cases of severe seborrhoeic dermatitis. In elderly, bald persons, the eruption of seborrhœic dermatitis often extends widely over the scalp and its colour tends to be a brighter red. Itching may be a prominent feature in the middle-aged and elderly. In younger subjects, except when the disease is acute and extending over the body, itching is not usual ; a sensation of heat or discomfort is more often their complaint, and the eruption is often paler, its pinkness having a fawny tinge. Hairfall does not occur, unless there is some complication.

*Diagnosis.* In acute, rapidly spreading *psoriasis*, the diagnosis may be difficult. Points to note are the position of the patches elsewhere ; in psoriasis these predominate on the extensor aspects of the limbs, and there may be found some chronic areas, covered with the silvery scales characteristic of psoriasis. The various forms, stages and causes of seborrhœic dermatitis are described under pityriasis (pp. 163 and 167). Often, and chiefly in young patients, it is difficult to differentiate a severe case of seborrhœic dermatitis of the scalp from *streptococcal dermatitis*, especially when streptococcal infection has begun to complicate it. The supervention of streptococcal infection is to be suspected when there is rapid extension of the rash, with swelling and itching, and when there is a retroauricular fissure (see VIII below). Infection with *Staphylococcus aureus* also may occur, especially when there is aural discharge. Then the folds of the body, where there are opposed surfaces, may become inflamed and ooze serum. Exfoliative dermatitis may ensue.

For *Ætiology, Prognosis* and *Treatment* see pp. 162 et seq.

II. In the common variety of RINGWORM affecting the scalp, erythema is the earliest symptom. This stage, which lasts about a day, is rarely seen by the physician ; as a rule, medical advice is not sought until there is a scaly patch, with broken hairs (see p. 184). In certain types of ringworm infection the skin of the face and neck and also that near the scalp shows small, discrete, rosy patches, with scaling. These occasionally show a double-ringed margin. The variety of fungus in such cases is usually a microsporon of animal origin—cat, dog or horse. The use of a mild mercurial or iodine ointment usually cures such patches.

III. LUPUS ERYTHEMATOSUS begins with one or more small red patches of irregular shape, under the hair. Gradually the hair falls and a fine atrophy replaces the erythema. The white scar tissue and erythematous edge form the diagnostic features of this slowly progressive malady. Whilst scales usually form a predominant feature when lupus erythematosus attacks the face, they may be absent when the disease affects the scalp. A horny point may be found in some of the dilated hair follicles. The patient may be unaware of the early stages of this disease, especially if it occurs in a woman who wears long hair. As a bald patch is the symptom for which the sufferer usually seeks advice, lupus erythematosus is described in the section on baldness with atrophy (p. 137).

IV. HERPES ZOSTER may begin with a red patch on which vesicles soon develop ; hence it is described under vesicular eruptions.

**V. Syphilis.** With the lenticulo-papular syphilide, the patient may seek advice on account of a red raised rash on a section of the forehead and margin of the scalp, the *corona veneris*, a manifestation of syphilis which usually appears during or after the second year. It may also appear on the neck, extending on to the scalp, on the face and other parts of the body, chiefly on the flexor aspects of the limbs. The papules are indurated, dull coppery red in colour, often showing at their edges a fine scaling ; they tend to run together, forming a patch either in a complete ring or with a festooned or polycyclical margin with a collar of scales and a depressed centre. The condition was frequently seen before the introduction of the arsenical treatment of syphilis, and often caused difficulty in diagnosis ; in the young adult, from *seborrhœic dermatitis*, the " *corona seborrhœica* " and in older persons, from psoriasis. In the " *corona seborrhœica* " the rash is more fawn coloured or pale red, usually of wider extent, not raised nor indurated, and with sticky yellow scales. When *psoriasis* affects the brow and adjacent scalp, the scales may not be so thick and silvery as on other parts of the scalp, but there is a history of chronic scaly patches on the knees, elbows and elsewhere ; the colour of the syphilitic rash is of a dull coppery red, the scales are grey, not white or silvery, and the underlying rash is infiltrated. See also scaly eruptions, p. 180. In *secondary syphilis*, at the time the erythemato-papular rash appears on the brow, there are usually present also enlarged cervical glands, mucous patches on the throat and some papules and macules on the body, especially well seen on the abdomen when the skin is slightly chilled from exposure. In *later* (tertiary) *syphilis*, the eruption is more raised and some of the papules may be crusted with typical serpiginous ulceration beneath, and later, papery white scars. The gumma is described under nodular eruptions (p. 254). All forms respond to anti-syphilitic treatment, which is not dealt with in this book.

VI. PITYRIASIS RUBRA PILARIS. In severe cases a widespread erythrodermia develops in the later stages of this disease. On the scalp, face and body may appear a vivid erythema ; the skin appears tightly stretched and dry, with thick adhesive scales. Some parts of the skin of the body usually remain healthy. Hairfall is not a noticeable feature till the late stage, when erythrodermia is marked. As the patient has usually had for some years scales on the scalp and scaly papules on the backs of the fingers, see the section on scaly conditions (p. 180).

VII. Erythema is even more prominent a feature than scaliness in the early stage of cases of **Generalized Erythrodermia,** such as occurs with exfoliative dermatitis, primary or secondary. The erythematous skin is congested and hot to the touch, although the patient feels cold. The redness may persist for months or years. Exudation of serum may follow, with complicating local infection.

In **Exfoliative Dermatitis**, whether primary or secondary, the scalp is usually involved and hairfall may be marked. The disease is acute or chronic. In the acute form the skin is vivid red, with large flakes of epidermis which are shed abundantly. PRIMARY EXFOLIATIVE DERMATITIS is due to some internal toxin of unknown origin. There is fever at times. The patients are usually of middle or advanced age. Chronic cases may last for years.

For a whole year I watched the severe case of a farm worker aged forty-eight. Periods of high fever alternated with weeks of comparative recovery. No cause could be found. The temperature dropped after the gradual extraction of many septic teeth.

During the bouts of fever the hair fell from the scalp and face. Life was despaired of after several relapses ; recovery came with penicillin injections ; the hair returned and the entire body began to look normal. Again fever began to rise, and all the hair fell out. Eventually a blood culture showed hæmolytic streptococci ; abscesses developed in the rectus femoris, then in the arm ; only when these were incised and dealt with did the patient slowly recover. The hair of his face and scalp returned.

SECONDARY EXFOLIATIVE DERMATITIS may follow diseases which affect the skin, such as psoriasis, seborrhœic dermatitis, pemphigus, acute lichen planus, mycosis fungoides and leukæmia—also the ingestion of certain drugs, such as the barbiturates, and injections of gold, bismuth and arsenic. With barbiturate poisoning the eruption may start as erythema, resembling scarlet fever, measles, erythema multiforme, and less often, with vesicles and bullæ. When exfoliative dermatitis with fever ensues, the condition becomes very grave, and a fatal issue is not unusual.

MEPACRINE DERMATITIS can be accompanied by loss of hair which usually returns later. The use of too strong local remedies, such as chrysarobin, may be the starting-point of exfoliative dermatitis. Darier drew attention to EQUINE SCABIES, a rare disease, without burrows or severe itching ; the erythrodermia may be universal, including also the face and scalp, or affecting only the face and scalp.

Darier summarized the forms of exfoliation seen in the *newly born* and in *infants* : (i) an exaggeration of the normal shedding of the epithelium, beginning about the third or fifth day and continuing for one to two months ; (ii) infantile eczema, which may affect the whole body ; (iii) exfoliative dermatitis in quite young breast-fed babies may follow seborrhœic dermatitis. Starting on the scalp, the inflammation may spread over the body ; intestinal complications are usual, and the outlook is serious. (iv) In Ritter's disease the scales and dermatitis are the remains of bullæ ; the scaling may be moist, the underlying skin angry purple red. This serious condition is probably due to a pyogenic organism, and is akin to pemphigus neonatorum.

*Treatment.* The general condition must be carefully considered : Rest, warmth, protection from draught or chill, free bowel action, restricted diet, according to the individual indications, ascorbic acid in full doses, up to 200 mg. t.d.s. ; glucose, alkalis or acids as required. Seek for septic foci ; a blood culture may reveal the infecting organism. Do not forget to look for arsenical poisoning. Autohæmotherapy and colonic irrigation have cured many cases of apparent primary exfoliative dermatitis. The desquamation leads to loss of cystine, which can be replaced by administering 1 G. daily by mouth, or 0·25 G. by subcutaneous injection.[1] Research is being carried out with amino-acids, plasma and protein hydrolysates for such cases. Locally, soothe with an inert powder, such as talc, or when scales predominate, apply zinc oxide powder in olive, castor or arachis oil, equal parts, or with 40 per cent. of the powder. A liniment with olive oil and liquor calcis is also comforting. The French School preferred to use talc or other inert powder, and followed with weak ichthyol ointment when there was much congestion. I find their method more pleasant than oily applications, both for the patient and the nursing staff.

Although MYCOSIS FUNGOIDES and LEUKÆMIA are mentioned here, it is improbable that sufferers from such diseases will seek advice on account of the erythema of the scalp. In the early stage of mycosis fungoides there is recurring erythema on any part of the body, accompanied by marked itching. The diagnosis can often be made by a biopsy. Later, tumours appear (see Chapter XVII). In leukæmia the erythema is dark red, tense, raised, and itching is very severe. The blood examination decides the diagnosis.

For these cases X-ray gives some relief and certainly calms the irritation.

GROUP C. *Erythema accompanied by exudation.*

VIII. **Subacute** and **acute streptococcal dermatitis** is usually due to infection with streptococci, but may also be complicated by staphylococcal organisms. It often starts as a complication of preceding disease, such as pityriasis steatoides, psoriasis, impetigo and " seborrhœic dermatitis " ; it may also arise without any preceding skin disease. Sometimes it originates from a fissure or other tiny lesion of which the patient is unaware. It is recognized when, as mentioned above under

---

[1] PETERS, *Lancet*, 1945, **1**, 264, and *Nature*, 1945, **156**, 616.

seborrhœic dermatitis (p. 203), and psoriasis (p. 173), there is a rapid extension of the existing erythema, and sometimes marked itching with tenseness or swelling. In acute cases exudation of serum soon follows, and the inflammation spreads along the surface of the skin. As the serum dries on the surface, it forms yellowish crusts. Formerly, the condition was regarded as eczema, but true vesicles and bullæ are rarely seen. In the sub-acute form there may be no crusts and oozing serum, but only scales, as in the chronic type (see p. 176). In both forms fissures usually develop behind the ears ; when the ear is pulled forward the whole area behind it, and up under the adjacent hair, is seen to be a vivid, glazed red, with crusts or scales. The fissure is torn open more widely as the ear-lobe is pulled up and a few drops of blood may be seen mingled with the serum. The eruption in severe cases occurs also on the body, especially where there are opposed surfaces, such as the umbilicus, the axillæ and under pendulous breasts, the conjunctival folds and even the neck creases in fat children, in the groins and along the intergluteal fold. What used to be called intertrigo is now known to be due to mycotic, or, more often, to streptococcal invasion of the skin. Therefore the diagnosis of this type of dermatitis of the scalp is aided by the presence of areas of erythema, crusts and fissures behind the ears and on other opposing surfaces of the body.

*Ætiology.* Children under ten form the majority of the sufferers. Amongst adults, women are more often affected than men. Sabouraud first established the streptococcus as the causal organism in impetigo and in the acute type of dermatitis now being considered. John Kinnear, one of his pupils, found that the streptococci which gave rise to this form of streptococcal dermatitis belong to the non-hæmolytic variety.

*Prognosis.* The disease may be very obstinate, lasting for months or years, even with careful treatment. Recurrences are frequent, and often severe, especially if the patient, believing the condition is cured, stops the local applications before the skin has become normal. When the scalp eruption recurs in adults I often find at the same time cervical discharge and eczema ani. Sometimes the hair falls out in very inflamed regions, but it returns after the inflammation has subsided ; hairfall is not a feature of this disease. Some degree of folliculitis, with staphylococcal infection, may complicate a severe case ; but the staphylococci do not usually gain much foothold.

*Treatment.* Washing with soap and water must be forbidden, and during the acute stage also all strong remedies, such as mercury or sulphur. Ointments should not be used in widespread dermatitis with much serous

exudation, because the oozing extends below the greasy application.
For young children Sabouraud recommended Eau d'Alibour every few
hours ; before each dressing epithelial debris had to be gently detached.
Protect the newly growing epithelium with zinc paste. In adults with
strictly localized dermatitis Sabouraud's favourite remedy was one per
cent. iodine in 70 to 90 per cent. alcohol, twice daily, followed by a zinc
paste. Where there is co-existing extensive dermatitis on the body,
with consequent sensitization, mild local dressings must be used, such as
the aqueous solution of gentian violet, 1 or 2 per cent., and talc powder
or a cream of zinc oxide powder in two parts of oil. I have often seen
how careful dressings carried out by a good nurse succeed when the
patient has failed. When the canal of the ear is involved, drop into it
Burow's solution (lead acetate gr. 24 ; solution of aluminium acetate
m. 60 in 1 oz. water), after syringing with normal saline. The same
solution, half strength, can be soaked into butter-muslin and pushed into
the folds of the auricle and behind the ear. The canal must not be
blocked up with a wool plug. Ung. quinolor with an equal part of pasta
zinci is another valuable remedy. A time-honoured application is 2 per
cent. silver nitrate in water or in spt. eth. meth. ; it is especially good for
fissures. Sealing the fissures with Tr. Benzoin Co. is effective in other
cases. Watch the effect of any fresh remedy ; take care with the
manner of its application, and do not change to a new drug when one
is succeeding. In the severe condition often seen in children, and
when extending to the scalp the hair has to be cut short. The crusts
must be removed ; for this purpose use the starch poultice, as described
under impetigo (p. 216). At first 1 per cent. iodine in spirit is used daily ;
gently but thoroughly rubbed on the scalp, and a dry dressing left on
all day. As progress continues, paint every other day, then twice a
week. In very obstinate cases, try an occlusive dressing such as visco-
paste, or Unna's gelatine once a week for about four to six weeks. For
long-standing and recurring cases Kinnear [1] recommends peptone
(Armour's No. 2·5 per cent.), subcutaneously, 1 c.c. followed by three
doses of 2 c.c. on alternate days. Autohæmotherapy is also useful, 5 c.c.
every other day for four doses ; but it and vaccine therapy may fail.
For adults, I use an intradermal vaccine in small doses. The recurrences
are shortened, and the coinciding uterine and anal signs respond to rest,
alkalis and B. acidophilus therapy.

When the hair is long, the removal of crusts may cause much difficulty.
Oil of cade 4 or 5 per cent. in almond oil may be left on for twenty-four
hours ; for very thick scales add salicylic acid 4 per cent. When the

[1] *Brit. Med. J.*, 1935, 1, 291.

scales are thus softened, they can be gently picked off. After their removal, coal tar 2 per cent. is effective.

When the retro-auricular fissures remain very obstinate, a few applications of ultra-violet light or of zinc ionization often set in motion the healing processes of nature. A layer of lint, soaked in a 2 per cent. solution of zinc sulphate, is gently pushed into the fissure. The electrode is attached to the positive pole, whilst the indifferent pole is placed at any convenient part. If the fissure is behind the ear, it is important that the indifferent pole is placed on the same side of the body. Then a current of 2 to 3 ma. is passed for three to ten minutes, according to the size of the crack.

For *treatment* of chronic streptococcal dermatitis, when scales predominate over erythema, see scaly conditions (p. 176).

**IX. Infantile Eczema.** Many forms of eruption occurring in infants have been called Infantile Eczema. True infantile eczema has these special features : the rash usually begins when the infant is 1 to 3 months old, and usually disappears at a year, eighteen months or two years. The lesions begin on the cheeks, and throughout the course of the malady the face is the part most affected. Then the forehead, scalp and ears become involved ; the median area of the face almost always remains clear. The rash begins with a vivid erythema which soon becomes swollen, vesicular and crusted. It may spread to the limbs and trunk, but only rarely becomes generalized. With the appearance of each tooth the rash is usually aggravated or fresh papules appear. The severity of the itching, especially in the evening and at night, is a characteristic feature. Scratching may lead to secondary infection and complications ; broncho-pneumonia, enteritis, nephritis, loss of weight, even sudden death may occur.

*Ætiology.* There is still controversy as to whether infantile eczema is due to a constitutional allergy, or is a contact dermatitis due to external irritants. Washing, soap, changes of temperature, cold winds, have been blamed by many dermatologists.[1] Others are equally certain that the condition is an allergic phenomenon. Eczema starting after the infant is six months old is probably a contact dermatitis ; if at the stage of walking or crawling, suspect rugs or other furnishings, furniture polish, rubber bands, or dyes from clothing. In some infants the stools appear to be normal, and the child is healthy. In others there is an abnormal intestinal flora [2] and a history of excess of food, especially of fat and

[1] *Proc. Roy. Soc. Med.*, 1925–6, Joint Disc. No. 5, Sect. Derm. and Dis. Children. A. H. M. GRAY *et al.*
[2] CHARLES WHITE, *Arch. Derm. and Syph.*, 1923, **7**, 50.

starch. In stout infants there is often bronchial and adenoid trouble, with rapid alterations of weight and glandular enlargement. In breast-fed infants the diet of the mother affects her baby ; when she takes beer, for example, the infant's eczema is aggravated. There may be too much fat or protein or an incorrect balance in the milk. Usually it is the lactal-bumen which is the erring constituent. When the eczema returns in childhood the foods most incriminated are milk, eggs, wheat, tomato and orange.

*Diagnosis.* *Infantile eczema* has a characteristic distribution on the cheeks, the middle line of the face being almost free. In *seborrhœic dermatitis* the scalp is first and chiefly involved ; often the condition of the mother and nurse reveals the infecting source. With a staphylococcal secondary infection there is an inflammatory reaction and eczematization of the skin.

*Treatment.* (1) The diet must be modified to suit the individual case. In breast-fed infants one must ensure that the mother's food contains no deleterious agent, and has adequate vitamins and lime. When the infant is on cow's milk, a simple change of milk may suffice for a cure ; in other patients, cow's milk has to be given up and goat's milk, soya bean and foods substituted ; or the remedy lies in altering the proportions of the sugar, fat and farinaceous elements. When the older child is also unable to take eggs or cereals, cure may be obtained by omitting these articles of diet ; or desensitizing may be necessary. The atopic dermatitis of the allergic constitution will often relapse. Allergic subjects react to many cutaneous tests. When there is water retention in the skin, restrict milk and fat, allow sugar and farinaceous foods, and give alkalis and calcium. Sudden changes of temperature must be avoided. Sometimes an intestinal vaccine has been successful.

(2) *Local treatment* is essential whether the cause be due to internal or external factors. Infantile eczema must be distinguished from " seborrhœic dermatitis " ; in the latter the scalp of the mother, nurse and infant should be washed and treated with a mild sulphur ointment. In all types of eczema the prevention of friction and of scratching is of prime importance ; the elbows and wrists can be effectively immobilized with a roll of newspaper bound along the flexor aspects of the arms. During the acute stage, use a soothing lotion such as calamine, and a zinc paste. No soap or water can be used. White's coal tar ointment has many advocates. Care is required for the proper preparation of this ointment. Its original formula was : crude coal tar and zinc oxide, 2 parts of each, thoroughly mixed, then 16 parts each of corn starch and of vaseline are added. Some years later, White preferred

to omit the corn starch. It is applied night and morning, on muslin or old fine linen, which must not be tightly bound on. Before each dressing the old ointment is dabbed off gently, with olive oil. Crude coal tar alone is also successful, but must not be used if pus is present. Many years ago I had several of such cases at the same time in the same ward in hospital and tried the effects of different pastes and lotions. I found the most all-round efficacious ointment was : Liq. picis carbonis ℥. viii, zinci oxidi. gr. xl, acidi boracis gr. x, amyli gr. 60 in an ounce of soft paraffin. The excellent article of Lewis Hill repays study ; his conclusions are based on twenty-six years' experience of many types of infantile eczema.[1] Atopic dermatitis is due to an allergic constitution, and that cannot be changed ; but local treatment and sedatives aid much.

X. DERMATITIS DUE TO TRAUMATISM falls within both groups of erythema, C and D, and is described in Group D, below. In mild cases only erythema, without exudation, may develop ; in severe and acute cases there are vesicles, bullæ and a profuse flow of serous exudation, with subsequent formation of yellow crusts.

GROUP D. *Erythema not necessarily accompanied by exudation in the early stage.*

X. **Dermatitis due to traumatism and to sensitization.** Erythema, sometimes with swelling and exudation, begins a few hours after the use of the traumatic agent, increases for a day or a little longer and begins to subside after a few days. The swelling may have vanished in a week and is followed by exfoliation. Too strong a dose of *ultra-violet light* may after a few hours cause itching, then erythema, swelling, blistering and serous exudation. Sometimes, as with the Kromayer lamp, a strong dose may have been intentionally administered, and the operator has omitted to tell the patient of the expected effect of the dose. Too prolonged or too vigorous application of the *high-frequency vacuum tube* can be followed by erythema. The use of *rubefacients* can bring about acute erythema, even swelling and vesicles, and later, especially in infants and old people, secondary infection with pustules. Of such agents may be mentioned chrysarobin, cignolin, ammonia, tincture of iodine, turpentine, mustard, acetic acid, liquor epispasticus, soft soap, too strong a solution of an antiseptic such as phenol or lysol. Cheap perfumes, used in soaps, lotions and powders, have caused dermatitis, especially at the scalp margin. Certain skins react with dermatitis after *sulphur* and many *cosmetics* in ointment, lotion or powder. Often the use of moderately strong local remedies would have produced only a simple erythema had

[1] *J. Amer. Med. Assoc.*, 1949, **140**, 139.

there not been present an abrasion or some minute vesicle. With such means of ready penetration into the skin, the traumatic agent may rapidly set up a widespread dermatitis with serous exudation. Some of the popular proprietary *shampoo lotions* contain ingredients which in certain people have set up itching and dermatitis : ammonium lauryl sulphate [1] and xylene are amongst several chemical preparations which injure some scalps. Recently I saw an elderly man whose doctor had tried many remedies for " seborrhœic dermatitis " on the bald vertex ; all in vain. The eruption had started when he began to use a new stiffening application to keep flat the few long hairs which concealed the hairless skin. Apparently the *resins* now added to these hair smoothing fluids can lead to sensitization ; many cases have been recorded. Dermatitis has been caused by the synthetic resin of hair lacquer pads ; and " hair tonics " with resorcinol have been followed by sensitization. A patch test should be made in doubtful cases. Under this heading also comes the dermatitis due to various *plants, chemical* fertilizers, lime, or frequent use of a " cold Perm ". This may have extended from the face, or the patient, whose hands are affected, may have rubbed his brow, ears or scalp. Contact dermatitis due to fumes or dust from various industrial processes often affect the hands, face and neck, and thence extend to the scalp.

The *diagnosis* is simple when there is a clear history of itching and burning a few hours after the use of a strong application or other traumatic agent ; but the patient is often quite unaware of having used anything which would do harm. For example : a patient has a scurfy, itching scalp, with a minute abrasion ; he scratches and then rubs in a remedial lotion or ointment which, unknown to him, contains some irritating or powerful ingredient. An erythematous reaction follows, perhaps even a streptococcal infection, and in a day there is lighted up an acute local inflammation of the scalp. When the dermatitis is severe, hairfall may follow, but this is uncommon.

With correct soothing *treatment*, the outlook for cure is excellent. Forbid the use of any accustomed " hair tonic," hair lacquer or other application. Do not allow washing with soap and water. Apply a soothing application such as lead lotion or simply olive or almond oil ; if the hair is short, calamine and zinc may be added. After a few days or a week the crusts and exudation may be removed with a starch poultice or with an egg beaten up in soft or rain water.

XI. The **dermatitis due to dyes** is a special type of allergic dermatitis. It may be of acute onset, with swelling, œdema and vivid erythema,

[1] BIEDERMANN, *New England J. Med.*, 1937, **217**, 1088.

sometimes even vesicles and bullæ. Or it may be of slow onset, and may be mistaken at first for " seborrhœic dermatitis " or a streptococcal condition. The history of the use of hair dyes gives the clue to the diagnosis. Often the patient at first denies all knowledge of a dye ; but close examination reveals the difference of colour of the hair shaft close to the scalp. Certain shades of dyed hair are unmistakable when the scalp is seen in a good light. In doubtful cases, a microscopical examination of the hair shaft reveals the presence of some dye. The patient's denial may be in good faith ; she may be using a hair " restorer," a hair " tonic " or " wash," without any suspicion that a dye is often present in such apparently harmless preparations. The subject of hair dyes is so important that it is discussed in a separate chapter (p. 272).

GROUP E. Certain NODULAR CONDITIONS, in their early stage, are regarded by the patient as a red rash, e.g. lupus vulgaris, lichenification of the scalp, syphilitic gummata and sarcoids. See nodular conditions, which are dealt with in Chapter XVII.

## CHAPTER XIV

## PUSTULAR CONDITIONS OF THE SCALP

Pustules may make their first appearance as pustules, as papules, or as vesicles which rapidly become pustular. They may discharge freely, or form thick yellow crusts. Both staphylococci and streptococci may be the causal infecting organism in pustular infections of the hair and scalp. Staphylococci invade the hair follicle and cause superficial or deep-seated folliculitis, with formation of pus. Streptococci prefer to travel along the epidermis, giving rise to serous exudation ; a secondary infection with staphylococci often follows up and leads to pus formation. An example of such a mixed infection is found in *impetigo contagiosa.* The sites invaded by staphylococci vary with the age of the patient. As a rule, pustules in children are found in the superficial part of the hair follicle ; in older patients, pustules tend to form in the lower part of the follicle.

The causes of pustules on the scalp, mentioned as far as possible in order of frequency of occurrence, are :

| *In Children.* | | *In Adults.* | |
|---|---|---|---|
| I | Impetigo contagiosa. | VII | Boils and Carbuncles. |
| II | Bockhardt's impetigo. | VIII | Sycosis nuchæ. |
| III | Traumatism. | IX | Acne varioloformis. |
| IV | Kerion. | X | Gummata and other nodular |
| V | Chickenpox. | | conditions breaking down. |
| VI | Secondary infection after pedi- | XI | Pyoderma (including |
| | culosis and with ringworm. | | ecthyma). |

| | |
|---|---|
| XII | Secondary infection of streptococcal dermatitis. |
| XIII | Smallpox. |
| XIV | Certain drug eruptions. |
| XV | Vegetative conditions. |

CLINICAL INVESTIGATION. When one is consulted about a pustular condition of the scalp, note, first, whether there is *erythema.* This is present when there is much surrounding inflammation, as in boils, carbuncles, kerion, ulcerating nodules, pyoderma and streptococcal dermatitis. When erythema is the predominating feature, turn to the chapter on erythematous eruptions (p. 201). When the pustular condition predominates, note, first of all, the *age* of the patient ; certain diseases are more common in children than in adults, and vice versa. At

215

a glance it is seen whether tiny discrete vesicles and patches of yellow crusts affect the face ; if so, suspect impetigo contagiosa. If the patient is an infant or a child, and many hairs pierce through a pustule, consider Bockhardt's impetigo. If there is a red swelling with holes in the skin through which pus oozes, one expects to find kerion in a child, a carbuncle in an adult. If the few lesions on the scalp are puzzling, an *examination of the body* may shed light on the subject by discovering the varied lesions of chickenpox ; or evidence of past syphilis. The *history* may be very important ; contagion at school, or in the home, may solve the problem of smallpox, chickenpox, and some forms of impetigo. Certain drugs, especially bromides and iodides, less often mercury, antipyrin and salicylates give rise to pustules. The history of X-ray epilation for fungus infection explains the semi-bald head of a child with many scattered pustules and papules. By *inspection of the patient*, an opinion can be formed as to the condition of the general health. Seek for septic foci, and test the urine for sugar ; if these are detected, the cause of recurring boils and carbuncles is clear. Is there anæmia, weakness and under-nourishment ? At all ages, in the debilitated, ecthyma and pyoderma may supervene on any previous pustular affection. In old people a superficial pustular condition may occur, resembling the Bockhardt's impetigo of childhood. In children the scalp is especially susceptible to infection with streptococci and staphylococci. Where no local cause of infection can be detected naso-pharyngeal, antral or sinus disease may be present, leading to sensitization, with pustules on the head. In such cases there are usually pustules also on the body, which yield no organisms on culture. The names of some diseases carry with them their diagnosis : e.g. sycosis nuchæ, acne varioloformis. A blood test is advisable in obscure cases. *Examination of the pus* is carried out for interest, but, except in vegetative and certain nodular conditions, it is rarely necessary for diagnostic purposes.

*A child is brought with rapidly forming, heaped-up yellow crusts, more on the face than on the scalp. Or an adult comes with bullæ and flat crusts, sometimes developing a circinate outline—the disease is usually* Impetigo Contagiosa.

I. **Impetigo Contagiosa.** On an average cursory inspection, impetigo contagiosa conveys the impression of being mainly a pustular condition on account of the heaped-up semi-transparent yellow crusts. Tilbury Fox originally described two forms of this disease : a bullous variety, seen in infancy, and the common type seen in children of school age. Of recent years another type has become prevalent ; it occurs most frequently in adults, but may also be seen in childhood. These two forms have distinctive clinical features. The usual one begins as discrete, tiny red points, rapidly becoming vesicles, affecting the superficial layer of the skin. The exuding serum in a few hours becomes turbid with leucocytes, and dries into the typical yellow crusts. When the physician is consulted, usually for the crusts, he may see freshly formed lesions passing through the brief vesicular stage. The appearance of the new vesicles can sometimes be foretold by a burning or itching sensation which leads the child to rub the site. On removal of the crust, the under-lying skin is seen to be pink or moist, with a thin layer of serum or pus ; a new crust forms as the exuding serum again dries. The lesions usually appear first on the face, most often near the nose and mouth, and rapidly increase in number ; adjacent spots coalesce to form large patches, so that the face may be almost covered with crusts. In the second type of this disease, so prevalent since the outbreak of war, the eruption shows more bullæ, which persist longer than the vesicles of the other variety. The exuding serum forms flatter crusts, and the lesions tend to develop a circinate outline. On the scalp the disease may at first pass unobserved, although it pursues the same course, with oozing serum drying into crusts. A number of hairs may remain stuck fast in the crusts ; as these drop off, after several weeks, the hairs fall also, leaving a temporary bald patch. The parents may have noticed nothing on the scalp until the bald areas developed (see p. 140).

*Ætiology.* On the face and body Impetigo may arise spontaneously, from an infected abrasion, or it may follow a discharge. The common type, affecting chiefly children, occurs most frequently in cold weather. The bullous form can occur in children, but is more frequent in adults, especially in the summer. The common form is due to infection with streptococci, usually hæmolytic, soon complicated by staphylococci. Scratching and pediculi on the scalp lead to secondary infection. In the bullous variety the staphylococcus is the primary invader ; very soon there is a secondary infection with streptococci which increases as time passes.[1]

*Course and Prognosis.* A simple case runs its course in two or three weeks. The crusts fall and the underlying epidermis looks normal in a few days. Though many small bald patches may be left on the scalp, the hair usually grows in again at once ; indeed, in some cases, a fine down is seen as soon as the crusts fall off. In severe cases, on the other hand, the disease may remain for weeks, extending to fresh regions as soon as

---

[1] STEPHAN EPSTEIN, *Arch. Derm. and Syph.*, 1941, **41**, 317, and *Wis. Med. J.*, 1941, **40**, 383.
See also full discussion in *Lancet*, 1943, **1**, 559.

the earlier lesions begin to heal. The disease may affect many children in a school—the condition popularly known as " scrumpox." When the backs of the ears and other grooves are affected, a fissure may develop, and may linger on unhealed for a long time ; from this source the impetigo is apt to go on recurring. Pemphigus Neonatorum (see p. 236) is bullous impetigo occurring in infants. Bullous impetigo is exceptionally contagious ; a whole household may be affected, and the disease may spread to any part of the body (of the original victim and his family) which has come in contact with the serum and crusts. Still another complication of severe impetigo may occur : ecthyma. In ecthyma the infection extends below the original pustular or bullous condition, and an ulcer forms below the crust ; on removing the crust, the ulcer oozes serum, blood and pus. Ecthyma appears chiefly on the body, on the lower extremities, buttocks and back. It is seen for the most part in those who have debility, who are under-nourished and exhausted, in the alcoholic or the diabetic, or in the very poor who are living in unhygienic conditions. It must be mentioned here, because it has been seen on the scalp of patients who appear to have little or no resistance. It may also be secondary to pediculosis and (on the body) to scabies. This form may appear in adults as well as in children.

*Treatment of Impetigo Contagiosa.* When the scalp is affected the crusts become entangled in the hair ; with careless nursing and low general health this may lead to obstinate and recurring pyoderma. The crusts must be removed before using any local application. Starch poultices [1] have long had a high reputation. When starch is hard to obtain use soap and water, one of the new cleansing agents (such as cetavlon), or oil and ointment with 16 grains of salicylic acid and sulphur in equal parts of vaseline and hydrous lanolin, or in an emulsifying base ; then mop over with 95 per cent. alcohol. The hair should be shaved and kept closely cut. Reports of sulphonamide sensitization, especially from countries with strong sunshine, have made dermatologists chary of ordering that group of drugs for local application. I still like 5 per cent. sulphathiazole cream for use on five nights, and Eau d'Alibour by day. Penicillin has not proved so successful as was anticipated ; it destroys

---

[1] Sir Norman Walker gave these directions for making a boracic starch poultice. One teaspoonful of boric acid, four tablespoonfuls of cold-water starch (Orlando Jones's or Colman's rice starch) ; add cold water to give the mixture the consistency of cream. Pour on a pint of boiling water ; stir the mixture constantly, until the starch bursts and a translucent jelly forms. Or pour the cream into the boiling water. When the jelly is quite cold, spread the amount required on cloth in a layer about half an inch thick ; cover with muslin and apply to the part. Renew the poultice about four times a day.

only the organisms which are penicillin-sensitive.  Recently a penicillin resistant type of infection has become common.  It is given in a spray or an ointment, and never for more than five successive days.  New bases and forms of administration and dosage are constantly appearing.  Contamination is avoided by the use of a sterilized spatula ; the lid of the container must be at once replaced after use.  Many dermatologists find that the remedies advised by H. G. Adamson in " Skin Diseases of Childhood " (1907) are of more value than the sulphanilamide group of drugs or penicillin.  Of these, ½ per cent. sulphur with 1 per cent. hyd. ammon. chlor. in a paste has stood the test of many years.  Silver nitrate 3 per cent., aqueous solution of gentian violet 2 per cent., or an ointment of equal parts of ung. hyd. nit. dil. and ung. zinci oxidi, succeed in most cases.  As a rule pastes are better than ointments because the exudation is thus absorbed.  On the face angry reactions may follow the use of mercury, but on the scalp stronger doses can be used, such as sulph. praecip. gr. 40, with hyd. sulph. rub. gr. 5 to the ounce of vaseline.  Good nursing is essential, so that the crusts are removed before the application of remedies.  Scrupulous cleanliness must be observed after apparent cure ; all may relapse if a tiny fissure is left from which the organisms may lead to reinfection.  A condition of infective eczematoid dermatitis may thus ensue, due to secondary infection.  Obstinate recurring types are described under Pyoderma (p. 227).  Pediculosis, an important and often overlooked cause of impetigo, is dealt with in Chapter X.

*A child or infant is brought with superficial pustules surrounding many of the hairs of the scalp—the most probable diagnosis is* BOCKHARDT'S IMPETIGO.

II.  **Bockhardt's impetigo** is a folliculitis affecting the superficial or upper part of the hair follicle, on the scalp or the body.  First a red papule is seen round the hair, but this has usually developed into a pustule by the time advice is sought.  The pustules increase rapidly ; a hundred or more may spring up in one night.  When the patient's resistance is low, the whole scalp may be covered with the lesions of folliculitis.  In severe cases, there are recurring outbreaks with preceding tenderness and enlargement of the occipital and cervical glands.

*Ætiology.*  Infants and young children are especially susceptible to this form of invasion of the hair follicles of the scalp by staphylococci.  The mild cases are usually due to the *staphylococcus albus*, a normal habitant of the pilosebaceous follicles, but harmless until some external traumatic agent renders it over-active.  The disease may follow rubbing and scratching, combined with the too vigorous application of some strong remedy, such as might have been used with the object of destroying fungus infection, or it may be set up by overheating and dampness of the scalp. An acute form in infants, almost the entire scalp being covered with tiny, superficial pustules round each hair, may develop with suddenness. Lee MacCarthy has seen such a condition appear in young adults after dietetic indiscretion. In severe cases the *Staphylococcus aureus* is at work ; originating from a small wound, an insect bite or sting, or a boil, the lesions rapidly extend over the scalp. Abscesses may form deep in the follicles and extend laterally.

*Prognosis.* In certain cases where the health is poor, this condition is very obstinate and recurs frequently. When fungus infection or pediculi are present, the pustular condition clears up rapidly after removal of these causal agents. In other cases the whole follicle may become infected, and when the pustules heal, after a few weeks, there are left behind small bald patches, usually transient, but in severe cases, where there has been necrosis of the dermis, the baldness is permanent, with scarring (p. 140).

The *diagnosis* is plain, but the cause may be difficult to trace.

*Treatment.* The hair should be cut short and clipped daily. The affected region should be swabbed once or twice a day with rectified spirit or absolute alcohol, then dressed with a 2 per cent. mercurial paste or lotion, or a powder, which keeps the region dry. Infants and children dread the stinging sensation of spirituous lotions, but they are effective. The pustules should be opened and painted with 5 per cent. silver nitrate or gentian violet. Tyrothricin applied locally gave promise ; streptomycin 5 mgm. per gm. of ointment base is used for penicillin sensitive cases. Epilation is the best method of cleaning up the follicles ; when the pustules cover much of the scalp, the hairs should be removed by X-ray. On Besredka's principle intradermal vaccine and special local preparations of the invading organism can be tried. Build up the health with ultra-violet light baths when an open-air life, seaside or mountain air are all out of the question.

III. **Traumatism.** Under this heading come wounds, from missiles or from falls and cuts. Less obvious causes are the application of too strong ointments and lotions ; this is especially frequent with infants and children.

IV. **Kerion** is a purple red, œdematous, boggy swelling under the skin of the scalp, with suppurating points in the skin and holes through which a sticky fluid discharges ; when the swelling is large the discharge is sero-purulent. The swelling is tender and, when large, is painful. Kerion is usually due to infection of the follicles and hairs with large- or small-spored ringworm; occasionally it accompanies favus. Kerion is generally single, but may be multiple. A generalized eruption and symptoms of toxæmia may be present when this inflammatory reaction complicates fungus infection (see p. 185). Baldness follows, but often there is no permanent scar and the hair returns.

*Diagnosis.* Kerion resembles a *carbuncle* with its multiple openings discharging pus. A carbuncle causes more pain, is full of pus, with a slough at its base, runs a definite course and is rarely seen except in an adult. Kerion is less painful than a carbuncle; the child complains of itching and burning in the early stage. With kerion, ringworm hairs are found in the swelling and there is usually evidence of fungus infection on other parts of the scalp or body. If incised, an *abscess* is full of pus, whereas kerion contains much sticky clear fluid mixed with pus.

*Treatment.* Incision is not advisable. Usually the pus loosens the infected hairs, so that they fall out and spontaneous cure results. Cure is hastened by epilation of the hairs and application of a mild antiparasitic ointment. As the ringworm is

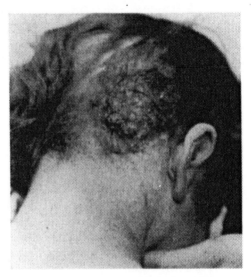

Fig. 47.—Kerion on head of a child.
(*Photograph kindly lent by Dr. L. Forman.*)

unlikely to be confined to the area with kerion, the scalp must be carefully examined and adequate measures taken (see Chapter XII).

V. The lesions of CHICKENPOX often affect the scalp. Their appearance may be preceded by marked itching. After the initial erythematous spot a vesicle quickly forms; its fluid soon becomes turbid, then purulent. After about three days the vesicles crust over and show umbilication, and often they leave permanent scars (see pp. 138 and 231). The diagnosis is made by the character of the lesions on the face and body, and by the fact that they come out in crops, so that all stages may be seen in adjacent areas at the same time.

VI. The SECONDARY PUSTULAR INFECTION following *pediculosis* is discussed on p. 154. After epilation with X-ray for ringworm it is not uncommon to see on the bald scalp many superficial pustular lesions ; pus can occur with *fungi* infections even in the absence of any secondary infection.

The following pustular conditions of the scalp occur chiefly IN ADULTS :

## VII.  **Boils** and **Carbuncles.**

The most common situation for a **boil** on the scalp is near the occipital region (see Sycosis nuchæ, p. 224).  A boil begins as a tender red papule over a deep-seated folliculitis ; the inflamed area varies in size from a pin-head to a large pea, and is usually very painful.  Occasionally the inflammation subsides (a blind boil), but as a rule the pus works upwards, the skin softens and breaks down.  In a few days a slough is discharged ; healing follows, often with a tiny scar.  When the cause lies in the blood, boils usually come in crops and may continue to appear for weeks or months.  I have seen boils appear when the scalp has been irritable ; in such cases it is probable that abrasions and infection were caused by scratching.

A carbuncle may be described as a group of confluent boils.  Hence it begins as a red, indurated, tender swelling, which soon involves the whole skin and the patient feels very ill.  After several days the boggy skin surface gives way ; pus wells out from a number of holes, and as these coalesce, a large slough is seen in the deeper layer of the skin and adjacent subcutaneous tissue ; it breaks up and is gradually discharged.  Carbuncles are frequent on the nape of the neck, but they may occur on any part of the scalp.  I have seen several on the scalp at one time ; in one severe case this followed itching of the scalp and therefore probable infection with the fingers.  Sometimes a permanent scar is left, but often the hair grows in again even after severe boils and carbuncles.

*Ætiology.*  The *predisposing* cause of boils and carbuncles lies in a lowered condition of the general health, which permits the local infection to make headway.  Of such causes may be mentioned glycosuria, Bright's disease, anæmia, septic foci, malaria and the defective metabolism which occurs in the stout and middle-aged who eat and drink too much.  The *exciting* cause of boils and carbuncles is a local infection of the deep part of the hair follicle by the *Staphylococcus pyogenes aureus.*  Rarely, *S. citreus* and *albus* are the causal organisms usually found in the milder type of infection.  The ensuing inflammatory process leads to deep-seated surrounding inflammation with a necrotic core.  Boils occur in both sexes and at any age, but they are most frequently seen in those who are debilitated or underfed and in males past middle age who are obese and over-fed. Those with a seborrhœic diathesis are less resistant to the staphylococcal invaders. The sites infected are usually those where there is apt to be lack of cleanliness of the skin or the clothing, e.g. the back of the neck, the axilla, the vulva, the buttocks and the anus. Where compresses have been used, and the general resistance is low, the local infection readily extends to neighbouring follicles and thus causes crops of boils in the vicinity.

*Treatment* must be both general and local. *General* : The patient should be thoroughly examined and any causal factor dealt with. Sinus trouble, septic teeth, gall-bladder, and residual jaw infection may be unsuspected septic foci. Every possible means must be taken to raise the general health. Diabetes must be appropriately and promptly treated. Except in the aged or diabetic, general ultra-violet light baths are usually of great value. Alcohol and sugar must be severely restricted, and constipation corrected. Abnormal intestinal conditions should be corrected with appropriate diet, antiseptics or bacillus acidophilus. Penicillin was the favourite agent for curing and aborting boils and carbuncles when it came into general use after the war. Some physicians have returned to older remedies, such as yeast, dilute sulphuric acid (m. 20 t.d.s. after meals), stannoxyl and calcium sulphide. Three or four injections of manganese butyrate or colloidal manganese, given at three-day intervals, often yield dramatic success. Edwenil is now unfortunately no longer manufactured. Penicillin is valuable when the organism is penicillin sensitive : 100,000 to 200,000 units are injected every eight hours. The dosage and the method of administration is under constant revision. For carbuncles give 200,000 units injected intramuscularly twice daily for five to eight days ; similar dosage in oil is not so successful.[1] Vaccines are still advised ; 30 million of stock staphylococcus aureus may abort a boil ; for recurring boils give a course of autogenous vaccine. Failure occurs when too large doses are given. Never increase dosage when reaction results. Intradermal vaccine and autohæmotherapy aid obstinate cases.

*Local.* Penicillin spray or cream, absolute alcohol, weak tincture of iodine, 2 per cent. gentian violet, and ichthyol can be used, on and around the inflamed area. The surrounding skin is thus treated because staphylococci are in most cases present in the follicles adjoining the active lesions. Inunction with thyothricin is on trial. Pure ichthyol and ultra-violet light, up to an erythema dose, may abort and aid the recovery of boils and carbuncles. These and other forms of acute inflammation can also be aborted by suitable small doses of X-ray, filtered through

---

[1] S. GOLDWATER, *Brit. Med. J.*, 1947, i, 309.

aluminium ; for details of technique, X-ray manuals should be consulted. Short-wave diathermy and the Kromayer lamp have given good results in expert hands. Boils should not be treated with hot fomentations or poultices, nor be incised before the pus is pointing ; instead of a knife, some employ the diathermy spark or the cautery for this purpose. The area must be immobilized ; for this purpose an occlusive plaster dressing is recommended. Some surgeons still excise carbuncles, but conservative treatment is now advised ; this is especially necessary when the carbuncle attacks the cheek, lip or head. When pus is visibly pointing, incision not only aids its exit but relieves the pain and tension which are so marked in these cases. When a boil or a carbuncle is freely discharging, it should be dressed with a saturated solution of magnesium sulphate, or of 10 per cent. ichthyol, in glycerine, or with the hypertonic (10 per cent.) solution of salt which proved of so much value in septic wounds. Boils and carbuncles must not be squeezed ; this merely injures the weakened adjacent tissues and vessels and spreads the infection. When surgery is indicated the necrosed core should be removed as a whole. Local applications with Besredka's staphylococcal antivirus used to be much employed.

VIII. **Sycosis Nuchæ,** as the name implies, is a disease in which pustules occur at the nape of the neck, in the form of folliculitis or boils. At the beginning, a few pustules occur round hairs on the neck ; these heal, leaving cicatrices which are thick and hard to the touch. The pustules recur from time to time. Sometimes also sebaceous cysts form, with pus around them.

*Ætiology.* The disease is due to an infection of the hair follicles of the neck and adjacent scalp, usually by the *Staphylococcus aureus.* It is seen chiefly in middle-aged men, especially when they have an oily skin ; when they are stout ; when they eat and drink too much ; and when they have a septic focus.

*Course and Prognosis.* As the malady has its origin in some faulty condition of the general health, and is usually neglected at first, it may continue, with remissions, for years. The pustules may extend to the occipital region of the scalp. In time, over the infected region are seen raised bands of hypertrophic scar tissue, pierced by a few sparse hairs and orifices from which deep-seated pus wells up. At this stage the condition is known as DERMATITIS PAPILLARIS CAPILLITII or ACNE KELOID, from the resemblance of the hypertrophic scar to true keloid (see p. 140).

*Treatment.* Cleanse the skin twice daily with soap and water and then rub over with a weak solution of iodine 1 per cent. in rectified spirit.

Use a lotion with sulphur, half a drachm to the ounce of spirit and water, Eau d'Alibour, or an ointment with 3 to 10 per cent. mercury or a similar percentage of sulphur. Washing over with cetavlon, which is effective against the staphylococcus aureus, is very useful. Avoid friction with the clothing ; the collar must be worn low. As in the case of boils, the general health needs attention. In the stout and middle-aged man the diet must be restricted. Substitute fruit and alkaline mineral waters for farinaceous food and alcohol. In the early stage intradermal vaccines are of value here as in other pustular conditions. X-ray, zinc ionization and ultra-violet light are all of use in skilled hands. Acne Keloid requires X-ray ; see section on scar tissue (p. 140).

IX. **Acne Varioloformis** (Syn. : Acne Necrotica) is the descriptive title given to a somewhat uncommon disease. It is due to a follicular pustule, with necrosis of varying degree, of the follicle and perifollicular tissue. Hence a hair is always present in the centre. Indurated papules are seen scattered chiefly over the forehead and adjacent scalp, especially along the hair border. Sometimes it also occurs on the face and chest, and occasionally on other parts of the body. Itching is a marked feature in the early stage. Slowly the papules become vesico-pustules, with an umbilicated centre topped by a reddish-brown crust. The crust forms so soon that the pustular stage is often missed. After about a week the inflammation decreases and the crust is thrown off, with the central hair, leaving a superficial ulcer and later a scar. If the pustule is scratched the appearance of the lesion is proportionately modified and complicates diagnosis. There may be left a permanent small or a large oval and pitted scar (see Fig. 42). The condition usually continues, with intervals of freedom, on and off for years.

*Ætiology and treatment.* The initial papule surrounds a hair ; in the follicle microbacilli have been found, with staphylococci (usually *S. aureus*) above. These findings do not explain the presence of the itching nor the cause of the disease. It is said to be more common in stout men about 50 years of age ; but I have seen it also in young men and in women from the ages of 18 to 50. Sometimes it appears to be due to alimentary toxæmia ; sometimes, in the thin and fatigued type of patient, to a septic focus. Teeth, tonsils and sinuses should be examined ; in women, the cervix is too often forgotten as a source of sepsis. When the patient belongs to the plethoric type, cut down sweets, farinaceous foods and alcohol ; for a time, the result is usually striking. Locally, mild antiseptics are effective : such as equal parts of ung. hyd. nit. dil. and ung. zinci oxidi ; or resorcin gr. x, or sulphur gr. xxv to the ounce of soft paraffin. In America ung. hyd. ammon. chlor is recommended. Others

H.S.                                                                                                          I have reported benefit from staphylococcal vaccines, oil of cade and a course of ultra-violet light. (See also p. 151.) Penicillin can be tried. Local treatment remedies the active lesions, but to prevent recurrence the general health has to be investigated and treated along the lines above indicated.

X. GUMMATA and OTHER NODULAR CONDITIONS breaking down. Before the introduction of the arsenical treatment of early syphilis it was

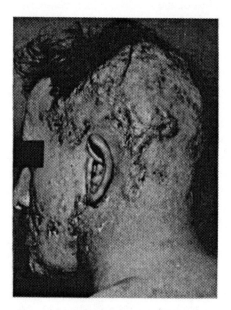

FIG. 48. Acne conglobata (Perifolliculitis abscedens et suffodiens.)
(*Photograph kindly lent by Dr. Hamilton Montgomery.*)

quite common to see gummata in the late stage, i.e., many years after the original infection. They not infrequently occurred on the smooth skin above the outer side of the frontal bone, and spread thence, invading the scalp. The nodule had a dark, coppery red colour, and ulcerated later, with the characteristic " punched out " steep edge of a syphilitic ulcer (p. 254). These ulcers often extended deep, even to the bone. Late syphilides may also produce frambœsiform swellings, with granulations and thin pus (see p. 254).

Nodules due to other diseases may appear on the scalp, and when these ulcerate cause a sero-purulent or a purulent discharge. Of such may be mentioned *iodide* and *bromide* eruptions, *mycosis fungoides* and *malignant growths. Actinomycosis, blastomycosis* and *sporotrichosis* rarely, if ever, appear on the scalp. In actinomycosis the pus has yellow granules which are typical, but all these fungi infections may defy diagnosis before examination of sections, or growth on culture. Except in the case of a gumma, it is rare indeed that any of the above-mentioned nodules affect the scalp alone. *Acne conglobata* (Fig. 48) is described on page 140. *Sebaceous cysts* which have grown to a fair size may be injured by the brush and comb, and a certain amount of pus may form outside the cyst. When this leads to exudation of the contents of the cyst the pus is mixed with sebaceous matter, and has a characteristic unpleasant odour (see p. 252).

XI. In conditions with generalized **Pyoderma** the scalp also may be affected. The infection may originate from a neglected latent source, such as a retroauricular streptococcal dermatitis ; secondary invasion with staphylococci follows. Superficial ulcers may form under thick

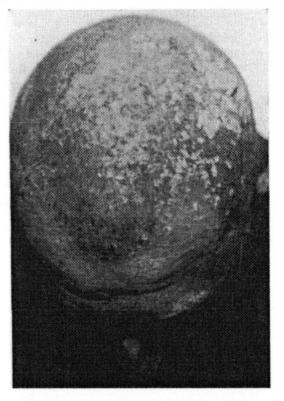

FIG. 49.—Chronic pyogenic infection of the scalp. In this case there was similar infection on many parts of the skin of the body, and a discharge from various cavities.

(*Photograph kindly lent by Dr. H. W. Barber.*)

crusts ; this condition is known as **Ecthyma**. Folliculitis and loss of hair are then apt to ensue (Fig. 49). Ecthyma occurs in debilitated patients, in the old or the young who suffer from neglect, dirt and malnutrition, with consequent lowered resistance. Pediculosis, traumatism and herpes zoster are common portals of entry of infection. Streptococcus pyogenes is the usual infecting agent, but staphylococci also may be the original organisms.

*Treatment.* Remove the local cause and use antiseptic measures similar to those employed for Impetigo Contagiosa (p. 216). Where the general health does not respond to diet and tonics such as quinine, iron and strychnine, an open air life at a seaside or mountain resort should be advised. When change of environment is impossible, ultra-violet light aids the young patient ; for older people give a prolonged course of autogenous vaccine.

XII. STREPTOCOCCAL DERMATITIS has a cloudy exudation which may be invaded by staphylococcal organisms. But, as a rule, the staphylococci only gain a temporary foothold and cause a certain amount of folliculitis. The acute form of the disease is described under erythematous eruptions with exudation (p. 207) ; the chronic form is dealt with under scaly conditions (p. 176).

XIII. **Smallpox** is rare and unlikely to affect the scalp alone. The vesicles become pustular about the ninth or tenth day of the disease ; the constitutional symptoms are usually marked. The distinguishing features are described under Chickenpox, p. 232.

The *diagnosis* is made by the presence of the eruption on the face and the body, and by the general condition. Varioloid (modified smallpox) must also be borne in mind.

XIV. DRUG ERUPTIONS are not uncommon on the scalp, especially in the case of infants. They are described under nodular conditions (p. 248), bullæ (p. 234), and vegetative conditions (below).

XV. **Vegetative Conditions.** Vegetative growths with heavily granulating surfaces, oozing with pus and serum, readily bleeding, sometimes with crusts, may develop on the sites of other lesions such as impetigo, pemphigus, iodide and bromide eruptions. All those conditions may appear on the body, face or scalp. On the legs, groins and body they frequently extend over a considerable surface. They are often readily amenable to simple antiseptic dressings. In obstinate cases the granulations should first be scraped (Bauwens), then zinc and copper ionization administered. It must not be forgotten that the later syphilides may develop this type of granulomata ; O'Donovan relates the case of a pustular syphilide of the scalp which had been treated for a year as impetigo, before its true nature was recognized. Where drugs are suspected, and are discontinued, the rapid healing of the lesions confirms the diagnosis.

## CHAPTER XV

## VESICULAR AND BULLOUS CONDITIONS

Some forms of skin disease belong especially to the scalp, e.g. various types of scaling, of erythema, of oily secretion and disease of the hair shafts. Other forms of skin disease may attack equally the scalp and the body, e.g. lupus erythematosus, seborrhœic dermatitis and pustular folliculitis. Vesicles and bullæ show a serous exudation situated in the epidermis ; vesicles are under 0·5 cm. in diameter ; bullæ are larger. They differ from the scaly and the erythematous skin diseases in that they are more common on the body and face than on the scalp. Therefore, when vesicles and bullæ are seen on the scalp, it may not be possible to make a diagnosis until the body has been examined.

### VESICULAR CONDITIONS

The following points are helpful in enabling one to form a diagnosis : Several of the diseases described in the chapter on the Erythematous conditions of the scalp show vesicles at one time or another, but the vesicles in these cases do not form a prominent feature. Vesicles occur in the early stage of ECZEMA, but on the scalp they are rarely seen before they break and exude serum, and they are accompanied by erythema and crusts. Hence eczema of the scalp is described in the chapter on Erythematous conditions (p. 210). Most cases of so-called eczema of the scalp in the adult have been found to be due to streptococcal or other form of dermatitis. A vesicular stage occurs in Varicella, Smallpox and, for a few hours, in Impetigo. DERMATITIS due to dyes, certain drugs, burns and strong rubefacients such as turpentine and croton oil, may show vesicles, with profuse serous exudation, as part of the general inflammatory condition. A few minute, discrete, soon-broken and crusted-over vesicles occur on the scalp in a condition, characterized by itching, which is described under acne necrotica miliaris on p. 151. Both vesicles and bullæ are present in DERMATITIS HERPETIFORMIS, which often invades the scalp, but on the scalp the eruption is only a part of that complex and widespread disease.

FALLACIES in the diagnosis of vesicles should receive brief mention. Hyperidrosis, excess of perspiration, should not be confused with serous exudation (see p. 81).

The rare conditions hydrocystoma and lymphangioma usually occur on the brow and may extend to the margin of the scalp. They may readily at first be mistaken for vesicles.

HYDROCYSTOMA usually occurs on the face and forehead. It shows deep-seated pin-head to pea-sized, firm vesicles, without any surrounding inflammation. It is due to a dilated duct of the sweat gland. The lesions often subside in cold weather, and appear in conditions of warm moist heat.

LYMPHANGIOMATA are white or pink, translucent swellings, formed of lymphatic vessels. They are not infrequently associated with vascular nævi. LYMPHANGIOMA CIRCUMSCRIPTUM forms thick-walled vessels which appear in groups.

Apart from the diseases mentioned in the introductory paragraph, vesicles form a *prominent* and *diagnostic* feature in I. HERPES ZOSTER ; II. CHICKENPOX ; and III. ANTHRAX.

**Herpes** (Syn., Herpes Zoster, Shingles) is an acute malady which, according to recent research, is slightly contagious. The eruption is often preceded by a day or two of malaise, slight fever and glandular enlargement, and often marked tingling and pain which later may be severe. Herpetic vesicles develop in one or more groups along the area of distribution of a sensory nerve root, and may occur on any part of the body. When the first division of the fifth cranial nerve, the supra-orbital or the ophthalmic branch, is involved, the vesicles are seen on the brow, the eyelid, the nose or the eye, and extend on to the hairy scalp. Herpes starts as a red patch or cluster of red papules which soon become vesicles. For a few days fresh groups form, or discrete, outlying vesicles may appear in the vicinity, or at a distance ; occasionally even on the opposite side of the body. The group of vesicles has a characteristic appearance, thin-walled, of uniform size, closely set together, usually small, but occasionally large as a pea. They contain clear serum which in a day or two looks opalescent. After a few days, sometimes without oozing or rupturing, the vesicles dry up, leaving crusts.

*Diagnosis.* Herpes is rarely difficult to diagnose. It is usually unilateral, and its root distribution simplifies diagnosis. The clear, close-set vesicles on a red base resemble no other skin disease. In severe cases, scars may be left, and thus cause bald patches with atrophy (see below).

*Course and Prognosis.* As a rule, a herpetic eruption has run its course within a fortnight. In a mild case, itching or tenderness on brushing or combing may be the first symptom to draw attention to the presence of the eruption on the scalp. Even in mild cases it is not unusual to find several fine scars when the cluster of vesicles has healed. In severe cases the vesicles become hæmorrhagic, or they slough and leave permanent and marked scars (see p. 142). When the patient is elderly and does not have complete rest in bed until the vesicles are healing up, severe pain may continue long after the eruption has gone. Complications are facial or ocular paralysis and destruction of part of the eye tissues. *Ætiology.* Herpes zoster occurs at any age, and in both sexes. Certain cases appear to be caused by a virus which affects the posterior spinal root ganglion and the corresponding ganglia of the cranial nerves. Apparently in some cases the virus is the same as that of varicella ; there is now abundant proof of the relationship of the two diseases. Other organisms, such as streptococci, appear to have played a causal part, and tuberculosis and syphilis have been definitely implicated in certain cases. Tumours, growths and inflammatory exudates involving the posterior root ganglia may all cause herpes zoster. In other cases the eruption is due to chemical poisons ; many cases were seen during the epidemic of arsenical poisoning which occurred in 1901, due to drinking beer contaminated with arsenic. Arsenical injections have caused herpes ; so also have other drugs, such as mercury and bismuth.

*Treatment.* In simple, uncomplicated cases, a dusting powder of talc or zinc oxide is all that is necessary. Complete rest in bed and skilled nursing are required for severe cases. The herpes which attacks adults who have escaped chickenpox in childhood is apt to be severe. Cut the hair and protect the vesicles. Liver and dekadexolin injections frequently administered hasten recovery. Recently success is claimed for aureomycin and terramycin.[1] For the pain pethidine, veganin or other analgesics are usually required. Quinine aids some greatly. For severe pain the galvanic current affords the most relief, when the positive pole is placed over the painful area. The electrode is of fine netting, and the padding has several layers of thick gamgee tissue. The negative pole should be on the arm or shoulder of the same side. Very slow turning on and off of the current is an essential feature of good technique. Some patients do best with a strong, others with a mild current (i.e. 50 milliampères or 15 milliampères for forty or twenty minutes) three times a week. Deep X-ray to the posterior nerve roots is also effective, in small repeated doses, as originally introduced in France for intractable sciatica —the so-called radicular therapy. Autohæmotherapy and pituitary extract injection ($\frac{1}{2}$ to 1 c.c.) given daily till the pain subsides have aided obstinate post-herpetic neuralgia. Marked exhaustion remains after the rash has gone.

II. **Chickenpox** (Syn., Varicella) is an acute contagious disease ; its

---

[1] Binder and Stubbs, *J. Amer. Med. Assoc.*, 1949, **141**, 105. But see Carter, *Brit. Med. J.*, 1951, i, 987, and ii, 1485.

eruption shows successive crops of vesicles, usually accompanied by slight exacerbations of fever. The rash consists of pink, slightly raised, ovoid papules, which in twelve to twenty-four hours become vesicular. The vesicle is at first thin-walled and translucent, containing a clear fluid, which after a day or two becomes opaque and cloudy. The vesicle dries up and its crust separates within ten days or a fortnight ; rarely leaving much scarring. The distinctive eruption comes out in successive crops, therefore different stages of the rash are seen on the same area of skin. The rash starts on the chest and neck, and spreads to the body, including the face and head, but it is sparse on the distal ends of the extremities.

*Diagnosis.* The following table, taken from Savill's *Clinical Medicine,* gives the chief points of distinction between chickenpox and smallpox. For a book which deals only with the hair and scalp, there is in the table sufficient information to render unnecessary any further description of smallpox. It must not be forgotten that Varioloid (modified smallpox) has been mistaken for chickenpox, because its constitutional signs are so mild.

| *Varicella.* | *Smallpox.* |
| --- | --- |
| No symptoms before rash. | Three days before rash, sudden onset of illness with backache. |
| Soft pink papules becoming vesicular. | Shotty papules becoming vesicular or pustular. |
| Chest, neck and trunk, fewer on face and limbs. Rash is centripetal. | First on the face and wrists ; more on limbs than on trunk. Rash centrifugal. |
| *Successive crops,* and thus find small papules beside vesicles of various sizes. | *All one stage* (papular or vesicular, or pustular) at one place. |

*Ætiology.* Varicella is a disease of childhood, but may also affect adults. It occurs in epidemics.

*Prognosis.* Chickenpox is usually over in a week or ten days, but it may, especially in adults, be followed by considerable weakness. Death may follow a confluent attack. Complications are few, the chief being impetigo. Hæmorrhage into and between the vesicles, and from the mucous membranes is rare.

*Treatment.* Itching is generally the chief trouble ; this is relieved by sponging with a lotion of phenol, 1 in 20. The child should be prevented from scratching the vesicles, as this leads to suppuration and consequent scarring which, on the head, causes characteristic bald patches with atrophy (p. 141).

III. **Anthrax** (Syns., Woolsorter's Disease ; Malignant Pustule), not infrequently occurs on the back of the neck and the adjacent part of the scalp, when an infected hide has been carried on the shoulder. At the site of invasion by the anthrax bacillus, after one to four days' incubation period, a papule appears and becomes a vesicle or bulla in a day. This breaks, oozing blood-stained serum or pus, and about the fourth day shows a gangrenous black slough ; around it is a zone of intense inflammation, with a ring of red vesicles ; pustules may also be present. Œdema extends for a considerable distance, and pus may form about the tenth day. The adjacent glands enlarge and may suppurate. Often only moderate pain is experienced. Constitutional symptoms may be slight, or severe, with high fever and prostration as other lesions develop on the skin or in the internal organs.

*Diagnosis.* The disease is now rare, but its early stage must not be forgotten. At first it may be mistaken for an insect bite, then later for carbuncle or erysipelas. The dark gangrenous slough is distinctive. The patient's occupation should set one on the track of anthrax infection. Wool-sorters and tanners are especially liable. At one time the disease was conveyed by cheap shaving-brushes imported from foreign sources, where the disease was more prevalent. Butchers and those dealing with cattle have also been victims. The bacillus is not always detected in smears taken from the lesions.

The *prognosis* varies with the position ; it is more serious when it occurs on the neck and face, when several lesions are present, when there are severe constitutional symptoms, and when treatment has not been instituted early.

*Treatment.* Locally, use penicillin and antiseptics. Systemic penicillin in large doses 1 to 4 million units intramuscularly or intravenously is so valuable that Sclavo's anti-anthrax serum (100 c.c. at start) is now reserved for cases where penicillin has failed.

## BULLOUS CONDITIONS

Owing to the presence of strong hair, it is difficult for bullæ to form on certain scalps, yet many of the bullous diseases which affect the body may also affect the scalp. In some of these diseases the bulla is not a prominent or frequent feature, and the malady is therefore described in another section. Always examine the body and make a *thorough medical investigation* when bullæ are present.

In IMPETIGO CONTAGIOSA large bullæ may show. This type used to be quite rare and is very contagious. The disease is described in the section on pustular conditions (p. 216).

STREPTOCOCCAL DERMATITIS not infrequently develops large bullæ when it occurs on the limbs. It is possible that such may occur on the scalp with an uncomplicated and severe streptococcal infection (see p. 207). More often there is seen on the scalp itself only oozing and crusts, and the bullæ appear on the face and body. The following case illustrates this point :

In 1926 I saw a man of 43 with serum oozing profusely over a large part of the scalp ; his thick hair was clogged with crusts and scales. At the margin of the scalp were a few small bullæ. As he had an evening temperature of 99° to 100°, he was put to bed and watched by a skilled practitioner who kept me informed of his progress. Every day during the following week fresh erythematous patches with rapidly forming bullæ appeared on the limbs and chest. Examination of the organs and excreta gave no clue to the cause of his condition ; but an examination of the blood revealed marked hypoglycæmia. With rest, mild antiseptic dressings and suitable diet, with plenty of glucose, he recovered in a month ; there was no recurrence before he died, ten years later. Soon afterwards I had under my care a middle-aged woman with hypoglycæmia. I could find no other cause for her widespread erythe-mato-vesicular rash ; the scalp also was involved, showing many vesicles and crusts. She made little progress until suitable treatment, with large doses of glucose, was instituted.

The history of those patients proves the importance of a thorough medical investigation when bullæ are present.

Bullæ may be seen on a patch of ERYSIPELAS, or may arise on the inflamed areas caused by the BITES and STINGS of insects such as mosquitoes, wasps and horse-flies. In severe HERPES ZOSTER, I have seen the vesicles run together and form large bullæ.

Bullæ may develop after strong RUBEFACIENTS, which have been used with a therapeutic object in view. Thus, for example, very large bullæ, with comparatively little surrounding erythema, may develop a few hours after a bald patch of alopecia areata has been painted with liquor epispasticus. Blistering doses of ULTRA-VIOLET LIGHT may give rise to bullæ situated on an inflamed congested base. When the dermatitis due to DYES is very severe, bullæ may be present at an early stage. Bullæ may appear with an IODIDE ERUPTION, which not infrequently invades the face and scalp. It is especially apt to take on a bullous form in children ; in the adult, a pustular condition is more usual. This eruption may be difficult to diagnose when it is not known that the patient is taking iodide. I recall having seen, when I was a medical student, a deplorable case, a woman who had been taking a popular and widely advertised " blood tonic," which contained potassium iodide. Bullæ may also appear with BROMIDE eruptions, but pus and granulomata are more usual. Both eruptions subside when the drugs are discontinued, the bromide more slowly than the iodide. See also page 260, where the papilliform and fungating nodular forms of drug eruptions are dealt with. A bullous condition may follow the administration of the sulphonamide group of drugs, the barbiturates, occasionally even mercury and quinine. When phenobarbitone (luminal) has been taken, as often ordered, over a prolonged period of time, many forms of rash may be seen, from scarlatini-form erythema to bullæ, with fever and generalized erythrodermia.

In addition to the above-mentioned forms of acute dermatitis, which sometimes have bullæ, the presence of bullæ forms a *prominent and a diagnostic feature* in the following diseases :

    I   Dermatitis Herpetiformis.
   II   Pemphigus.
  III   Bullous Syphilide.
  IV   Pemphigus Neonatorum.
   V   Epidermolysis Bullosa.

**I. Dermatitis Herpetiformis** has a polymorphic eruption, presenting on an erythematous base, and at the same time, papules, vesicles and bullæ, sometimes also pustules. The disease has relapses of varying severity which continue over many years. Itching is so intense that it forms a diagnostic feature. The eruption may affect any part of the body, tends to be symmetrical, and to occur in patches or groups. Pigmentation may follow. Even the scalp and the mucous membranes of the mouth and throat may be involved ; but in some patients the scalp, face, palms and soles escape. The fresh outbreaks may be accompanied by gastro-intestinal disturbance, and each crop lasts about a week to a month. Yet the general health often remains good, provided the intense irritation does not lead to prolonged insomnia.

*Prognosis.* The disease continues for years, but can sometimes be held in check by treatment, so that the attacks are less frequent and intense.

*Diagnosis.* Pemphigus causes much difficulty in diagnosis ; some believe that transitional forms occur ; a prolonged period of observation may be necessary.[1] In pemphigus the bullæ have as a rule no preceding erythema ; itching is rare, and the general health suffers more.

*Ætiology.* The disease is more frequent in men. The cause is obscure ; some believe it is due to a virus.

*Treatment.* Arsenic has for long been the most reliable drug ; it is still used, especially in the form of Fowler's solution or Asiatic pills, when sulphapyridine in small doses has not controlled the malady. Arsenical medication must be watched if it is taken for long, but cancerous development in these patients is rare. Andrews found benefit from vaccines made from the stool organisms which had given skin reactions to previous tests. Lumbar puncture relieves itching. Autohæmotherapy and autoserum therapy relieve itching in many cases. Adequate vitamin intake must be ensured. Rest in bed is advisable during acute outbreaks.

[1] GRANT PETERKIN, *Brit. J. Derm. and Syph.*, 1951, **63**, 1. A. ROOK and WHIMSTER distinguish these diseases by the histology of the bullæ, *Brit. J. Derm. and Syph.*, 1949, **62**, 443.

Locally, the hair should be cut ; precipitated sulphur ½ drachm, with oil of cade 1 drachm to the ounce of vaseline, is a valuable application. Lotions, powders and spirit suit best when bullæ form.

II. **Pemphigus** is the chief bullous disease. It may appear on any part of the body. Though comparatively rare, every form of pemphigus —bullous, foliaceus and vegetative—may affect the scalp. The large crops of bullæ coming out over extensive areas of the body, the absence of erythema and itching, the frequent involvement of the buccal mucous membranes, with increasing ill-health and prostration, all are characteristic of this malady. The physician will not be consulted for the scalp in a disease so widespread over the body. As the disease is usually fatal, arsenic in many forms is justifiable : germanin and stovarsol have prolonged many lives. The new antibiotics are now in favour and have had many successes. In bullous conditions keep the hair short, and it is a good rule to use powders and lotions rather than ointments.

III. A **bullous syphilide** used to be not infrequently seen with congenital syphilis. The infant might be born in a marasmic condition, with various cutaneous manifestations of congenital syphilis ; or the skin lesions might appear within a few weeks or months of birth. The bullæ of congenital syphilis are usually symmetrical in distribution ; they may be small or large, usually flaccid, with blood and serum contents. They contain many spirochætes. They usually appear on the buttocks, palms and soles, and on the lower limbs, but may be widespread, in which case they also affect the scalp. They are situated on a reddish-brown base and soon ulcerate. The prognosis is grave. To save life, anti-syphilitic treatment must be prompt and thorough.

IV. **Pemphigus Neonatorum** is bullous impetigo affecting the newly-born within four to twenty days after birth. Although rare, the disease is of much importance because it so often runs a fatal course. The rash begins with vesicles and bullæ which come out in crops in one region until, probably by contact, rubbing or chafing of the delicate skin, they begin to spread all over the body, including the face and the scalp. Crusts rarely form.

*Prognosis.* In mild cases the bullæ cease to appear in about three weeks and heal in the fourth week. In severe cases they continue, and as they rupture, a widespread exfoliative dermatitis sets in, usually with fatal result, the infant dying with profound toxæmia.

*Ætiology.* For over thirty years there was dispute regarding the cause, whether it is of streptococcal or of staphylococcal origin. Tilbury Fox, Sabouraud, Gilchrist, Whitfield, Adamson and others found that streptococci are the usual cause of bullæ. In many bullous diseases, after the initial streptococcal infection, the secondary invasion of the serum by staphylococci occurs so rapidly that only by the most delicate technique can the presence of streptococci be detected. Staphylococci usually lead to a pustular infection of the follicles, rather than to the infection of the epidermis which forms bullæ. Pemphigus neonatorum is a form of bullous impetigo, which falls into two groups, one due to staphylococci, the other to streptococci. Recent investigations prove that both streptococci and staphylococci may be responsible for outbreaks of epidemics of pemphigus neonatorum. The infection reaches the infant by direct contact, being conveyed by those of the personnel of the nursery or the hospital who have a septic sore, such as a suppurating finger, a purulent discharge, or *S. aureus* in the throat or nasal secretions. Investigation of an outbreak of the disease in a maternity ward revealed the presence of various strains of staphylococcus pyogenes in the noses of many of the nursing staff, of the healthy infants, and in the blankets, bedding, gowns, dust and air of the nursery. The infecting reservoir lay apparently in the noses of the nurses and thence spread to their hands and to the skin of the infants.[1]

*Diagnosis.* Bullous *chickenpox* is rare and there is a history of contagion. The differentiating points of the *bullous syphilide* have been described above.

*Treatment* is largely preventive. As the fatal infection has been sometimes conveyed by doctors and nurses with boils and whitlows, it is of the utmost importance that no one in charge of an infant or of its linen or furnishings is suffering from a septic wound of any kind. In mild cases quite simple antiseptic dressings and powders have been effective. Open the bullæ and apply 2 to 5 per cent. argent. nitrate to the base, especially the periphery under the loose epidermis. Then paint over with 2 per cent. gentian violet, and dust with a powder containing bismuth subgallate and boracic acid, āā gr. 60, in one ounce of talc. Or use sulphadiazine or sulphathiazole for 5 days 5 per cent. in powder, jelly or cream ; or 3 per cent. mercurochrome. In streptococcal cases sulphanilamide can be used both by mouth and externally, but watch lest sensitization occur. Penicillin is used when the infecting staphylococci are penicillin sensitive. Great care must be taken to prevent undue friction when rubbing or drying ; skin abrasions form fresh portals of entry for the organisms.

V. **Epidermolysis Bullosa** is a hereditary condition which may affect many members of a family. It usually starts in infancy or early childhood, but sometimes may not appear till later in life. Painless bullæ form below the horny layer within an hour or so after the skin has received the slightest blow or knock. Even the mild degree of traumatism caused by the pressure of the clothing is sufficient to raise the bullæ. Provided no infection takes place, these bullæ subside. The parts of the body most affected are, naturally, those exposed to traumatism, such as the elbows and knees, hands and feet, even the mucous membrane of the mouth. In one form of epidermolysis bullosa, bullæ are continually appearing on areas exposed to the slightest pressure or traumatism, and the affected areas gradually become covered with atrophic scars. The lesions frequently appear on the scalp. In cases with obscure lesions on the body, the fact that the scalp shows bullæ and scarring may lend important aid in diagnosis. In some cases of congenital alopecia (Chapter VII), epidermolysis bullosa has also been present.

As regards *treatment*, protective dressings on exposed regions are indicated. In certain cases, ergot and endocrine therapy have given good results.

---

[1] ALLISON, V. D., and HOBBS, BETTY, *Brit. Med. J.*, 1947, **2**, 1.

## CHAPTER XVI

## DEFECTS OF THE HAIR SHAFTS

Certain conditions of the hairs themselves, apart from the scalp, present definite, distinguishing characters, which are readily recognized by the naked eye or with the aid of a lens.

These conditions are :

|      |                                      |
|------|--------------------------------------|
| I    | Trichorrhexis Nodosa.                |
| II   | Fragilitas Crinium—Trichoptilosis.   |
| III  | Monilethrix.                         |
| IV   | Trichonodosis.                       |
| V    | Plica Polonica.                      |
| VI   | Idiopathic Trichoclasia.             |
| VII  | Trichokinesis.                       |
| VIII | Trichomycosis nodosa.                |
| IX   | Trichostasis Spinulosa.              |
| X    | Progressive kinking.                 |

The broken hairs of RINGWORM, the " exclamation " hairs seen with ALOPECIA AREATA and sometimes after X-RAY and THALLIUM EPILATION, the short and coiled hairs seen with FOLLICULAR DISEASES, have been mentioned under their respective leading symptom in other chapters.

Their differentiating features are shown in the accompanying illustration, Fig. 50. The " exclamation hair " of alopecia areata may or may not have a root sheath attached ; the root and the adjoining part of the shaft is atrophied and lacks pigment ; the free end is deeply pigmented, club-shaped, and may be pointed, but often has the frayed appearance of trichorrhexis. The " exclamation hairs " which may occur after epilation with X-ray and thallium acetate are very similar to those of alopecia areata, but the free ends are usually less club-shaped. The hairs of Brocq's pseudo-pelade usually have an attached sheath ; the root and adjoining part of the shaft is pigmented and has an irregular outline, as if it had been pressed upon and modified by the causative inflammatory process.

Below are described those few conditions in which the hair shafts show characteristic modifications. MONILETHRIX is also mentioned under baldness (p. 136) and keratosis (p. 183) because in some of the patients, at first sight, it is the absence of hair and the keratosis which strikes the observer. Of the ten conditions mentioned above, Trichorrhexis

FIG. 50.—A. " Exclamation hair " from
case of alopecia areata.  Note atrophied
root, thin and depigmented lower part
of shaft, and swollen and pigmented
free end.  The free end is often frayed.

B.  " Exclamation hair " after X-ray
treatment.  Atrophied root, pale and
thin shaft and usually a normal appearance of the cut free end.

C.  Hair from case of pseudo-pelade.
Note attached sheath, irregularity of
the shaft and root.  The free tip often
lacks pigment, but the shaft has
normal degree of pigmentation.  (After
Sabouraud.)

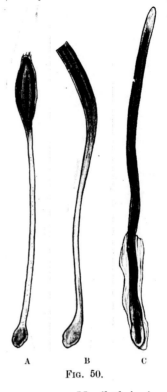

A            B            C
FIG. 50.

Nodosa and Fragilitas Crinium are very common ; Monilethrix is uncommon, and the remaining four are rare.

I.  **Trichorrhexis Nodosa** is a condition of the hair rather than
a disease.  Nodes are seen, grey, white or dark, along the shaft of the
hair, especially at the distal end.  Several nodes may be present on one
hair.  They can be felt as rough swellings on the hair.  Under the microscope the nodes are seen to be regions where the hair shaft is split.  The
splitting up of the shaft occurs in such a way that it looks as if the bristles
of two brooms were so placed that they faced and interlocked with each
other.  Heaped-up masses of pigment granules are seen where the hair
shaft branches.  If the hair is drawn down at the position of the node, it
remains bent at that angle, having no elasticity to enable it to return to
its natural straight line in a normal manner.  Or the hair may break off
or split up when the node is brushed, combed or knocked.  Trichorrhexis
nodosa may affect the hair of the head, beard, moustache or pubis.  The
condition is often seen when women have the hair bleached with peroxide

of hydrogen ; then a number of hairs near the temples may look as if covered with little grey pearls.

*Ætiology.* Trichorrhexis nodosa was first described in 1853, and during the ensuing years many descriptions appeared in medical journals and in the reports of medical societies. The condition was attributed to many diseases, even to a special type of bacterial invasion of the hair shaft. Early in the century the brilliant dermatologists of the French school traced the cause to be mechanical traumatism, acting on hair which has been rendered too dry and brittle with over-frequent washing, especially with strongly alkaline soaps. H. G. Adamson [1] independently came to the same conclusion. The same condition is often seen in shaving-brushes, not necessarily very old ones. Hair which is frequently washed with soap, which contains soda, and especially soft soap which contains potassium, is liable to become affected, because strong alkalis weaken and can dissolve the hair cells. When the hair is thus rendered fragile, slight traumatism, such as occurs with brushing and combing, even rough drying with a towel, can cause injury sufficient to lead to trichorrhexis nodosa. Dyed hair is especially susceptible to this form of injury. Sabouraud pointed out that many of the alkaline hair washes and lotions in common use, even those prescribed by physicians, are liable to cause both trichorrhexis and trichoptilosis. A familiar example is the popular hair lotion which contains strong ammonia ; this should never be employed over a prolonged period of time. As already mentioned, bleaching the hair with hydrogen peroxide has often apparently caused trichorrhexis nodosa ; this may be due to the ammonia with which hydrogen peroxide is usually combined.

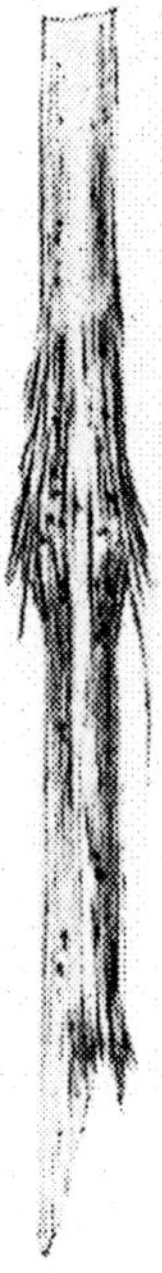

Fig. 51.—
Trichorrhexis
nodosa.
Sketched
from an
actual hair.

*Diagnosis.* The diagnosis can present no difficulty. Although at first sight the grey or white nodes have been mistaken for the ova of pediculi, the breaking off at the node, on pulling the hair, is characteristic of trichorrhexis nodosa, and the microscope shows an unmistakable picture (see Fig. 51).

*Treatment* consists in the avoidance of the cause and in the free use of oil until the hair has grown afresh. For the sake of appearances, the hair may be cut off above the region of the node.

[1] H. G. ADAMSON, *Brit. J. Derm.*, 1907, **19**, 99

II. **Fragilitas Crinium** and **Trichoptilosis** have often been described separately, but appear to be identical. Fragilitas Crinium is a condition in which a number of hairs are so dry and brittle that their shafts split. The splitting is often seen at the free ends of the hairs, but it may occur higher up. There may be so many splits that the hair shaft looks like a tree with many fine branches ; a severe form with the divided ends turning up along one side has been compared to the feathered top of a quill pen. The simple form used frequently to be seen when the hair was worn long ; many of the free points were so affected that the end of a long tress of hair showed a greyish hue.

*Ætiology.* When long hair is worn, splitting of the hair occurs when the general health is below par. It is often seen after all kinds of fevers, in cases of anæmia and chronic toxæmia due to a variety of causes. Before 1914, when hair was usually worn long, I used often to see it associated with an unhealthy state of the scalp in women who had apparently normal health, especially when there was a marked degree of pityriasis sicca. Anything which causes dryness of the hair can lead to breaking of the hair. Thus the use of alkalis, dyes, and too frequent washing tend to cause splitting of the hair. Twisting, curling and rough combing, used singly or together for cosmetic purposes, can all result in splitting of the cortex of the hair. Hence it is especially seen on the hair over the brow and temples. At the present time, with the prevalence of the permanent wave, splitting of even quite short hair is common, because the free ends are too dry. Fig. 23 shows the fraying of the cuticle which can occur after a badly-executed permanent wave.

Some have described an *idiopathic* form of fragilitas crinium, in which no disease, local or general, can be found to account for the splitting of the hair. The breaking of the shaft is at the free end, the middle, or it may even occur at the bulb. The long split parts of the hair may curl up or branch out and break off. Even the short hairs of the beard may show splitting. When women comb the long hair thus affected, thin broken parts of the hair shaft break off. Many years ago I watched a severe form occurring in two sisters, who had very long hair with a natural wave. They had never had the trouble before. I never discovered the cause. They said they had never injured the hair with excessive washing, brushing or combing. Stimulation of the scalp in these cases with ammonia and cantharides increased the brittleness of the hair, even although an ointment was freely used on alternate nights. Treatment with oil and massage brought about a steady but slow cure. The oil was thoroughly rubbed into the scalp and also along the free ends of the hair.

*Diagnosis.* When ringworm or favus *fungus* invades the hair shaft, splitting of the shaft is common, but it occurs where the hair breaks off, close to the scalp, and cannot be confused with the simple splitting of the free end of a long hair. The microscopic examination settles the point if any difficulty in diagnosis occurs, as might happen in the case of the splitting of very short hairs.

*Treatment.* Any disease of the scalp which is present must be treated, and consideration of the general health should never be omitted. Oil should be used freely on the split ends of the hairs, and all causal agents must be avoided, such as alkalis, spirit lotions which bring about dryness of the hair shaft, too frequent or erroneous permanent waving methods, and excessive washing. When girls wear long hair, the unsightly split ends can be cut off. Unless oil is used, however, and the state of the scalp is improved, cutting will not cure, because almost at once there appears a splitting of the new free ends. Massage and friction of the scalp play an important part in improving the circulation and therefore the nutrition of the hair in these cases. It is useless to singe the free ends ; splitting soon occurs higher up the hair shaft.

*The patient, usually a child, comes on account of baldness since the first hair fell out. There is keratosis on the bald area and the defective hairs show characteristic beading. The disease is* MONILETHRIX.

III. **Monilethrix** (moniliform hair) is a condition in which the hair shaft shows nodes or swellings with intervening constrictions ; thus the hairs have a beaded appearance. The hairs break off readily at the thin atrophic portion, which is very fragile ; this may occur even within the follicles.

The usual history given by the parent is that the child was born with apparently normal hair, most of which fell from the scalp after six weeks, whilst the eyebrows and eyelashes remained normal. No normal hairs have grown in again, and the region with defective or absent hair is extending. The hairs are seen broken off near the scalp and the denuded area feels rough to the finger, because at the site of each hair is a conical projection, which is sometimes slightly red, sometimes more like " goose skin " or keratosis pilaris. The condition is most marked near the neck, over the occipital region (see Fig. 52), where the bald area showing rough scaly papules usually begins ; the few hairs present on it are about an inch long. Sometimes an extensive area of the scalp is involved, causing widespread baldness.

*Prognosis.* Monilethrix has a natural tendency to disappear about the age of puberty. Sometimes the disease undergoes spontaneous improvement, the keratosis diminishing as the years pass ; in such cases there may be short hairs of irregular lengths all over the head.

The *diagnosis* is not difficult if the physician is aware of the existence of this rare disease. At first sight he may mistake it for *ringworm*, but on closer examination he sees that the scaly elevations are not due to the epidermal heaping up of scales invaded by fungus, but to keratosis pilaris. The family history aids the diagnosis, because several members are usually affected similarly ; the microscopic examination of the hair reveals the characteristic beaded appearance (see Fig. 53).

*Ætiology.* Although the disease is rare, the physician who sees one case

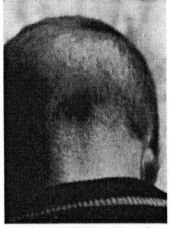

FIG. 52.—Monilethrix. Shows loss of hair and horny cones at mouths of follicles.

(*Photograph kindly lent by Dr. Goodwin Tomkinson.*)

will soon meet with a number, because monilethrix usually occurs in several members of a family. Both sexes are affected equally. The condition usually appears after the normal first hair of the infant has fallen, about the sixth week of life, but cases have been recorded in which it began in youth and even in adult life. Sabouraud found seventeen cases in five generations of one family ; McCall Anderson reported fourteen cases in six generations ; Dr. Goodwin Tomkinson found twenty-two cases in five generations of one family. The condition appears to be due to some defect in the development of the hair ; no micro-organism has been found associated with it. One theory of causation is the existence of a rhythmic pulse of increase and retardation in the rate of growth. Alternate constrictions and swellings in the wall of the hair follicle have been seen ; the illustrations of Dr. Goodwin Tomkinson's case shows this very clearly

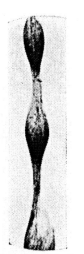

FIG. 53.—Monilethrix. Shows beaded shaft.

(*Microphotograph kindly lent by Dr. Goodwin Tomkinson.*)

(see Fig. 54).[1] A healthy woman of twenty-one was shown at the Royal Society of Medicine in 1949. Her brittle dry hair had never been cut ; its length was 10 to 15 cm.

[1] J. GOODWIN TOMKINSON : *Brit. Med. J.*, 1932, ii, 1009.

*Treatment.* The patient usually goes from hospital to hospital, from doctor to doctor. The usual remedies for keratosis, sulphur and

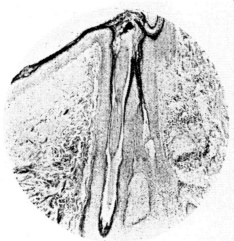

salicylic acid, should be given fair trial together with frequent washing, in order to remove the keratosis. Deep massage, together with stimulating lotions and oily applications to the hair and scalp, is advisable. Epilation with X-ray brings about temporary improvement, and cases have been recorded of permanent improvement, even cure, after several epilation doses given at safe intervals. Few dermatologists see enough of these patients to be able to carry out or to test methods of treatment for a reasonable length of time.

FIG. 54.—Section of scalp with monilethrix. Shows constriction in follicle and in hair shaft within follicle.

(*Microphotograph kindly lent by Dr. Goodwin Tomkinson.*)

IV. The name **Trichonodosis** means knotted hair. The hairs appear short, but on examination are found to be knotted just above the mouths of the follicles. Directly the hair has shown above the surface of the scalp it becomes knotted or looped. There may be one or more knots on each hair. The hairs are usually dry and tend to split or have brush-like ends. The condition is usually traumatic in origin, as from rough tugging with broken combs or stiff brushes. Scratching of the scalp, the use of alkalis, frequent washing, hot irons or other causes of dryness of the hair, all contribute towards the formation of knotted hair. It may affect all the hairs on the body as well as those on the scalp. It is said to occur chiefly in hairs which have a flat transverse section ; such hairs curl over more rapidly than do normal round hairs.

This rare condition was described by Galewsky[1] in 1906 ; and by MacLeod[2] in 1907. Possibly the tendency to curl and loop may begin in the follicle and root ; see Fig. 59, of a condition I have often seen with regrowth of hairs after electrolysis or frequent plucking.

V. **Plica Polonica** is the name given to describe a condition in which the hair is matted together in coils or masses, of various thicknesses and lengths, occurring close to or at some distance from the scalp. The felted mass of hair may be covered with dust and dirt, and often also pediculi.

[1] GALEWSKY, *Arch. Derm. u. Syph.*, 1906, **81**, 195.
[2] J. M. H. MACLEOD, *Brit. J. Derm.*, 1907, **19**, 40.

The scalp itself may be normal, but if the plica is near the head the surface of the scalp is moist and has a rancid smell. When the clotted hair forms one long mass, it is called *plica caudiformis*, because it has the appearance of a tail. With shorter hair, many coils may form, to which the descriptive name " caput medusa " has been given. Several observers have noted the formation of the *plica neuropathica*. In such cases the matting of the hair occurred after illness, or in hysterical women, and took the form of tangled lumps or tails which developed rapidly and could not be unravelled.

*Ætiology.* The condition was formerly believed to be a disease, but Hebra discovered that it was due to deficient care of the hair. Any disease of the scalp aids the formation of plica. It used to be common in Poland, where there was much uncleanliness of the head, and where disease of the scalp was aggravated by the custom of wearing tight fur caps. In some of the neuropathic cases, microscopic examination of the hair showed that the cuticle of the shaft was torn from the cortex and split up ; hence the tendency of adjacent hairs to adhere together and form a thick mass.

*Treatment.* The plica should be cut off. The scalp is soaked in oil, carefully washed and thereafter brushed and combed daily. Directions must also be given regarding the destruction of lice (see p. 155).

VI. **Idiopathic Trichoclasia.** Sabouraud described under this name a rare condition ; he had seen only eight cases in forty years. On the vertex or the brow are found one or more almost bald, oval areas, small or large. On examining closely one finds that all the hairs are present, but broken off, usually about 5 or 6 millimetres above the skin. The hair root is healthy ; the free end is split, presenting a brush-like appearance, like the broken node in trichorrhexis nodosa, but forming close to the scalp, with the remainder of the hair shaft broken off at the node. The areas extend, and may remain stationary for a long time before the hair begins to grow normally again. The condition might continue for a year, and recur again after several years. The microscopical appearance is not that of cut hair. In some cases the skin was lichenified and intense irritation was present. The condition occurs in both sexes and may appear at any age. Sabouraud was not convinced that the condition was due to traumatism, but scratching might be a cause.[1] Trichoclasia appears to resemble the cases described by Bowers : his patients had been over-vigorous in massaging the scalp (see p. 96).

VII. **Trichokinesis** (Twisted Hair ; Pili Torti [2]) is a rare condition in which the hair shaft is twisted throughout its length, usually at regular intervals, but some may be longer than an adjacent part. The hair has a shimmering appearance, owing to the reflection from the twists. The patient is usually born without hair and it remains short when it begins to grow. The scalp is dry, often scaly, sometimes with hyperkeratosis. Sometimes no hair is seen till the child is one or two years old. The alternating dark and light spindle-shaped swellings, the short shafts and the keratosis

---

[1] The case exhibited in June 1935 by Dr. W. N. Goldsmith, at the Dermatological Section (Roy. Soc. Med. London), was probably an example of this condition.

[2] GALEWSKY, *Arch. fur Derm. u Syph.*, 1935, **75**, 173 ; ORMSBY and MITCHELL, *Arch. Derm. and Syph.*, 1920, **12**, 146 ; RONCHESE, *Arch. Derm. and Syph.*, 1932, **26**, 98.

make the condition so like monilethrix that the two maladies are readily mistaken. In some patients the eyebrows and eyelashes are affected. The hair may grow longer after puberty. Montgomery's patient recovered in three years.

Astbury and Hellier have reported on the X-ray of the molecular structure of the Twisted Hairs.[1]

*Ætiology.* The disease may occur in several members of a family ; and the same person may have both monilethrix and twisted hair. The hereditary factor of ectodermal defects is seen ; ichthyosis may be found in other members of the family. No cause has been traced. For some unknown reason only fair-haired people seem to be affected. When the twists bear some relation to the monthly amount of hair growth, ovarian dysfunction has been suspected.

VIII. **Trichomycosis Nodosa** (syn. **Lepothrix**, Fig. 55) is a condition in which hard nodules adhere to the hair shaft associated with a fungus of

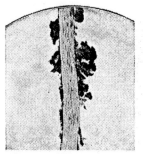

FIG. 55.—Trichomycosis Nodosa.

which there are several forms. On the pubis and the axillæ red or yellow concretions occur when washing is infrequent and perspiration prevented from evaporating by woollen clothing close to the skin. In native women in South America it affects the scalp and in men the scalp, beard, moustache and eye-lashes. The nodules may be as minute as the head of a pin, oval or round, adhering to or surrounding the shaft like a collar. They are usually dark brown and hard, like a stone ; hence the name *Piedra* (a stone). Combing the hair may therefore be a noisy process. The hair tends to split in their neighbourhood. Under the microscope, after having been softened by soaking in liquor potassæ, the nodules are seen to consist of fungus spores encased in a viscous matter.

*Diagnosis.* The condition must be distinguished from the nits of pediculi, which is simple ; but the type of fungus is difficult to determine.

*Ætiology.* The red and yellow concretions affecting the axillæ and pubis may occur in any social class and nation. The hard nodules known as *black piedra* are found in South America, East Indies, Java, and Cochin China. *White piedra* occurs in South America, Europe and Japan. The sticky substance used by natives for dressing the hair encourages fungus contamination.

*Treatment.* As the removal of the nodules is difficult, it is best to cut off the hairs. Afterwards, use a mild anti-parasiticide and keep the hair free from sticky dressings.

IX. **Trichostasis Spinulosa** (Pinselhaare) is a condition seen in some persons, usually over fifty years of age. Black dots are visible on the vertex, brow, nape of the neck, the cheeks and the upper part of the back and chest. On close examination these are seen to consist of short hairs in groups emerging

[1] *Brit. J. Derm. and Syph.*, 1940, **52**, 173.

from a single follicle mouth choked up with horny matter like follicular keratosis. The hairs may be few, five or six, or as numerous as fifty ; they are usually lanugo hairs a few millimeters long, with rounded, tapering free ends, and bulbous roots held together in an encasing horny plug.

*Ætiology.* Various causes have been adduced in an attempt to explain the presence of so many hairs in one follicle, with hyperkeratosis. No inflammatory reaction is found in the adjoining tissues, but the region is seborrhœic. The condition is possibly less rare than has been believed.

X. **Progressive kinking** of the Hair (Woolly Hair). A few cases of kinking, leading to an appearance as of woolly hair, have been reported.[1] The condition was an acquired one, affecting only part of the scalp. The hair was also altered in colour. The shafts were very thin, deeply pigmented, and the ends were split. The cause is unknown.

---

[1] WISE and SULZBERGER, *Arch. Derm. and Syph.*, 1932, **25**, 99 ; SANDERS, *Genetica*, 1936, **18**, 97 ; C. P. SCHOKKING, *J. Hered.*, 1934, **25**, 337.

# CHAPTER XVII

# WARTS, SWELLINGS, NODULES AND TUMOURS

The patient may come complaining that there is a swelling on the scalp. Many surgical conditions may, in their early stage, be regarded by the patient as a swelling or tumour. A consideration of such would take us too far afield for a dermatological text-book. Here will be passed in review only those swellings which are connected with the skin of the scalp. The most common of such is undoubtedly a wart. In such a case, very often the patient arrives with the diagnosis already made, either by himself or by one of the relatives. Warts and their treatment are therefore dealt with first, on p. 249.

INFLAMMATORY SWELLINGS are for the most part described under pustular and erythematous conditions, in their respective chapters. The cutaneous manifestations of SYPHILIS come within the category of erythematous eruptions and also of swellings, and are therefore described under both these headings. CARBUNCLES, KERION, inflamed CYSTS and TUMOURS show swelling, erythema and often alopecia.

BROMIDE and IODIDE ERUPTIONS may appear on the head, especially in children ; they usually develop granulomatous swellings with thin pus. In both adults and children, bullæ may also appear, especially with iodides. The fixed eruptions, usually raised red plaques, due to certain drugs, may cause difficulty in diagnosis ; of these may here be mentioned phenolphthalein, cinchophen (atophan), phenobarbitone (luminal) and other barbiturates. Other similar swellings on the face, body and legs are usually present, and these assist the diagnosis ; so also does the history of taking the drug.

GROUP A. SWELLINGS which have a VERY CHARACTERISTIC APPEARANCE ON THE SCALP are :

    I   Verruca.
    II  Sebaceous cyst.
    III Epithelial cysts.
    IV Tertiary syphilis, especially a gumma.
    V  Vascular nævus.

GROUP B. Certain nodules apt to become MALIGNANT, or ALREADY MALIGNANT, are :

    I  Rodent ulcer.
    II Epithelioma, primary and secondary.

III Sarcoma.
IV Meningioma.
V Carcinoma of the sweat glands.

GROUP C. Nodules and tumours which may affect the scalp and, in the majority of cases, are diagnosed by the presence of SIMILAR LESIONS ON OTHER PARTS OF THE BODY : a list of these is given on page 259.

GROUP D. This includes several rare conditions which are described on page 264.

I. **Warts** are not uncommon on the scalp; therefore they are described before the other causes of swellings, nodules and growths.

The WARTS (verrucæ) which affect the body may attack the scalp ; some only at its margin, others on the vertex. These are :

The small, PLANE or " juvenile" wart, is occasionally found on the margin of the scalp or even on the scalp itself. They are smooth, skin-coloured, slightly raised, flat or dome-topped, small, with angular margins and almost a glossy surface. Though usually seen in children, they can also occur in adults. In men they may affect a large area of the chin and cheeks, probably being carried by the shaving-brush.

*Treatment.* Magnesium sulphate internally is the usually recommended remedy, and certainly appears to help some cases. Ionization with a magnesium or zinc salt succeeds when each wart is pricked and the drug introduced under the positive pole. Diathermy fulguration is successful, and has less danger than X-rays ; in expert hands, however, X-ray gives excellent results when there is a group of warts. Others prefer to use carbonic acid snow, but this causes considerable, though temporary, reaction. Locally, to prevent extension of the warts, it is advisable to use a lotion of mercury in spirit, e.g. hyd. biniod. gr. ½ in an ounce of absolute alcohol.

The ordinary wart, VERRUCA VULGARIS, such as is often seen on the hands, can infect the scalp and face. On men between thirty and fifty years of age the digitate type of common wart is not uncommon on the scalp. They appear to spread in groups, on the chin, cheeks and scalp, as if carried by the razor and shaving-brush on the face and the brush and comb on the head. The warts may coalesce into rough patches. Because they originate in the deeper layers of the skin, they can be very troublesome ; the comb and brush catch in the rough tops of the warts and bleeding ensues.

*Diagnosis.* Senile Keratoses and verrucæ are described with clinical and histological illustrations by Sachs and others.[1] Two rare conditions may be mentioned here.

EPIDERMODYSPLASIA VERRUCIFORMIS is a rare disease, usually affecting the backs of the hands and feet, occasionally the face and the scalp. It is really a nævus, which begins in infancy or about puberty. It resembles a cluster of verrucæ planæ which have formed a plaque. In later life it may become malignant.[2]

ACROKERATOSIS VERRUCIFORMIS (Hopf) is a form of epithelial nævus which is very rare ; it may occur on the scalp, but is more often seen on the palms and soles as well as on the backs of the hands and feet. Clinically, it is like a plaque of flat warts or keratoderma.[3]

Both diseases are distinguished by the history of onset in early life, resistance to treatment and by the histological appearance.

*Treatment.* The warts must be destroyed. X-ray is effective, but the dose which is sufficient to destroy the wart will also epilate the hair. When the warts are few in number, a good method of dealing with them is to transfix the base with a zinc needle attached to the positive pole, and pass a current of 1 to 2 ma. for two minutes. The wart dries up and falls off. When the warts are numerous, each wart must be pricked with a sterile needle ; then a large pad, soaked in 2 per cent. zinc or magnesium sulphate is placed so as to cover the whole group, and the current used is proportionately larger. The drug is driven in from the positive pole. Diathermy fulguration or the galvanic cautery can also be used ; Sabouraud used the latter. The last mentioned methods of treatment are painful ; if there are a large number of warts, this must be taken into consideration when choosing the method of treatment. A local anæsthetic is usually necessary ; procaine, novotux or other similarly acting drug may be injected intradermically ; the warts can then be dug out with a curette. Fuming nitric acid provides another method for the destruction of warts, but unless it is skilfully applied severe scarring may result. Care must be taken to prevent the acid flowing on to the adjacent skin ; for this purpose oil or vaseline may be smeared round the base of the wart. A small quantity of cotton-wool is tightly twisted round a sharp-pointed wooden stick, which is dipped into the acid. The point is continuously and gently pressed on the top of the wart, but *only for a few seconds.* After the fluid has been absorbed by the wart another application may be made. In about a minute the wart looks yellow and coagulated, and becomes painful ; no more acid should be applied that day. A few

[1] *Arch. Derm. and Syph.*, 1949, **59**, 179.
[2] WAISMANN, MORRIS and MONTGOMERY, H., *Arch. Derm. and Syph.*, 1942, **45**, 259.
[3] MONTGOMERY, H., *Minnesota Med.*, 1935, **18**, 735.

days later, the top of the wart is a hard crust ; when this falls off, the wart may be gone. With very large warts, two or three applications may be necessary. Not a single wart must be left, or a fresh set will soon form ; this is so discouraging that it is wise to warn patients that the course of treatment may be lengthy. Other acids can be used : trichloracetic and glacial acetic or phenol followed by nitric acid. A moistened stick of silver nitrate rubbed in vigorously twice daily destroys most warts.

The *Senile wart* used to be called the flat seborrhœic wart. It does not have any connection with seborrhœa. It may appear in elderly people, on any type of skin. The wart usually appears first on the face, but may originate on any part of the body. Few develop on the hairy scalp itself, but often on its margin, especially on the temples. On the bald scalp of old people many small warts may develop near a large one. Beginning as a small, round or oval, rough macule, the wart becomes slightly raised and extends along the skin surface ; its surface is ridged rather like a papilloma. Adjacent warts join, to form quite a large disfiguring patch with a characteristic surface—yellowish grey or dark brown, almost black in colour, with a thick crusted surface which is easily scraped off, but it soon forms again. This type of wart does not undergo malignant transformation (see p. 249).

*Treatment.* The thick surface may be softened by using strong salicylic ointment (90 to 120 grains to 1 oz.) for a few days. It is then easily scraped off, and the base can be destroyed by fulguration with diathermy or by the galvanic cautery. Scrape off gently the charred remains of the wart. Sabouraud for thirty years obtained excellent results with the cautery used at white heat for the thick warts, and at less high temperature for the thinner warts. If the white heat cautery is used it is apt to be too hot ; when the finger scrapes off the black residue a white stain below indicates that a scar will be left. It is advisable to use only a dull red heat till one has attained the expert's skill in using the cautery. In modern days diathermy is preferred.

*Methods of Diathermy Fulguration.* The destructive spark may be obtained in several ways. (1) A needle in an insulated handle is attached to one terminal of the machine. The operator brings it near the edge of the wart till a fine spark is seen. Then he turns off the current and pushes the needle in to the base of the wart, approaching the middle from several angles. The current should be turned off before the needle is removed, and turned on when introduced again in a new position. The operator keeps up a gentle but steady pressure, so that the wart is gradually loosened ; often it is suddenly raised up, leaving a moist, bleeding or charred surface. A boracic acid ointment dressing is applied and fixed by zinc oxide plaster or elastoplast.   In a week or ten days the base should have healed.   (2) In another method the patient holds a metal handle attached to one terminal of the apparatus, and sits on the condenser couch, or on a plate attached to the other terminal.   The operator approaches with the insulated needle, which is earthed, either by a wire to a gas pipe, or simply by the operator standing on an uncarpeted floor, and holding in his bare hand the metal of the needle ; this provides the means by which it is earthed.   An air cushion is placed in a convenient position, so that the operator will not touch the patient whilst he carries out the sparking as in the first method.   It is useless to try to destroy the top of the wart if it is dry and hard ; hence the need to undermine it by passing the needle through its base.   (3) Diathermy coagulation (see below) is not advisable for the destruction of warts on the scalp. Except for insensitive subjects, local anæthesia should be used with all these procedures.   Procaine may be injected intradermically, or Bonain's solution [1] painted over the part.

As terminology varies, it is well here to explain the methods of destruction by diathermy which are employed in dermatological procedures.   *Surgical diathermy, diathermy* or *electrocoagulation* destroys tissue by causing coagulation of the part.   There is œdema, inflammation, and a slough separates off, leaving a fine scar.   In both forms of treatment the indifferent electrode is placed at some convenient part of the body, or a condenser couch may be used.   The active electrode is a needle, a button or a disc.   The needle is introduced under the skin, the button or disc are placed in close contact, with slight pressure.   The current is not turned on before such preparations have been made.   With *electrodesicacation* (or *fulguration*, is it is termed in Europe) the active electrode is usually a needle which is not placed in contact, but a short distance from the surface ; when the current is turned on, sparks fly to the skin and char the part.   This blackens and falls off, leaving no mark.   Full details can be studied in the classical volume of Cumberbatch,[2] a pioneer of diathermy in Britain.

These types of swelling merit special consideration : the SEBACEOUS CYST ; the EPITHELIAL CYST ; the TERTIARY SYPHILIDE (less frequently seen since the introduction of arsenical medication) and the VASCULAR NÆVUS.

II.   **Sebaceous Cysts** are common in youth and early middle age. They form round or oval swellings in or below the skin, hard or soft according to the condition of the sebaceous matter within.   On the scalp

---

[1] Bonain's solution consists of cocaine hydrochloride, menthol, phenol, āā 4 gm., adrenalin ·0004 gm. in glycerine, 1 oz.

[2] " Diathermy," by ELKIN CUMBERBATCH, Heinemann, London, 3rd edition, 1937.

one or several may be present.    Careful examination shows the tiny opening of the sebaceous gland, black or grey ; probing the orifice or pressure on the swelling causes the sebaceous, cheesy-looking contents, smelling unpleasantly rancid, to ooze out of the follicle.    Apart from showing a degree of hairfall, the skin over the cyst may be normal, so that the swelling may cause no trouble for years ; then one day the cyst begins to enlarge and the skin above it becomes inflamed.

*Diagnosis.*    A *fibroma* and a *lipoma* may at first be mistaken for a sebaceous cyst.    However, there is no central orifice through which sebaceous matter can be squeezed.    The lipoma feels elastic and may be lobulated.    Both can be moved under the skin.    They can be excised if causing trouble by pressure.    *Epithelial cysts* are described below.

*Treatment.*    The cyst should be excised in entirety.    After bringing about local anæsthesia with an injection of novocaine and adrenalin, make an incision along the surface of the skin.    With fine forceps the cyst wall is gripped and pulled up, and if possible the cyst is dissected out whole.    Care must be taken to remove the entire wall of the cyst, or it will fill up again with sebaceous matter.    If any part of the wall is left behind, twist a little cotton-wool round a fine wooden stick or probe, and with this rub in tincture of iodine ; then apply strong pressure over the part.    By this method the opposing sides of the inflamed inner wall very often adhere and prevent the cyst filling up again.

III. **Epithelial Cysts** may develop in middle life on the scalp as well as on the face and the body.    They appear as single or multiple painless small nodules, movable with the skin and varying in size up to about a centimetre.    They are diagnosed from *sebaceous cysts* (for which they have long been mistaken) by their greater firmness on palpation, the absence of the orifice and, on puncture, none of the characteristic cheesy secretion of the sebaceous cyst.    The histological appearance at once distinguishes them.[1] They enlarge slowly and usually follow a benign course.    If malignancy develops it is of the squamous cell epithelioma type.

*Treatment* consists of excision if in an inconvenient site, or when malignancy threatens.

IV. *Severe, late or* **tertiary syphilis** is not often seen to-day. The nodular or tubercular syphilitic eruption can appear on any part of the body.    Usually there are few lesions, concentrating on one region of the body.    A common position is on the forehead, at the margin of the scalp.    The nodules are large, infiltrated, flat, and of dark coppery-red hue, smooth or with a slight scaly collar, occurring in groups, often with circinate margin or forming the segment of a circle.    If untreated, the centre becomes depressed, pigmented and atrophic, and new nodules

[1] W. LOVE and H. MONTGOMERY, *Arch. Derm. and Syph.*, 1943, **47**, 185.

appear around. They may ulcerate below crusts, and when healed leave irregular cicatrices. Pustular crusted lesions may also be present, and mistaken for pyoderma. Apart from the blood test, the diagnosis is made by the characteristic dark coppery-red colour, the hard infiltration and the circinate outline of the lesions which have undergone serpiginous ulceration. As a rule there is no itching, and progress is comparatively rapid. All forms and stages of severe syphilitic eruptions may occur on the skin adjoining the scalp.

Another late syphilitic eruption is the **Gumma** ; it forms a swelling which may grow to be the size of a small walnut. When a gumma appears on the head, its usual position is on the frontal bone ; I have seen them on the occiput also. The swelling reddens, darkens, then forms a deep, steep-edged ulcer, with a sticky, bloodstained discharge, and, if untreated, with a yellow slough reaching to the bone. Several may develop together over a large area. Gummata used to be frequent on the scalp as well as on the body, but they are rarely seen since the introduction of the arsenical treatment of syphilis. *Frambœsiform swellings* may cover the scalp ; these are mentioned amongst the pustular conditions (p. 226). Large *vegetative* growths may be seen on the scalp as elsewhere ; their possible connection with an iodide eruption must not be forgotten, especially as the patient may have been taking potassium iodide.

The *diagnosis* is not so easy to-day as in the days when every student was well acquainted with the appearance of all forms of late syphilides, including gummata. There is no difficulty in diagnosis when other forms of syphilitic eruption or the scars of former syphilitic manifestations are present elsewhere on the body, when there is a clear history of infection and a secondary rash, or after the comparatively rapid formation of the crusted, serpiginously spreading ulcers. The ulcer of a gumma is circular, and has a characteristic, punched-out, steep edge ; before the ulcer develops, the swelling may be mistaken for sarcoma or sarcoid. The serum reaction is often absent in late syphilis. As Sabouraud expressed it, " the eye of the experienced clinician is the best diagnostic aid." The treatment of syphilis is too complex to be considered at all adequately in a volume dealing with diseases of the scalp.

V. The **Vascular nævus** or **Angioma** is congenital, or appears soon after birth, and is due to hyperplasia of vessels of the skin and, in certain types, of the subcutaneous tissue, either alone or in combination with the more superficial form. Angiomata are of various extent, from a pin point to several inches diameter. They are vivid red, purple or dusky in hue, flat, or raised above the level of the surrounding skin.

The flat nævus is described under alterations of colour of the scalp (p. 268). Angiomata may occur on any part of the body and often on the scalp. The RAISED or HYPERTROPHIC NÆVUS shows purple swellings with a lobulated surface ; it can be compressed, but immediately swells up again. It is inadvisable to leave it, as local injury might cause dangerous hæmorrhage. Sometimes these two types of nævi occur together as localized raised, "red currant" or "raspberry" looking swellings on a large port wine stain. The CAVERNOUS NÆVUS arises from the deeper tissues ; it is lobulated, often deep purple, sometimes with interspersed areas of almost normal skin, or it may be situated so deeply that the overlying skin is white.

The *diagnosis* is usually simple, except in the case of the deep-seated cavernous nævus in infants, before the bones of the scalp have united. To the palpating finger the cavernous nævus conveys the sensation of a sponge under the skin. It enlarges when the venous pressure rises, as when the infant is crying.

*Treatment.* Many methods of treatment have their respective advocates. Unless they are actively spreading, the modern teaching is that nævi should be left alone. The majority of nævi tend to disappear spontaneously, few grow after the infant is eight months old. Carbon dioxide snow used to be a popular means of destroying the slightly raised angiomata of medium size. The stick of snow was trimmed to cover the whole of the nævus ; then held in contact, with strong pressure, for about forty seconds. The inflamed part was kept free from contamination until healed ; this took a few weeks. The scar which remained was white and firm. The snow method is not to be advised for a nævus on the scalp of an infant before the bones have united. Even in an older child, this method should be reserved for the nævi near the margin of the hairy scalp ; in view of the proximity of the meninges, the danger of infection is too great. Another method was the injection of one of the solutions employed for dealing with varicose veins on the leg ; with quinine and urethane I have seen excellent cosmetic results. In the case of infants, injections are inadvisable near the sutures. The galvanic current is a satisfactory means of destroying raised vascular nævi. General anæsthesia is required ; with one or several zinc needles attached to the positive pole, and the indifferent pole placed on any convenient region of the body, a current is passed till the whole part is blanched. X-ray and Thorium X have succeeded with selected cases.

Diatheramy coagulation is not advisable on the scalp, especially of an infant ; diathermy fulguration also is not given for the raised and cavernous nævi. Cumberbatch pointed out that with diathermy fulguration the surface has to be destroyed, whilst with the galvanic current the skin is destroyed only at the points of entry of the needle ; and even these small scars can be reduced to vanishing-point if the needles are insulated with enamel at the skin-level. Fulguration, *in skilled hands*, produces an excellent result, with a fine scar, in small-sized raised and cavernous nævi. The expert arranges that only the spark, and never the needle point, touches the nævus. If the needle touches the nævus, charred tissue comes away when it is removed, and severe bleeding may follow.

For cavernous nævi, radium, excision or contact therapy with X-ray are the methods of choice. With the last-named the exposure is brief and easily performed by a skilled radiologist. Other forms of radiation are to be expected in the near future.

GROUP B. Certain nodules apt to BECOME MALIGNANT, or ALREADY MALIGNANT, are :

    I   Rodent Ulcer.
    II  Epithelioma, primary and secondary.
    III Sarcoma, primary and secondary.
    IV  Meningioma.
    V   Carcinoma of the sweat glands.
    VI  Moles and Nævi (see pp. 264 and 271).

I. A **Rodent Ulcer** (Basal cell epithelioma) begins as a small hard papule, which may have existed some time before the patient seeks advice. It spreads so slowly that some years may pass before it attains the size of half an inch in diameter, showing a depressed centre and a characteristic, hard, " rolled-edge," pearly-coloured margin. On the scalp and brow the usual form is cicatricial and superficial, with an ulcerating centre, and hard border ; this may enlarge gradually, with progress so slow that it is easily differentiated from syphilis and from lupus vulgaris. After some time, if left without treatment, the ulcer often takes on more rapid growth ; it may extend over half the forehead and face, and over the temporal region, destroying muscle and cartilage and may even erode through the bone.

*Ætiology.* The growth originates in the basal cell layer of the epidermis. Transitional forms are found between the frank rodent ulcer and the basal cell squamous epithelioma ; the latter is more serious and can give rise to metastases. Men are more affected than women, and usually over forty or in old age.

The *prognosis* is always anxious, because no one can foretell when active growth may set in. Basal cell epitheliomas are only malignant *in situ,* and do not have metastases.

*Treatment.* Carbon dioxide snow may cure an early case. X-ray, radium and surgical excision have all been tried and have had many cures to their credit. If the ulcer is seen at a fairly early stage, diathermy coagulation provides an excellent means of dealing with it ; the ensuing scar is very fine. Fulguration is sometimes successful, but is not so effective as coagulation. All apparently cured cases should be kept under observation for years.

II. **Epithelioma.** Primary growths are rare on the scalp. EPITHE-LIOMA, usually basal cell in type, occasionally develops on the lesions of multiple benign cystic adenoma (p. 264), but more often supervenes on scar tissue, especially that of old burns, xeroderma pigmentosa and radio-dermatitis. In such instances there is usually squamous cell epithelioma, although in xeroderma pigmentosa there may be a basal cell growth. Epithelioma may also develop on nævi which have ulcerated, in some cases as a result of injury with the comb. A particularly rapid form may occur on pigmented nævi, even in young people. The irregular outline, the hardness and the exuberant excrescences on the surface of carcinomatous growths are quite characteristic ; their rapid development necessitates early intervention. Many believe that melanoma develops when there is nævus cell activity at the dermo-epidermal junction, but Hamilton Montgomery (private communication) has seen hairy pigmented nævi, with nævus cells extending deep into the cutis, undergo malignant change. The subject is fully discussed by Lund and Scobbie in a study of 200 cases.[1] Sophie Spitz and other Americans find that melanomas in children under puberty rarely metastasize.[2] For the pigmented NÆVO-CARCINOMA (melano-epithelioma), Darier insisted on the superiority of the galvanic current (negative pole), to all other of the usual methods of dealing with these malignant growths. However, when the pigmented melanoma takes on malignant growth the metastases spread so rapidly that a fatal issue is usual. Grey Turner gave a remarkable paper,[3] which should be consulted by all who have to deal with this serious condition. If seen early enough, these cases can be saved by careful surgery which follows out the whole length of the lymphatics and glands along which the secondary deposits have travelled. Occasionally multiple primary growths occur simultaneously in the skin and the internal organs. As SENILE KERATOSES are apt to take on epitheliomatous growth, it is important to deal with them before such can occur. They

[1] *Amer. J. Path.*, 1949, **25**, 1117.          [2] *Ibid.*, 1948, **24**, 591.
Other articles on this subject are by : TRAUB, *Arch. Derm. and Syph.*, 1940, **41**, 214, and SACHS, *et al.*, in *J. Amer. Med. Assoc.*, 1947, **135**, 216.
[3] GREY TURNER, Prosser White Oration, *Trans. St. John's Hosp. Derm. Soc.*, 1939. Senile keratoses and verrucæ are described with clinical and histological illustrations by Sachs and others in *Arch. Derm. and Syph.*, 1949, **59**, 179.

are rarely if ever seen on the scalp, but are not uncommon on the brow, near the scalp margin, on the face, neck, ears and the backs of the hands. SECONDARY EPITHELIOMATOUS GROWTHS on the scalp are not uncommon. When several secondary nodules are present, before ulceration occurs the hair falls and the skin of the scalp may be stretched and glossy (see p. 134). Plaques such as are seen with *cancer en cuirasse* are rare except as a secondary manifestation. When these occur as multiple nodules they may at first sight be mistaken for Turban tumours (Cylindroma, p. 265). It is important to realize that a metastatic nodule on the scalp may be the first indication of the existence of internal carcinoma. When the clinical course of a disease leads one to suspect internal cancer one should examine the skin of the whole body. The presence of a cutaneous metastasis, especially on the scalp, may provide the diagnostic clue.[1]

III.   **Sarcomatous tumours** of the skin may be primary or secondary. They are rare in comparison with carcinomatous conditions. The scalp as well as other regions of the body may be involved. *Primary* growths are not common ; they may arise associated with many tissues. When connected with angiomata or myxomatous tissue the nodules are soft, but as a rule sarcomatous tumours are hard, with a definite edge, and smooth on the surface until the later stages, when ulcerating and fungating. In colour they may be dark red or blue, and often take long to break down. *Secondary* sarcomatous tumours may arise in connection with various dermatological diseases, sometimes after radiotherapy. When only one tumour is present, the diagnosis may be impossible without a histological examination. A blood examination distinguishes them from leukæmic nodules and syphilides.

IV.   **Meningiomas** are extra-cerebral or intracranial tumours which rarely metastasize. Laymon saw a meningioma which eroded the skull. The patient, aged 72, noticed a swelling in 1941 ; by 1947 it had grown large. He had had attacks of loss of consciousness. After his death in 1948 the tumour was found to be a non-cornifying epithelioma which had eroded the skull. Their origin is disputed. Most neoplasms on the scalp are Turban tumours (p. 265). When the diagnosis is difficult this article should be consulted, as it discusses the histological features of many scalp tumours.[2]

V.   **Carcinoma** of the **sweat glands** is exceedingly rare. Most of the cases thus diagnosed have proved to be the benign condition, cylindroma. The nodules are small, yellow, without any characteristic feature, occurring chiefly on the neck, axillæ, and the scalp.[3]

**Adenocarcinoma** of the sebaceous glands may occur as metastases.

---

[1] HAMILTON MONTGOMERY and R. KIERLAND, *Arch. Surg.*, 1940, **40**, 672.
[2] CARL LAYMON, *Arch. Derm.*, 1949, **59**, 626.
[3] *Mayo Staff Clinic Meetings*, 1939, **14**, 481.

GROUP C. Few swellings are peculiar to the scalp. The majority of the nodules and tumours which appear on the scalp are part of some general disease which is characterized by nodules or tumours on or in the body. Hence the subject will be dealt with very briefly here. Over most nodules and tumours, alopecia is present (p. 134); indeed, in many of these cases the patient may seek advice on account of localized hairfall. Swellings or nodules which may affect the scalp, and are often diagnosed by the PRESENCE OF SIMILAR LESIONS on the face or body, are :

    I Scleroderma.
   II Xanthoma.
  III Drug Eruptions.
   IV Molluscum Fibrosum.
    V Sarcoid.
   VI Molluscum Contagiosum.
  VII Leukæmia.
 VIII Mycosis Fungoides.
   IX Tuberculosis, Actinomycosis and other ulcerating granulomata.
    X Granuloma Annulare.
   XI Gouty Tophi.
  XII Multiple Benign Cystic Epithelioma.

I. **Scleroderma,** so often seen on the trunk, may also affect the scalp. It can appear in various forms—a plaque, a band or a spot. Localized, small-sized lesions of scleroderma are usually known as morphœa. Bands or spots of morphœa are not difficult to diagnose when they appear on the scalp. The affected region is hairless and hard, as if the skin were infiltrated or replaced by a piece of hard white wax or porcelain. Often there is a lilac-coloured rim, due to capillary congestion ; a few enlarged vessels often stray over the white patch. Sometimes the patch has been preceded by itching, a mild degree of erythema or pigmentation. When morphœa occurs in small spots, like drops of water, it is often referred to as " white spot " disease. As the regions affected by morphœa have no hair, this disease was alluded to in the section or bald patches with atrophy, in Chapter IX. Sometimes the band type seems to follow the course of a nerve, such as the supraorbital, but this is by no means always definite. The band form of circumscribed scleroderma is not infrequently seen along the median line ; when this occurs on the forehead it often extends on to the scalp, and resembles its description as *coup de sabre.* This linear distribution sometimes passes down the whole length of the upper or lower limb. Half of the face may be affected ; this may be followed by, or may be associated with *Hemiatrophy facialis.*

*Diagnosis.* Morphœa may be mistaken for *rodent ulcer* before ulceration has occurred. In morphœa other lesions are usually present on the face or body ; the subsequent course makes the diagnosis clear.

*Prognosis.* The disease may be stationary for a prolonged time, even for years ; or it may soften and become absorbed, leaving behind it atrophy or pigment. This is particularly clearly seen on the scalp, where the white atrophic patches may be mistaken for other causes of scars, such as lupus erythematosus, or when on the body, for lichen planus atrophicus. The *Cause* is unknown. The disease is more common in women, and in the first half of life.

*Treatment* varies. Many forms of treatment have been tried for this serious and usually progressive malady ; endocrine therapy, according to other indications, such as thyroid, œstrin, pituitrin injections,[1] mecholyl, gold and bismuth, have also had success. Locally, warmth, massage with oil, negative galvanism, negative electrolysis, inductothermy and radiant heat have all given good results.

II. **Xanthoma** nodules may appear on the scalp as well as on the body. They begin as a brownish macule, and in a few weeks grow to a hard shiny papule, and then become a soft orange- or lemon-coloured swelling, varying in size to a nodule or larger—XANTHOMA TUBEROSUM. They are usually multiple ; several adjacent nodules may coalesce. They all have a characteristic yellow hue, resembling chamois leather. There is no itching nor surrounding inflammatory reaction. They are associated with cholesterin metabolism ; usually there is excess of cholesterol in the blood. Fats and lipoids are often found in xanthoma nodules. Xanthoma tuberosum often affects the scalp of children. The xanthoma which appears in diabetic individuals often has nodules without the characteristic yellow hue, but with a red halo ; they develop more rapidly than the other type of xanthoma tuberosum and if familial are serious.

*Treatment.* In the diabetic cases, correct diet with insulin is curative. In other types the result of treatment is not so marked ; the avoidance of animal fats and yolk of egg is indicated. For both forms the administration of hyd. c̄. cret. and salicylate of sodium aids the free flow of bile. The cautery, the galvanic current (with negative needle in the lesion), diathermy fulguration or excision are effective locally.

III. **Drugs** can give rise to eruptions over the whole body, of mild or severe character, varying from erythema, urticaria, raised flat plaques, weeping vesicular and bullous conditions, to papilliform and fungating excrescences of alarming appearance, exuding pus from cribriform gaps

---

[1] OLIVER and LERMAN, *Arch. Derm. and Syph.*, 1936, **34**, 469.

resembling the surface of large carbuncles. The severe types of drug eruption are most often associated with bromides and iodides. In infants and children especially, fungating swellings may develop on the scalp and be long unsuspected as connected with drugs. Usually the pustule, especially with acne, is the form taken by a bromide and an iodide rash. With iodides, hæmorrhagic development is common—petechiæ, purpuric patches and bullæ.

The *diagnosis* may be difficult when the history of taking the drug is obscure. In some cases an infant has the rash whilst the nursing mother, from whom it has been acquired, remains free. Apparently sensitization to iodide has sometimes been due to the ingestion of iodized salt. The possibility of the presence of bromide and iodide in proprietary preparations is often overlooked by the physician ; a parent seldom volunteers the fact that she is dosing herself or her child with some favourite cough or " blood purifying " mixture.

Other forms of drug eruptions are referred to under their predominant feature : erythema, bullæ, etc.

IV. In **Molluscum Fibrosum** the tumours may be superficial and cutaneous, or deep-seated, connected with a peripheral nerve in the true skin or the subcutaneous tissue. They are multiple, and vary in size from a tiny seed to an egg, an orange or even larger. The small type are chiefly seen on the face and neck. The larger ones become pendulous and pedunculated and may become heavy. They are soft to the touch and can be invaginated ; one can push the swellings through an opening of skin which feels like a hernial opening. At first skin-coloured, they become red or purplish as they distend the skin in growing. When they form part of the triad of symptoms of **Von Recklinghausen's disease** they may be scattered abundantly over the entire body and scalp. In this condition the diagnostic points are spots of pigment and tumours associated with nerve trunks, in *addition to* the presence of multiple subcutaneous tumours.

*Treatment.* When small, these tumours can be destroyed with negative galvanism, the cautery or diathermy fulguration. When large, they should be cut off with surgical precautions of asepsis.

V. **Sarcoids** may affect the scalp. Several types of cutaneous lesions are included under the term **Sarcoidosis** or **Schaumann's disease,** which is at present believed to be a chronic infection of the reticulo-endothelial system. The old distinction of the lesions is being discarded as the clinical types are considered to be manifestations of the same disease. Formerly the names used were Boeck's sarcoid, lupus pernio, the subcutaneous nodule of Darier-Roussy, and the benign granuloma of Schaumann, with involvement of the internal organs, lungs, heart, lymph nodes and the bones. On the scalp the papules are pea to walnut size and as they unite they leave a pitted healing centre. They may form annular or semicircular patches which extend from the brow to the scalp.

*Ætiology.* The cause is unknown. Women are more often affected than men. The malady is associated with a special form of tuberculous infection.[1]

*Diagnosis.* In all cases with chronic reddish yellow papules or plaques which come and go, it is advisable to X-ray the lungs, liver, heart, and the bones of the extremities.

*Prognosis.* This is good in the majority of the cases.

*Treatment.* Success has been obtained with injections of gold salts (Barber), sodium morrhuate (Gray), arseno-benzol and calomel (Darier), etc. Good results have also been obtained with long continued arsenical treatment. Irradiation and endothermy have helped other cases. One woman under my care (diagnosed as lymphogranuloma by Darier in 1922) had typical large nodules on the upper arms, face and shoulders. With glandular treatment and diet she recovered completely. Some years later she had extensive lupus erythematosus over the cheeks, which became cured after the removal of septic tonsils, followed by skilled local massage to the face and neck.

VI. **Molluscum Contagiosum,** with its characteristic small, rounded papule of waxen appearance, with central depressed opening, may affect any part of the body. It does not often appear on the scalp itself, but it can do so. Recently, I have seen three women in whom only the scalp was affected. In rare instances, from the coalescence of the nodules, large masses have formed and caused difficulty in diagnosis from malignant growths. Each papule must be incised and swabbed out with a strong antiseptic; or one may use diathermy fulguration or the galvano-cautery. Care must be taken to avoid the towels, sponges, brushes and combs, and hats which were used before the nodules were destroyed. I have found recurrences due to the patients having retained their favourite sponge, hat or brush.

VII. The cutaneous nodules of **Leukæmia,** and the rare disease (VIII) **Mycosis Fungoides,** may affect the scalp. The early stage of both diseases is associated with, even sometimes preceded by, much irritation. The whole scalp in mycosis fungoides may be erythematous, scaly and devoid of hair (see p. 207). Years may pass before the appearance of the typical tumours of mycosis fungoides. The diagnosis is arrived at by a blood examination and a biopsy. Leukæmic tumours may be small, blueish papulo-nodules; irradiation and nitrogen mustards are now advised.[2]

IX. **Tuberculosis, Leishmaniasis, Actinomycosis, Blastomycosis** and **Sporotrichosis** may also, but rarely (especially in the latter three diseases) affect the scalp. In all of the above, ulceration develops. It is unlikely that in any of these diseases the nodules, ulcers and tumours will affect the scalp alone. The diagnosis may rest on examination of microscopic

---

[1] The subject is fully discussed by H. MICHELSON in *J. Amer. Med. Assoc.*, 1948, **136**, 1034.

[2] E. POHL and J. JUHL, *Journ. Amer. Med. Assoc.*, 1949, **48**, 223. Alpert, Greenspan *et al.*, *Ann. Int. Med.*, 1950, **32**, 393.

sections and scrapings, or on the cultures made from the ulcers.  Calciferol has had great success in the treatment of lupus vulgaris.[1]  Recently some failures have been reported.[2]  **Lupus Vulgaris** is rare on the scalp alone, but may extend there, and leave scars and alopecia with atrophy (p. 147). For actinomycosis, penicillin in full doses should be tried for two to four weeks.

X.  **Granuloma Annulare** is rare on the scalp.  It more often affects the hands and the limbs, and is more frequent in children.  It is disputed whether it is a tuberculide or a streptococcide.[3]

XI.  **Gouty Tophi** have caused swellings on the scalp.

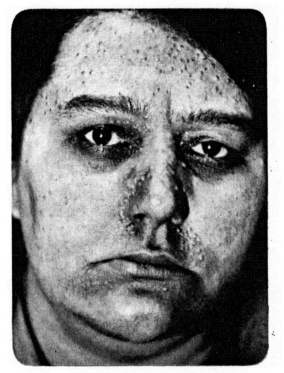

Fig. 56.—Multiple Benign Cystic Epithelioma.
(*Photograph kindly lent by Dr. Louis Savatard.*)

XII.  When the small nodules of MULTIPLE BENIGN CYSTIC EPITHELIOMA affect the scalp, they may be diagnosed by the presence of lesions on the face (see Group D (II) and Fig. 56).

[1] CHARPY, DOWLING and LOMHOLT, *Brit. J. Derm. and Syph.*, 1948, **60**, 121, 127, 132.
[2] *Brit. J. Derm. and Syph.*, 1950, **62**, 15.    [3] *Ibid.*, 1942, **54**, 75.

GROUP D.   A few rare conditions with distinctive appearance and histology remain to be described :

I.   **Lichenification** of the scalp is mentioned here, but it usually follows some disease, such as psoriasis.   The skin is thickened, raised, reddened, the natural grooves of the skin are exaggerated, and there are often fine dry scales on the surface.   Itching is a marked feature, and the constant scratching leads to thinning of the hair, or the hairs are rubbed off short.   The condition is most commonly seen near the neck or ears ; but when neglected, a large part of the scalp may be involved.   The diagnosis is difficult when the case has not been seen before it has reached an advanced stage.

II.   **Multiple Benign Cystic Epithelioma** (Syns., Epithelioma adenoides cysticum, Brooke's disease) is a rare but definite clinical condition. The name epithelioma in this connection does not imply any tendency to malignancy, but only an epithelial overgrowth.   The lesions are usually small, pin-head to pea-sized ; pinkish, pale yellow or yellowish-red in colour, or somewhat like vesicles in their translucency.   They are embedded in the skin, rounded or oval, firm to the touch and painless (see Fig. 56).   Occasionally larger lesions develop, almost like the early stage of a rodent ulcer.   These little growths tend to be symmetrical on the face, affecting the brow, eyelids cheeks, nose and chin ; they also appear, although less frequently, on the scalp, breast, neck and arms.

*Ætiology.*   The disease usually sets in about the age of puberty and is more frequent in women.   The apparent infrequency in the male may be due to the fact that men do not seek advice unless the lesions are very numerous or disfiguring.   It is often hereditary and familial.   It originates in the basal layer of the epidermis [1] and similar cells of the hair follicles (tricho-epithelioma).

*Diagnosis.*   The position of the little nodules on the face and scalp is characteristic.   The date of the onset of the disease and its presence in several members of a family or in several generations aids the diagnosis.   The small nodules may be mistaken for multiple rodent ulcer ; but rodent ulcer occurs in older people and does not remain stationary for so long.   The larger scalp tumours have been mistaken for sarcoma and for cylindroma (see below). A biopsy may be necessary before one can be certain of the diagnosis.   When there are few lesions on the face they are readily mistaken for non-pigmented moles.

*Prognosis.*   The lesions may persist for years unchanged ; only occasionally do they become epitheliomatous later.   Some of the larger growths disappear spontaneously.

*Treatment.*   Some recommend X-ray, excision or electrolysis.   Adamson states that any tumour can be surgically dealt with which gives rise to inconvenience, owing to its size or position ; but as a rule the growths are too numerous for removal to be practicable.

---

[1] This disease is fully discussed by H. G. Adamson, *Brit. J. Derm. and Syph.*, 1918, **30**, 130, and by Louis Savatard, in the same journal, 1922, **34**, 381, and 1938, **50**, 333.

III.  **Cylindroma** (Syns. Turban tumours, tomato tumours, Nævus epitheliomato-cylindromatosus, Benign epithelioma, Endothelioma capitis). The number of synonyms gives some indication of the rarity of these swellings and of the difficulty in deciding the cause of their appearance.  They are believed to be a variant of Epithelioma adenoides cysticum, described above.

Clinically, they present rounded, smooth, bluish pink nodules, pea to egg-sized, usually in groups, like bunches of grapes or tomatoes (Fig. 57);

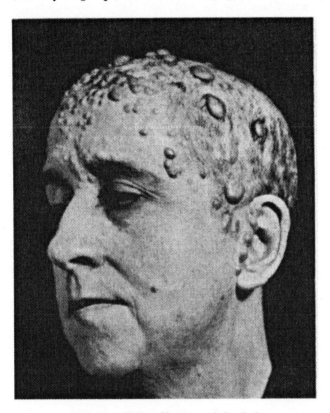

FIG. 57.—Turban Tumours of the Scalp.
(*Photograph kindly lent by Dr. Louis Savatard.*)

firm, never ulcerating.  They begin sometimes in childhood, more often about puberty, or in adult or middle age.  They may increase as age advances ; their growth is usually very slow.  They appear chiefly on the scalp, which they may cover like a turban.  The hair falls out as the tumours enlarge.  The brow, face and neck, even the upper part of the body, may be invaded.  Rarely, there is only a solitary tumour.

*Ætiology.*  The malady is hereditary and familial.  They rarely begin after 40 ; women are affected more often than men.  The tumours are due to basal cell epithelioma of benign form.    A capsule of firm connective tissue dips in between groups of cylindrical epithelial cells, closely packed in lobules surrounded by a hyaline sheath and proliferating in a hyaline matrix. Savatard[1] concluded that Turban tumours and Epithelioma adenoides cysticum are variants of the same condition, a basal-cell type originating from the surface epithelium or from the hair follicles, not from the sweat ducts or glands.    Montgomery[2] and others state that even in the same patient all transitions may be met with between cylindroma, epithelioma adenoides cysticum, syringoma and adenoma sebaceum.

*Diagnosis.*    Sebaceous cysts have a central orifice from which pultaceous matter can be squeezed ; they are less numerous and their colour is paler, more like normal skin.

*Prognosis.*    They are disfiguring, but as a rule harmless, malignancy developing seldom, and only after frequent irritation or incomplete removal.

*Treatment* is excision when the tumours are so large as to be troublesome ; or destruction by electrical methods.

IV.    **Cutis Verticis Gyrata,** as the name implies, is a condition in which the skin of the vertex appears to be thrown into folds.    The disease may appear to the patient as a swelling ; therefore it is described here.    The swelling is usually of very slow development and may be accompanied at times by itching.    In other cases the patient seeks advice because he finds a bald and raised ridge on the scalp (see p. 134).    Like thick folds of a curtain, the scalp lies in radiating furrows and grooves.    At first sight, in certain cases, the disease may be taken for alopecia, as the hair is absent over the raised ridges when these are fully developed.    This condition is very rare, and may be congenital or acquired.    It is quite distinct from elastic skin.    Its appearance has earned for it the name " Bull dog scalp." Stratton[3] reports a collection of 158 cases written by eighty-seven authors ; in his article are many vivid illustrations of the different types of the condition. These can be classified under four headings : (i) true cutis verticis gyrata, a congenital anomaly, a giant nævus ; (ii) a pachydermatous state such as is seen in acromegaly, myxœdema, and with chronic inflammatory tissue changes, as in leukæmia and syphilis ; (iii) a form associated with tumours, fibromas, neurofibromas and cellular nævi ; and (iv) a type which is consequent on trauma or acute inflammation affecting the sebaceous glands and their vicinity.    In this variety the folds can be manipulated and their position altered.    In type iii there is localized sensitiveness of the skin of the scalp to the pituitary growth hormone.[4]    In the cases recorded under type iv the patient has sometimes not observed the ridges and swollen regions for some months or even years after the originating cause.[5]

---

[1] L. SAVATARD, *Brit. J. Derm. and Syph.*, 1933, **50**, 333.

[2] HAMILTON MONTGOMERY, *Arch. Surg.*, 1940, **40**, 472.

[3] E. K. STRATTON, *Arch. Derm. and Syph.*, 1933, **27**, 392.

[4] " Endocrine Tumours," 1936, Lewis, London. ZEISLER and WIEDER, *Arch. Derm. and Syph.*, 1940, **41**, 1092 ; and H. W. BARBER in " Modern Trends in Dermatology," 1948.

[5] HARRY E. ALDERSON, *Arch. Derm. and Syph.*, 1932, **26**, 1021 ; A. TOURAINE, *Bull. Soc. Franç. de Derm. et Syph.*, 1938, **45**, 1638.

*Diagnosis.* The malady may be difficult to recognize in the early stage, especially when the hair is thick. In 1926 I saw a young man aged 23, who presented only a few small lumps resembling sebaceous cysts, but no orifice could be found. I expressed uncertainty as to the correct diagnosis. After ten years the patient returned, complaining that there were now more nodules. The diagnosis was obscure until his thick hair had been shaved; what had felt like firm swellings were then rendered visible, and easily recognized as ridges, disposed in the typical distribution of cutis verticis gyrata.

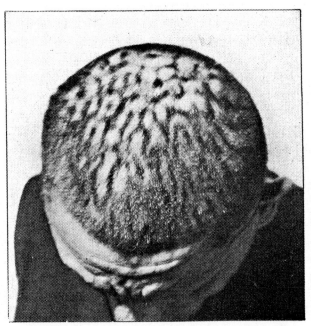

FIG. 58.—Cutis Verticis Gyrata (Dr. M. G. Hannay's Case).
*British Journal of Dermatology and Syphilis.*

*Treatment* consists in surgical removal of the redundant tissue, if and when the patient suffers discomfort from its weight.

V. A rare cause of small nodules is LEIOMYOMA.

The nodules of **leiomyoma** are firm and distinctly elevated above the surface of the skin, smooth, pink, often with dilated vessels at the periphery. They cause pain and are tender on pressure and on exposure to cold. They occur in large numbers, discrete or grouped, symmetrically situated on neck, face and forehead, occasionally on the scalp. They may also be numerous on the trunk and limbs. A biopsy reveals the smooth fibres which form the leiomyoma nodule. The nodules should be excised if causing much pain.

# CHAPTER XVIII

## ALTERED COLOUR OF THE SCALP

Certain distinctive alterations in the colour of the skin of the scalp are met with.

The ERYTHEMATOUS ERUPTIONS are described in Chapter XIII. PETECHIAL and PURPURIC rashes may occur after the administration of some DRUGS, such as iodides, the sulphonamide group, phosphorus, quinine, iodoform, mercury, and after injections of the heavy metals and animal serum.

The lilac or pink coloration around or over a MORPHŒA band or spot must be borne in mind ; the diagnosis may be difficult before the patch develops (see p. 259).

The flat nævus is described in this section of altered colour of the scalp, because the patient, usually an infant, is brought by the parents, who complain that there is a RED PATCH on the scalp. Almost always they know it is a " birth mark," and believe that it is due to some mental shock sustained by the mother during pregnancy.

**Capillary** or **Flat Nævus** (Nævus Flammeus). On the scalp, especially on the occipital region, there is often seen a patch of colour which close examination reveals to be a nævus. In infants it is common ; it often disappears spontaneously. Adults may be quite unaware that throughout life they have had a nævus on the occipital region of their scalp. It is usually covered with hair. The flat nævus may resemble a diffuse stain, varying in colour from pale pink and vivid red to the well-known purple " port-wine stain." In shape it may be a patch with irregular margin and uniform hue, or show as punctiform, discrete, small stains, with here and there definite telangiectases. The other forms of nævus are described on page 254.

*Treatment.* The flat nævus on the occipital region rarely requires any treatment. If it should tend to spread or if its colour is objected to, Thorium X is the modern method of treatment. A varnish containing 1500 E.S. Units per c.c. is painted over the nævus every fortnight or month till it gradually fades away. It can often be concealed by a cosmetic paste.

*The skin of the scalp has an abnormally white patch or patches, surrounded by pigmentation, and the same phenomenon is present on the face or body. The condition is* VITILIGO.

**Vitiligo.** (Syn., Leukoderma.) This somewhat uncommon disease does not affect the scalp so often as the body. When it spreads from the neck or brow to the hairy scalp, the epidermis of the scalp shows a white patch, just as when the disease affects the smooth skin, with a surrounding area of pigmentation deeper than that of the normal skin. The pigmentation shows a characteristic concave outline bordering the central white region. The hair on the white or depigmented patch on the skin of the scalp may retain its colour ; on the other hand, in some cases the hair is as blanched as the skin from which it grows. The hair on a leukoderma patch may remain healthy, or it may fall, especially when the patch is increasing in size. The disease makes slow progress over years, first extending, then healing spontaneously in time.

*Ætiology.* Vitiligo may develop at any age, but is rare before ten and usually begins before thirty. It affects both sexes. The cause remains obscure. Not infrequently it has been associated with alopecia areata, scleroderma, syphilis and Graves' disease. It has also occurred in conditions of organic disease of the nervous system, such as subacute combined degeneration and locomotor ataxy, and with disease of the vertebræ involving the nerve roots.

The *diagnosis* usually presents no difficulty. The concave outline and the polycyclical margin of the zone of pigmentation next to the white patch are very characteristic.

*Treatment* is not very satisfactory, although from time to time a wonderfully rapid cure is obtained by some method which does not succeed with the next case. Success has been obtained with injections of gold salts (Barber) ; and Burgess reported cure in a patient to whom sanocrysin 0·05 gm. injections were given intravenously once a week for seven weeks whilst at the same time exposure to ultra-violet light was given twice a week to the white regions, which had been well rubbed, twice daily, with a 10 per cent. solution of bergamot in alcohol or oil. The method of treatment by ultra-violet light after the application of bergamot had already had considerable trial, with a proportion of good results. Before exposure to the mercury vapour lamp it is important to rub in the bergamot oil thoroughly. Various sensitizers are being tested ; they are injected intravenously or intramuscularly before exposure to ultra-violet or to infra-red rays. The pigmented margin must be protected before ultra-violet light exposures. Sieve [1] reports success with para-aminobenzoic acid. One of my patients (aged 26) had many patches of alopecia areata and also extensive vitiligo. Examining for the cause, I found she had microcytic anæmia, a profuse uterine discharge dating from girlhood, and much nervous tension. She made rapid progress

[1] B. F. SIEVE, *Southern Med. and Surg.*, 1942, **104**, 135 ; *Virginia Med. Month.*, 1942, **69**, 487 ; and 1945, **72**, 6.

with ultra-violet light to the whole body as well as to the scalp, iron, full doses of Vitamin B (whole complex) and a course of copper ionization to the entire interior of the womb. Within seven months the discharge had gone, she felt renewed energy, the hair had returned, and to my surprise the vitiligo had practically disappeared. The trunk lesions gradually vanished ; after three years there remained a few white areas on the legs. She had continued with small doses of Vitamin B until about six months before seen again in 1945. In 1947 pigmentation began to return ; in 1948 she wrote that arthritis and chronic catarrh had had a bad effect on the skin. She lived too far from London to see me.

Many of the forms of pigmentation which appear on the body do not affect the scalp. Deficiency of Vitamin C appears to lead to pigmentation. Some **Conditions with Pigmentation** may affect the scalp as well as the body. Of such may be mentioned :

Pigmentation after exposure to real or artificial sunlight.

Pigmentation after exposure to X-ray when the tube has been activated by a current of high voltage.

Pigmentation of old age frequently seen on the hands can affect the bald scalp.

Urticaria pigmentosa.

Radiodermatitis.

Von Recklinghausen's disease.

Moles and the Blue Nævus.

Xeroderma pigmentosa.

Riehl's disease.

In Addison's disease the scalp becomes pigmented, though usually less deeply than the body. The hair also in some cases becomes more pigmented.

Pigmentation may be simulated by dark-coloured hair dyes which have accidentally soaked on to the scalp (p. 276).

Morphœa may show some degree of pigmentation.

After any prolonged inflammatory lesion, a degree of pigmentation generally follows, more or less lasting according to the degree and extent involved. Thus, for example, it is seen after the fixed raised erythema plaques which sometimes develop after prolonged administration of phenophthalein. The brown hue of Pityriasis furfur has been mistaken for pigmentation when it affects the scalp.

Argyria, pigmentation due to silver, causes a deep grey, slate-coloured pigmentation of the exposed parts ; the scalp and hair have also in some cases been impregnated with the metal. Silver compounds have been found in the epidermis and in the hair follicles (cp. p. 42). Pigmentation is common after long-continued ingestion of arsenic, especially where there has been exposure to friction or pressure. The pigment can be present in the corium or any part of the epidermis, but is not seen in the mucous membranes. On the skin tiny white regions are found like drops on the pigmented region.

**Urticaria Pigmentosa.** The lesions of the juvenile type of urticaria pigmentosa may affect the scalp. The disease usually starts in infancy, often decreases or vanishes at puberty, or persists throughout life. The rash shows as round or oval papules or macules, fawn to dark brown coloured. When rubbed or scratched, they become red wheals.

In RADIODERMATITIS, after an overdose of X-ray or radium, atrophic changes in the skin develop, with formation of pigmented spots, telangiectases, warts and later on epithelioma (see p. 147). Any hairs which happen to be left on the atrophic area are usually white.

VON RECKLINGHAUSEN'S DISEASE is discussed on p. 261.

**Pigmented Hairy** and **Verrucose Moles** occasionally are seen on the scalp alone, and not infrequently extend from the face to the scalp. The pigmented mole which may develop malignant growth, the so-called NÆVOCARCINOMA, is considered on page 257.

The **Blue Nævus** is a papule which may occur on the scalp and forehead as well as on the body. It is usually found soon after birth, forming a slightly elevated papule, blue or steel blue in colour, firm, even hard on palpation. Its course is benign, but with age or with traumatism there may be malignant development, usually in the form of a slow growing melanosarcoma.[1]

*Diagnosis.* H. Montgomery believes that the Blue Nævus is probably less rare than is supposed, because it is usually mistaken for a mole. Moles are more brown or fawn in colour ; a deep-seated hæmangioma is soft and bleeds on being punctured. A malignant melanoma is blue black, and is distinguished by its histological features.

The serious (and happily rare) disease **Xeroderma Pigmentosa** spreads from the face and neck to the temporal regions of the scalp. The disease also affects other parts exposed to sunlight, such as the backs of the hands and outer sides of the arms. It begins in childhood ; pigmented spots develop with exposure to light. These and the intervening skin gradually atrophy and shrink. Telangiectases and, later, warty growths and epitheliomata may appear.

**Riehl's Disease,** a rare condition which appears to be the same as the POIKILODERMA of CIVATTE, may extend from the arms, neck and face to the temples. It shows reticulated areas of pigmentation, slight telangiectasis and atrophy, and sometimes scaling at the mouths of the follicles.

---

[1] HAMILTON MONTGOMERY and J. KAHLER, *Amer. J. Cancer*, 1939, **36**, 527.

# CHAPTER XIX

## HAIR DYES

The use of hair dyes dates from antiquity. Allusions are found in the literature of Egypt, Assyria, Greece and Rome. The physician is frequently asked whether dyes are advisable. Most of us reply that dyes are dangerous, but it must be confessed that the majority of the medical profession base their opinion on the rare instances of dermatitis which have come their way. Many of us are also prejudiced because we have seen women take to dyes from worthless motives, or our artistic sense has been outraged by the hair which has an obviously unnatural shade, the dark strands showing green, purple or red tints in a bright light. Everyone also objects to the unnatural appearance of a shade of hair next the scalp differing from that which is seen half an inch beyond it.

Neither the dermatologist nor the general practitioner can possibly know all the chemical details of hair dyes and the dangers of wrongly applied ingredients, but it is useful to have some general knowledge of the main principles underlying this age-old practice. Probably it is best to counsel the middle-aged and older woman, with already visibly grey hairs, that any form of dye is inadvisable. The problem of the younger woman with many grey hairs is somewhat different; her plea for the use of a dye requires consideration in the individual case. Her livelihood may depend upon her being able to retain a youthful appearance. Or she may have a husband younger than herself, and the happiness of her married life may be at stake. In such cases the preservation of colour in the hair may play an important part in determining the whole course of their lives.

Before a woman seeks the advice of a hairdresser, she should be fully aware of all the dangers and drawbacks of dyes. Before she takes the irrevocable step, she should have obtained full and correct knowledge from some unprejudiced authority who has nothing to gain or lose by her decision.

As a rule, the only information a woman can find on the subject of dyeing her hair is obtainable from the firm who will apply the dye. It ought to be possible for her to seek advice from someone who can speak from a totally disinterested standpoint. I have known quite young women, with only a few grey hairs, persuaded to try dangerous dyes, without having received any warning. They believed they were merely "in the fashion," using harmless bleaching lotions, when they had in reality begun with a dangerous aniline dye, and would for appearance sake be compelled to go on with it indefinitely. One lady told me she had been assured that there was never any danger, so long as the skin of her scalp was healthy. This provided a loophole of escape for her hairdresser ; in the event of dermatitis, she would have been told that she had, though unaware of it, some slight scalp lesion, and would have believed that the fault lay with herself. Moreover, I have known women who used " restorers " and " tonics " without having any idea that they were in reality using dyes. Many lotions used for washing the hair really colour or bleach the hair ; on analysis, my chemists have detected lead in several apparently innocuous shampoos.

Few women realize beforehand that hair dyeing involves an immense amount of time, with frequent visits to the hairdresser. The shade has to be matched precisely at the subsequent " touching up," and when a woman is travelling it entails much trouble to arrange for this procedure every six weeks. In addition, a complete dyeing must be carried out twice or thrice a year. Again, some shades are very difficult to match ; when a woman is unable to have her usual hairdresser to perform the task, she may find that a new operator, however skilled, has given her quite a different shade of hair. The mixing of the ingredients, e.g. the strength of the peroxide, may have been just a little different and the resulting colour may be displeasing. Every now and then a mistake may be made, and the hair shows an unnatural green or purple shade. The hair also loses its natural strength and becomes friable ; occasionally a hairdresser, new to the client, may overdo one part of the treatment, and therefore the hair breaks off in short lengths all over the scalp. Again, at some early or distant date, the painful situation has to be faced, that the dye has to be given up ; the transition stage is never pleasant and necessitates withdrawal from social life for weeks or months.

If the physician can describe dispassionately all the above disadvantages, then his patient has at least some knowledge of what she is undertaking when she considers that there are in her life reasons vital enough to justify her decision to dye her hair.

In ancient times, as to-day, the use of hair dyes was not favoured by medical profession. Galen remarks that the application of compositions for the hair does not belong properly to the physician, but that he may sometimes be obliged to furnish them to *royal ladies*, whom under certain circumstances he cannot venture to disobey.[1] Antimony was much in use for painting the eyebrows black. Thapsus is often mentioned in old

[1] Quoted from *Paulus Æginata* (Sydenham Soc. Trans.), 1894, 1, 344.

writings ; it appears to have been a wood used for dyeing the hair and other substances. It was called " the red herb " by the Romans ; but it is not now possible to be certain to which wood or tree the name refers.

In the following mixtures there are noted certain ingredients which have been in use up to modern times. A black dye for the hair had this prescription : galls 1 sextarius,[1] sumach 2 pints, privet 2 pints, black myrtle leaves 2 pints, cinnaris and poppy heads a handful, lake water 12 pints, cimolian earth and quicklime an acetabulum.[2] Another prescription contained green walnuts 3 oz., roots of ilex 3 oz., dark wine 3 pints ; mix and boil to one-third quantity ; then strain and pound up with a pint of myrtle oil. Use daily.

For making brown hair yellow, an oxide of lead was recommended.

For making golden hair, alum and red arsenic, saffron and thapsus wood were mixed with lixuvial ashes. Sumach and galls, and thapsus wood were also used, mixed with wine, allowed to soak, strained and rubbed on the hair.

The medical objections to the practice of hair dyeing are threefold : (1) injury to the hair ; (2) insidious poisoning of the system by certain metals or drugs included in the dye ; and (3) the danger of local dermatitis.

Dyes and bleaching substances render the hair fragile. Every woman knows that when a dress is dyed, it loses a certain amount of its substance, and that when it has been dyed several times, it is thin and readily torn. The same fact is true of the human hair ; when often dyed, it breaks readily. Methods used for bleaching are especially liable to cause crinkly hair which breaks in many places when pulled. As regards the poisoning of the system with which metallic dyes are often credited, this is seldom seen to-day, because the dyes most favoured in former days, lead and silver, are comparatively seldom employed in modern times. Indeed, some dermatologists have never seen a case of lead poisoning due to hair dye. The risk is certainly present, however. The dermatitis caused by aniline dyes can be very serious ; no one who has seen it can forget it, and no patient who has been its victim will desire to repeat the dye. The general symptoms of lead and of aniline dye poisoning are often unsuspected for a long time. (See pp. 276 and 279.)

To be effective, a dye should penetrate between the scales of the hair cuticle and colour the cortex of the hair shaft. To facilitate the penetration of the dye, the natural oil of the hair has first to be removed by washing and by application of various grease dissolvents, such as ammonia, salts of soda and potassium. Alkalis must be used only by those skilled

---

[1] A sectarius was a little over a pint.　　　[2] About 2½ oz.

in their application, because the hair is destroyed by solutions which are too strongly alkaline.

Under the microscope a dyed hair is readily recognized by those accustomed to examine hairs. *Henna* makes the fibres very dark and details of the hair structure are thus obscured. Dyes which penetrate into the structure of the hair cause a heavy uniform tinting, instead of the varied and irregular appearance of the colouring matter of natural hair (p. 23).

For the purpose of bleaching or lightening the colour of the hair, *hydrogen peroxide* is the agent most commonly employed. Hydrogen peroxide by itself does not always injure the hair, but when the ammonia (usually combined with it) is too strong, the hair is rendered brittle and even destroyed. *Potassium permanganate* in weak solution bleaches the hair, but it may also be used to tint the hair. To decide which strength of permanganate is required to produce the desired shade, tests should be made with a lock of hair which has been cut off. After the dye is used the hair is washed, and 10 per cent. sodium thiosulphate is applied, if necessary, several times.

*Camomile* is a popular and harmless vegetable dye which produces a rich auburn tint with dark hair, and a golden tint with fair hair. It is found in some hair washes and shampoo powders. Many of these powders are now made so skilfully that they do not injure the hair.[1] Unfortunately, however, the old-world name of camomile has sometimes been used to disguise the true nature of less innocent chemicals. Henna is another vegetable dye, but as it is often combined with other ingredients it is dealt with later. Walnut extract is mentioned in many books as a safe vegetable dye. It can be added to ointments and to oils, but it is little employed by expert hairdressers, because it is a dye difficult to apply and the colouring effect is not really satisfactory. This name also has sometimes been chosen by manufacturers as an attractive title under which harmful dyes can masquerade with an air of old-world simplicity.

*Iron* is one of the ingredients found in some of the so-called hair " restorers " which the individual can use at home, brushing it on herself. Two per cent. pure ferrous sulphate crystals are dissolved in red wine, such as claret. This is not a satisfactory method of obtaining a good dye, but has the advantage of being harmless.

The two most well-known agents for producing dark shades are *lead* and *silver*. The ancients used to employ lead, copper and silver for hair dyes. Wine or vinegar was kept in lead or copper vessels, sealed and warmed in the sun. Thus, in due time, acetate of lead or copper was

---

[1] H. S. REDGROVE and G. A. FOAN: *Hair Dyes and Hair Dyeing*, London, 1934.

formed ; when the liquid was used on the scalp the sulphate gradually developed and dyed the hair dark. Analysis shows that lead is present in many of the hair " restorers " which dye the hair gradually. Lead acetate, sulphur or sodium thiosulphate are dissolved, and concealed in the " restoring " lotion. As these lead dyes do not stain the fingers or scalp, they are popular with the public, who do not realize that the " restorer " is a dye. These lotions can be applied by comb or brush and the hair passes progressively from white to yellow, brown and black. Another method of applying lead is by using combs made of lead ; these bring about a slow formation of sulphate of lead, which darkens the hair. Although lead tetræthyl readily penetrates the skin, the lead which is used for dyes does not enter unless abrasions are present.[1] Headaches, tremors, anæmia, colic, albuminuria, and apparently causeless fatigue are some of the symptoms of lead absorption. In cases of plumbism due to hair dyes containing lead, the metal probably reaches the system by means of the fingers. The hands may have been used, uncovered, to dab on the solution, or they may have touched the hair when damp with the lead lotion, and thus food has become contaminated with the lead.

*Silver nitrate*, with pyrogallic acid as a reducing agent, can be used to produce many tints varying from light brown to black, according to the strength of the solution of silver nitrate. Usually pyrogallic acid is applied first, in a solution of about 1 per cent. This is brushed in after the hair has been cleansed of all grease or oil. Then the nitrate of silver, together with ammonia and water, is applied. This salt once enjoyed a high reputation. Dr. Pincus, the skilled dermatologist, recommended silver nitrate as a dye which was harmless and also simple to use. By his method all oiliness was first removed from the hair with a solution of bicarbonate of soda, rubbed in with a sponge or shaving-brush. Then the hair was dried quickly and thoroughly before using silver nitrate, 1 to 4 grammes, in distilled water, 20 to 30 grammes. This was applied with a soft tooth-brush, rubbing the hair shafts towards the roots and also towards the free ends. Under the influence of light, a silver salt is broken up and oxide of silver is deposited on the hair and penetrates between the cells of the cuticle to the cortex. Silver salts blacken the scalp unless due care is taken. If the scalp becomes stained, apply a solution of potassium iodide (1 grm. in 50 of distilled water) or sodium hyposulphite (2 in 50 of distilled water). The latter removes the silver salt stain without affecting the dye on the hair, but it must be used very soon after the application of the silver to the hair, whilst the scalp is still wet and before the action of light has rendered insoluble the salts on the scalp. The hair should be

[1] *J. Indust. Hyg.*, 1948, **30**, 256.

dried whilst hanging loose, care being taken to prevent any of the moist silver solution touching the skin of the scalp, face, and neck. Silver dyes are not always successful in producing a good even colour, but as they have the merit of being fairly safe, they are still employed. The dark shades produced by silver salts have rather an unnatural appearance ; the paler tints procured by hairdressers with silver salts show a fine ashen blond colour.

*Bismuth* was once popular and is still sometimes employed, made up with dilute nitric acid and a watery solution of tartaric acid. It provides shades of black, dark brown and chestnut.

Metals rarely used, except for colouring wigs, are *cobalt, cadmium* and *manganese.* The sulphate of cadmium can produce a bright blond hue.

Cases of involuntary dyeing of grey hair have occurred during the process of permanent waving, after the use of a hair lotion containing *perchloride of mercury* (1 grain to the ounce) ; sometimes the hair has turned green. In one patient, after the application of an ammoniacal spirit lotion, the hair was heated ; on removal of the curling metals, the hair was brown. A chemical investigation revealed mercuric sulphide ; apparently the heating process caused the darkening of the hair by the formation of mercuric sulphide.[1] In a recent case grey hair after a permanent wave turned brown. A microscopic examination suggested the presence of a dye. A photo-spectrograph identified lead in the metallic contents of the ash of the hair.

*Pyrogallol*, although extracted from gall nuts, is not a safe dye. It must be cautiously used because it is poisonous, and if used in a stronger proportion than 5 per cent. it renders the hair brittle.

*Henna* is a vegetable dye obtained from the Egyptian privet, *Lawsonia alba* ; it has long been employed in the East for colouring red the hair and nails. It reached Western Europe about 1890. In the East it is often followed by a preparation of indigo ; the combination is known as henna-reng. Various proportions of the two plants can be made, producing shades from light brown to a blue black. Apparently the henna-reng acts satisfactorily in warm moist climates, but this safe dye is very difficult to use in colder countries. Natural indigo is harmless, but at present a synthetic indigo has replaced it. Other ingredients can be combined with henna, such as catechu, lucerne, rhubarb, gall nuts, and salts of iron and copper. Pastes of henna, mixed with other ingredients, were long used in Arabia and Turkey for dyeing the hair ; such pastes were known as rasticks. Rasticks used to have a basis of gall nuts, which were

[1] A. M. GRAY and ROBERT KLABER, *Brit. J. of Derm. and Syph.*, 1936, pp. 97 and 193.

powdered, heated and mixed with iron or copper filings, then scented with musk. A good dye is made by the oxidation of pyrogallol (obtained from gall nuts), combined with iron or copper salts ; this preparation can be used in association with henna. In modern times the term " henna-rasticks " denotes those dyes which consist of pyrogallol and salts of iron or copper, combined with henna powder. From France comes the " liquid rastick." This was accomplished by adding a reducing agent to a solution containing pyrogallol and metallic salts. When such a solution is used for the purpose of dyeing, oxidation occurs on exposure to the oxygen of the air ; with the " liquid rastick " the oxidizing reaction between the two ingredients is delayed.

Henna can be profitably used alone on dark hair which has only a few grey hairs ; it then lends copper tints to the dark hair. But when all the hair is grey, henna produces a red coiffure. When henna is used alone, it makes hair red ; the other shades between red and brown, although usually declared to be due to henna, are in reality caused by the presence of the above-mentioned ingredients mixed in varying proportions with the henna. Some modern hairdressers mix the henna powder in varied amounts to suit the original colour of the hair ; they estimate by calculating the proportion of white, grey and remaining hair not affected by canities.

About the year 1883 there was introduced, in Paris, a synthetic dye which is now known popularly as " para." It has become a favourite dye because it is easy to apply and gives an artistic and most natural appearance to the colour of the hair. It can be used to produce shades varying from fine auburn through many tints of brown to black. It is a crystalline base, being an amino-derivative of benzene, and is soluble in alcohol and water. The substance itself darkens on exposure to the air, due to absorption of oxygen from the atmosphere. Various methods have been invented to provide the necessary oxygen, such as the addition of peroxide of hydrogen in different strengths. Details of the formulæ can be consulted in the chemical books which describe the action of this dye. The dangerous effect which has given this dye so unfortunate a notoriety is believed to be due to the quinone diimine which is formed when there is insufficient absorption of the oxygen by the paraphenylene-diamine. In spite of the fact that hairdressers know its reputation, this dye continues to be used and is continually appearing on the market under a new proprietary name. Stanley Redgrove quotes M. Schueller, a French specialist in hair dyes, whose investigations showed that 3 to 5 per cent. of those to whom the dye is applied are susceptible to paraphenylene-diamine poisoning. And see p. 281 for further proof.

This does not conclude the matter.  Hairdressers are advised to test each patient before using the dye, but few realize the importance of repeating this test before every application.  A patient who has used paraphenylenediamine with safety for years may suddenly develop intolerance to it. It is not known what causes this acquired sensitiveness to the drug. Sabouraud in his later work stated that he had not encountered such acquired sensitiveness to the dye, but I have seen several patients who had used this dye for many years, and then developed dermatitis immediately or soon after an application by their usual hairdresser.  In two cases the eruption was mild and patchy at first, and became severe at a subsequent application.  At present the client's susceptibility to the dye should be tested every time it is proposed to use it.  The Sabouraud-Rousseau test affords assistance.  The dye and the oxidant are kept in separate bottles, and an equal quantity of each is mixed and applied to a small area of skin behind the ear, allowed to dry, and covered with collodion.  After twenty-four hours this collodion film is removed and the skin washed with soap and water.  In a susceptible individual the skin is then seen to be red and inflamed.  In France some hairdressers take the extra precaution of making the test on the tender skin in front of the bend of the elbow, over the median basilic vein, or on the thigh over the internal saphenous vein.  The patch must not be left on longer than twenty-four hours ; sensitization has been caused in some people after an even shorter time.[1]

The *symptoms* of **paraphenylenediamine dermatitis** may be slight or severe.  In a mild case itching is felt a few hours after the application of the dye.  Except at the margin, the scalp is less affected than the face, which becomes blotchy and erythematous, with papules or vesicles. In severe cases, within forty-eight hours the whole face is enormously swollen, the eyelids cannot be opened, the lips and mouth are so œdematous that speaking and swallowing are difficult.  Albuminuria may be present.  There is rarely fever, though there may be general prostration. This distinguishes the case from erysipelas, which is usually suspected when the physician is unaware that a dye has been used.  The swelling usually reaches its maximum in three days, but the patient may be confined to the house for a fortnight or three weeks ; as a rule the inflammation subsides within six weeks.  Albuminuria may last for some weeks or months.  In severe cases the eruption may extend over the body, with scaling, urticaria, papules, vesicles and sometimes secondary infection, with resulting boils and adenitis.  Constitutional effects may endure for weeks or months.  A fatal case was recorded in which a woman

[1] *Brit. J. Derm. and Syph.*, 1940, **52**, 155, and 1948, **60**, 184.

had suffered rapid local and general symptoms soon after the application of the dye to the eyelids and eyebrows. In other patients the symptoms of systemic poisoning have developed so gradually that for long the dye has not been suspected. Causeless giddiness, " gastric influenza," dyspepsia or tachycardia have often been complained of by elderly men, but it is unlikely that the physician will associate such symptoms with the use of a dye unless he notices that the beard or moustache are uncommonly dark. A hairdresser, who had often applied the dye without protecting his hands, came near death ; on ceasing his work, he began at once to recover.

False hair and furs which have been dyed with paraphenylenediamine can cause dermatitis. In the winter of 1922 and the spring of 1923 there was an outbreak of a curious form of inflammation of the skin of the cheeks, neck and chin. About 1,000 such cases were reported at the time and very soon the cause was traced to wearing cheap fur collars of beaver coney. In all the furs there was detected the presence of a member of the paraphenylenediamine group of dyes. Dr. Alan Parson's report on the outbreak of dermatitis occasioned by the wearing of furs in 1922 and 1923 was published by the Ministry of Health in 1924. A notable feature in these cases was the latent period ; before dermatitis set in, the majority of the patients had worn the furs for six to eight weeks. In some cases it appeared that a greasy skin, in others that moisture, as from rain or the breath, was the exciting cause. The presence of the aniline dye was definitely discovered to be the main cause of the 1,000 cases of dermatitis.

The report contains information about the methods of dyeing furs, which provides useful comparison with the methods of hair dyeing with the same drug. When paraphenylenediamine is treated with an oxidizing agent, several chemical bodies are formed : quinone diimide first, then Bandrowski's base ; the further changes are obscure. Hydrogen peroxide is the oxidizing agent usually employed ; in the trade this is known as a " mordant," because it causes the dye to " bite " into the hair or fur. The skin irritant is apparently due to the presence of incompletely oxidized intermediate products, such as quinone diimide. Bandrowski's base— known by hairdressers as " the para "—may not be, but probably is inert. In the dangerous furs of 1922-3 there were found in some cases the intermediate products of the dye, also metaphenylenediamine and paraphenylenediamine. With defective oxidation, during the process of dyeing, one of the irritant products formed is soluble. Hence the importance of thorough washing after the use of the dye, in order to remove the soluble irritant. When oxidation has been incomplete, and the washing process has been scamped, dangerous toxic effects can occur in many people.

Variations in the amount of the oxidizing agent determine the shade of the dye. With oxidation the colour becomes darker, and this chemical effect had its parallel in the fact that the lighter shades of fur caused the more severe forms of dermatitis. When the dyeing technique is thorough, oxidation is complete and none of the intermediate irritating products are left in the fur. There must have been many thousands of women wearing the beaver coney furs so fashionable in 1923, therefore a comparatively small number of persons appear to be injuriously affected by the dye. Sometimes the skin of the individual who uses the dye may remain normal, but members of the household become sensitized. H. W. Barber and others have seen sensitization of this type in the husbands of women who themselves had remained unaffected by the use of this hair dye.

John Ingram of Leeds found that only a few of the workers in the industries connected with the dyeing of fabrics ever suffered from dermatitis. Moreover, this dermatitis only developed after some years of work. Therefore it appeared that the dermatitis was due to an acquired sensitiveness, on the part of the individual, to contact with the chemicals used in his daily work. To establish this point Ingram [1] carried out experiments on 1,000 volunteers and found that approximately 4 per cent. of normal individuals show a natural idiosyncrasy towards the phenylenediamines. This figure agrees with that quoted from the French hair-dye expert (p. 278). Ingram's research led him to conclude that hair-dye and fur-dye dermatitis were in the nature of an allergic skin reaction. It is of interest that the reactions obtained in the 1,000 volunteers occurred at varying periods of time. Some developed trouble at once ; others after a week or fourteen days, and a few after as long as eighteen and twenty-four days. Recently the dermatitis of a worker in fur was found to be due to traces of bichromate of potash which had been used in the dyeing process, and not to the paraphenylenediamine. [2]

*Tests* for the presence of paraphenylenediamine can be made. If the bottle containing a hair dye is a clear solution which darkens on the addition of an equal quantity of hydrogen peroxide, the presence of paraphenylenediamine may be suspected. Pour dilute acetic acid on a stick which has been dipped in this solution. If paraphenylenediamine

[1] JOHN INGRAM, " Dye Dermatitis in Relation to Idiosyncrasy," *Brit. J. Derm.* 1932, **44**, 422.

[2] C. E. HERCUS, *Lancet*, 1935, **1**, 985.

is present, the stick becomes bright red ; on the addition of ferric chloride it becomes violet.

*Treatment.* The treatment of paraphenylenediamine dermatitis is along the general lines of any acute skin disease. In mild cases wash off any excess of dye, rinse with hydrogen peroxide solution, then soothe with boracic acid solution and simple calamine lotion, in order to subdue the pain, swelling and irritation. In severe cases the hair may have to be cut off. The patient must be confined to bed and the face and scalp bathed frequently with cooling lotions ; sodium thiosulphate 1 in 4 appears to give most relief. This can be followed by a lotion of calamine with a drachm to the ounce of liquor plumbi subacet. dil. It is of importance to use the best calamine, which contains no gritty powder. The absence of glycerine and the roughness of the powder during World War II rendered useless the time-honoured soothing properties of calamine lotion. We were then obliged to employ substitutes such as zinc oxide with castor or arachis oil, equal parts. The bowels must act freely and the diet in serious cases should be a fever diet, water and fruit juice for a few days. Look for the presence of albuminuria and treat if present. The dye must never again be used by those who have once shown susceptibility to it.

Sometimes it is necessary to remove a dye from the hair, on account of irregular diffusion of the tinting, unsuccessful colouring, or injury to the hair or scalp. In this case experimental tests should be tried on a lock of hair cut off the head ; it is dangerous to try the decolorizing agents directly on the scalp. Sodium thiosulphate in 5 per cent. solution, acidulated with 2 per cent. strong sulphuric acid, is a decolorizer which can be used in the case of metallic dyes. The most effective decolorizer is hydrogen peroxide used with ammonia. Redgrove recommends the proportion of 1 part of 0·800 ammonia to 20 to 30 parts of 20 vols. strength of hydrogen peroxide ; this method is useful for the coal tar product series dyes. Lest the hair be made brittle, this should be followed by the rubbing in of oil. Weak oxalic acid, not over 4 per cent., is used to remove dyes containing iron. The decolorizing process usually takes a quarter of an hour. It is scarcely necessary to state that this delicate process must be left to hairdressers who are accustomed to carry it out.

Hairdressers find that certain dyes are difficult to apply to hair which has been permanently waved. The henna-reng dye is difficult to apply even on normal hair, but it is harmless, gives a fine range of colours from red to black, and can be used with permanently waved hair. After the use of metallic dyes, it is difficult to give the hair a permanent wave ;

hence the difficulty of using the henna rasticks dye when so many women to-day have permanently waved hair. Henna and camomile are excellent dyes for fair and brown hair ; for grey hair they are not so effective.

Which, if any, dye is harmless ? The perfect dye leaves the hair uninjured, is not poisonous to the individual, and does not cause local dermatitis. Some dyes are harmless, but none possess the three qualifications which can pass the claim to perfection.

Most vegetable dyes are harmless, because non-toxic. Pyrogallol, a vegetable dye, is the exception to the rule. Henna reng comes nearest to the ideal dye, being harmless, and of plant origin. But henna alone merely produces a red colour, and Western Europe has not learned to combine it with the indigo dye advantageously. " Henna rasticks " produce fine brown shades, but as above-mentioned, it is not available as a dye for permanently waved hair. Certain high-class chemists make up various preparations of vegetable dyes which may be used by women at home without danger. In this way henna powder may be applied to dark hair in order to produce reddish tints. Some shampoo powders contain also a small proportion of both camomile and henna ; such " shampoos " can be used on hair of all shades. One of my patients retains much of her youthful appearance because, after her originally golden hair had become grey, she began to use a henna powder diluted in water and brushed over her hair. After trial of varying proportions, she discovered the precise amount of powder and water which best suited her appearance. Another patient, a young woman, by using a camomile shampoo, has rendered her mouse-brown hair vivid with golden high lights.

Other non-poisonous dyes are hydrogen peroxide, potassium permanganate, dyes made from carbon (e.g. some form of kohl) and iron. Dyes which have poisonous properties are, in order of harmfulness : paraphenylenediamine, lead, silver, copper and pyrogallol. With the exception of lead, the toxic properties of the last three dyes are reduced to a minimum if a weak enough solution is made and the dye is applied by an expert. The dye which produces the best range of colouring is unfortunately the most dangerous, the coal tar product. Many hairdressers apparently believe that paraphenylenediamine is dangerous only when the scalp has some abrasion, pimple or skin disease. Many women have repeated to me this statement, so comforting to both operator and client, but unfortunately so far from truth. Most of the lawsuits in connection with hair and fur dyes have been due to the use of this drug. , It is concealed in many of the dyes and restorers with fancy names. Unfortunately, some manufacturers of this dye take on all responsibility, guaranteeing to refund to the hairdresser any financial claims made by clients who have suffered from dermatitis. The bottle may be labelled " dangerous " ; but the client never sees the label. It is not necessarily the unscrupulous, but rather the ignorant and careless hairdresser who makes use of such new variants of the aniline preparations. He feels no anxiety or responsibility ; he uses the preparation lightheartedly, because he knows that in the event of injury to a client all legal and financial expenses will be met by the manufacturer. Having given all these warnings, it is only fair to add that I knew one lady who used a paraphenylenediamine dye for more than twenty years and never suffered any symptom of dermatitis ; her sole objection to its use was the difficulty of finding someone to apply it when she was travelling far from large towns.

# CHAPTER XX

## HIRSUTIES

Hirsuties, or hypertrichosis, is the medical term for the condition of excessive growth of hair on regions of the body where it is natural to have lanugo or downy hair. Patients describe this disorder as " superfluous hair." In a few cases congenital hypertrichosis has been so extreme that the body and face have been covered with hair. Several dermatological text-books publish two well-known illustrations of such hairy subjects. One is a Russian man, with a face so hairy that he resembled a dog ; the other, recorded by Duhring, in 1877, is a woman with a long thick beard. A thick lock of hair is often seen over the spine, associated with spina bifida. Many illustrations of hairy men and women are given by C. H. Danforth in his book on Hair.[1] Moles are frequently covered with strong hairs ; thus an extensive mole may resemble an area covered with fur.

Hirsuties on the face is the cause of much mental distress in women. Many degrees of hypertrichosis are met with, from a few facial hairs to the extensive involvement encountered with Virilism. This condition is described under ætiology (p. 288). Hirsuties of the usual moderate type appears to run in families and to be more common in certain races ; the Jews and Spanish are particularly prone. Soon after the menopause many women develop a moustache, and two tufts of hair on each side of the chin. When hypertrichosis occurs in young women, beginning about puberty or early womanhood, the condition, when marked, may have really tragic consequences. The amount of unhappiness which is caused by hirsuties on the face of girls and women is known only to the physicians whom the sufferers consult. The character of many of these women is adversely affected ; their mental outlook is often abnormal. Elderly women who have had the blemish from youth will confide to the physician their wish that some young niece similarly affected would come for treatment, but the presence of the hairs cannot be mentioned to the younger woman. Although you point out that the relative must be aware of the excessive hair on her face, and that she must also see that her aunt has had the hairs successfully removed, the older woman will usually reply that she never speaks of the hairs to her niece, nor would the niece dare to mention that she had noticed the improvement in the appearance of

[1] " Hair : with Special Reference to Hypertrichosis," American Medical Assoc., Chicago, 1925.

her aunt. Such nineteenth-century reticence can be met with even in these modern days of outspoken realism.

A young girl with a fair and fine moustache may treat the matter lightly if she be otherwise of attractive appearance. But when she has also a coarse skin, she tends to become introspective, to shun society, and to imagine that everybody is speaking about her. Much depends on how the mother and other members of the family treat the young girl who develops hair upon the upper lip, chin, and cheeks. When there is a healthy family atmosphere, no harm may result ; the girl seeks advice, treating the cosmetic blemish as she would any other physical malady. Where the atmosphere is unhealthy, the attention of the sufferer becomes concentrated upon her blemish, and her whole mental horizon is filled with the fact of her excessive hairiness. She becomes depressed, and may even drift into an asylum with melancholia.

*Ætiology.* I have been unable to find any proof of the popular belief that the use of face creams can provoke the growth of hair on the face. Many of the most devoted adherents of face creams show not a trace of hair on their skin. On the other hand, I have seen many women with mild and pronounced degrees of hypertrichosis who have never used any ointment or lotion on their faces. Any cause of local inflammation of the skin (e.g. a wound) may temporarily stimulate the growth of hair in its vicinity. Exposure to wind and sunshine is for this reason often credited with causing hirsuties. Patients have told me that the growth of hair on their legs and arms began with sun and sea bathing,[1] but the worst cases of hypertrichosis in my experience have developed in city women whose lives have been spent in schools, in offices, and underground travelling.

In the majority of patients who consult the dermatologist for a moderate growth of hair on the face there is no trace of ill-health. Transitory hirsuties of face and body has occurred associated with menstrual irregularity, during pregnancy, after pregnancy and with periods of amenorrhœa. Some have lost the hirsuties when they married and became mothers ; others have developed hairiness during successive pregnancies and this has disappeared or diminished in one to six months after the birth of the child. After the menopause many women have a slight growth of facial hair on the upper lip and chin ; various theories have been advanced to explain this common feature, but the endocrine changes discovered have not been constant. The hirsuties is sometimes

---

[1] In spite of a thorough investigation which failed to confirm the popular belief in the hair-stimulating properties of sun and wind. MILDRED TROTTER, *Arch. Derm. and Syph.*, 1923, vii, 93.

due to sensitivity of the adrenal cortex to the ovarian hormone.[1] Hirsuties, a transitory increase of seborrhœa, loss of hair on the vertex and temporo-frontal areas, sometimes even acne may develop about this time of life, probably due to increase of the male androgen. About puberty the increased activity of the pituitary sometimes causes temporary excessive production of the adrenogen hormone in the young girl, with accompanying acne, seborrhœa and a hirsuties which is not progressive. The average patients are normal young women, without menstrual abnormality ; they marry and have children ; they declare they feel quite strong. Brocq wrote much on this subject and states that most of his patients were healthy young women.[2] It is my impression that progress of hirsuties has sometimes been arrested by treatment of dyspepsia and constipation. Nasopharyngeal catarrh is so common in these patients that I have wondered whether the proximity of the pituitary gland has led to its dysfunction and hence to adrenal cortex stimulation.

During the past twenty years profound research has been carried out on the inter-relationship of the various endocrine glands. It is not possible in a book of this size to give more than a brief summary of the endocrine factors which are associated with hypertrichosis. Every day fresh experiments and reports are published which either confirm or seem to contradict the conclusions formed by other laboratory workers. Mild degrees of hirsuties have been referred to above. The dermatologist may not see many of the severe types, but should be able to recognize the outstanding features of the diseases which can be appropriately sent on to the surgeon or physician for adequate treatment. The chief causes are hyperactivity, with or without a tumour, of the adrenal cortex, of the pituitary gland, ovary or testis, a pineal tumour, anorexia nervosa, vitamin deficiency and a hereditary tendency to hairiness.

The most common of the serious causes is that known as the *Adrenogenital syndrome*. Clinically, this condition is known by the fact that there is generalized hypertrichosis associated with a definite group of signs—obesity, cutaneous striæ, delayed or absent menstruation and virilism. Most often the patient is a female. When the disease starts in early life there has been prenatal influence which leads to pseudo-hermaphroditism or doubtful sex : the clitoris is enlarged, the ovaries may be normal, so that the patient has a feminine appearance, or she may be masculine in type. Other members of the family are often affected. When the malady begins before puberty, there is precocious sexual

[1] *Journ. Clin. Endocrinology*, 1949, **9**, 795.
[2] *Ann. de derm. et syph.*, 1897, 3<sup>me</sup> Sér., **8**, 825, 1010, 1077.

development. When at puberty, the endocrine imbalance may cause delayed or absent menstruation and transitory hirsutism. When it starts soon after puberty or in adult life, other features assume importance : hirsuties of masculine distribution (on face, trunk, especially the lower abdomen, the breasts, chest, shoulders, arms and legs), amenorrhœa, involution of the breasts, enlargement of the clitoris, red and purple striæ on the abdomen, thighs, and buttocks, and considerable or even very great obesity, chiefly of the face, neck, buttocks, thighs, shoulders, breasts, but leaving slim the forearms and legs. In some cases the bodily outline assumes a more masculine aspect, with slim hips, broad shoulders and strong muscles. In others the patient develops even more masculine characters, such as a deep voice, loss of hair on the vertex and temporofrontal regions—the so-called Virilism—and changes of the personality, even amounting to homosexualism. It is accepted that the above described adreno-genital syndrome is due to hyperactivity of the adrenal cortex. Apparently this may be associated with simple hyperplasia, with single or multiple adenomata, or there may be only one growth which later tends to become malignant. Cancer of the adrenal cortex usually leads to the same condition ; it should be suspected when one sees a rapid development of the adreno-genital syndrome, especially in older women.

A somewhat similar group of signs was first described by Cushing. They constitute an entity known as *Cushing's Syndrome*. All stages of transition between these two maladies are encountered. Cushing's original cases had a lesion in the pituitary gland, a basophil adenoma in the anterior lobe, and secondary involvement of the adrenal cortex. It is now believed that even in Cushing's syndrome the original trouble sometimes begins in the adrenal cortex and that the pituitary change follows. There is still much discussion on the pathology of the condition. The patient is usually undersized ; has obesity of face, neck and trunk, but slim extremities ; purplish striæ on the abdomen are present, the skin is dry, often hyperpigmented. The problem is even more involved. The famous " bearded women " of Achard and Thiers had severe facial hypertrichosis (with beards, whiskers and moustaches resembling those of very hairy men), menstrual defects, hypertension and glycosuria, together with obesity as in Cushing's syndrome. Although some of the Achard-Thiers cases had a degree of adreno-genital signs in earlier life, Leonard Simpson suggests that they should be placed amongst the cases of marked post-menopausal virilism.

Another pituitary lesion, the eosinophil adenoma of the anterior pituitary, is associated with *Acromegaly*. During the stage of hyperactivity there is thickening of the hair of the scalp, face and body ; in the later phases of the disease, the hair falls out at the same time as asthenia, pigmentation and apathy set in. The diagnostic features of this malady are the enlargement of the face, hands and feet, and the gradual encroachment of the bony changes. Sufferers with tumour of the *pineal gland* show hirsuties, with profuse pubic hair; the condition is very rare and usually occurs in boys. The hirsuties of *Anorexia Nervosa* is of a downy type, affecting the face, arms and trunk; on the face there may also be some coarser hairs. This strange malady is found chiefly in young women; it is associated with amenorrhœa and is supposed to be due to a psychic trauma acting through the pituitary and the hypothalamus. *Vitamin deficiency* can cause hirsuties. The dietetic errors probably act by bringing about endocrine changes of the pituitary and adrenal glands. Thus, during the potato famine in Ireland long lanugo hair grew on the face and whole body. A man of sixty-one had three gastrectomies. After the second he developed lanugo long hair over the body and thick hair on the scalp which had been bald twenty-eight years.[1]

*Diagnosis.* The diagnosis can often be made from the clinical appearance alone. In less obvious cases X-ray examination aids, as with tumours of the adrenal or the pituitary glands. A negative report does not rule out the presence of hyperplasia or tumour, but a positive report may provide invaluable assistance. A shadow above the kidney suggests adrenal trouble; an enlarged sella turcica points to involvement of the pituitary, as in acromegaly, or with tumour or hyperplasia. With virilism it is important to decide whether the endocrine derangement lies in the adrenal or the pituitary. Examination of the urine sometimes gives guidance; with an increased androgen secretion, hyperplasia of the adrenal may be deduced. The increased activity of the adrenal cortex causes a rise of the 17-ketosteroid excretion from the daily normal of 2·5 to 12·5 mg. to 21 to 40, or in the case of a tumour, even to 100 mg. This excretion is also raised in Cushing's syndrome and in cancer of the adrenal cortex. Associated symptoms are discussed above, under Ætiology.[2] Urinary examination may also reveal, from the excretion of pregnandiol, that even with apparently normal menstruation, ovulation may be absent.[3] In idiopathic hirsuties the ketosteroid excretion levels measured weekly during complete menstrual cycles show maximum excretion at the time of ovulation; in normal women the excretion is more constant.[4]

[1] *Proc. Roy. Soc. Med.*, (1951), **41**, 155.
[2] " Endocrine Man," L. R. Broster, Heinemann, 1945.
[3] RAYMOND GREENE, " Androgen and pregnandiol excretion in hypertrichosis," *Lancet*, 1940, **ii**, 486, and *Brit. Med. J.*, 1940, **ii**, 561.
[4] *Journ. Clin. Endocrinology*, 1949, **9**, 795.

*Prognosis.* Apart from those cases due to endocrine disturbance, the prognosis of hirsuties depends upon the strength and number of the hairs, and the extent of the area affected. Still more does the prognosis depend upon the skill of the physician. Strong hairs are more difficult to destroy than fine hairs. On the other hand, when fine hairs grow extensively over the face, the duration of time necessary for their eradication is apparently interminable. A sitting once a week for one or two years is usually necessary for extensive cases. Brocq estimated that there were 15,000 to 19,000 hairs in a beard ; 1000 to 9000 could be found on the chin, and 700 to 1200 on the upper lip. To remove such a large number of hairs, one by one, is necessarily a time-consuming process, especially with electrolysis. With patience on the part of the operator and the patient, no case is incurable; but both the expense and the endurance required are usually too much for the young woman whose cheeks, upper lip, chin, and neck are covered with hairs. If the requisite patience and money are available, the prognosis of even the thickest growth is excellent as regards the destruction of the hairs. The prognosis of the final cosmetic result also depends upon the skill of the operator and the possession of appropriate apparatus. After over forty years' extensive experience, I have become cautious of promising a perfect result in the case of an upper lip covered thickly with fine hair. No matter how carefully the treatment of the upper lip is carried out, when a large number of hairs have been destroyed, there is seen, after a variable length of time, a fine white atrophy, or at least a depression, of the tissues. Hence, in the case of the upper lip, it is inadvisable to remove all the hairs with electrolysis, except when these are few and wide apart. On the chin, cheeks, or neck, on the contrary (after the initial reaction to the removal of the hair), even after the passage of many years, no depression or scar develops ; the skin looks as normal as if no operative procedure had been performed. I have seen patients after ten and twenty-five years, and hence can speak with confidence.

*Treatment.* (*a*) *General.* From the facts described in the paragraph on ætiology, it is clear that the management of endocrine therapy may be a complicated process, demanding expert medical and surgical care. Disappointing results followed inhibitory X-ray dosage of the adrenal gland. Surgery has had striking success in cases of virilism due to adrenal tumour ; complete restoration to health has followed removal of these growths.[1] The hypertrichosis vanishes with the other signs, but returns in the event of metastases or regrowth of a malignant tumour. With pituitary growths, X-ray has aided many cases and surgery has had some

---

[1] R. L. BROSTER, *Lancet,* 1934, i, 830.

remarkable results. With arrhenoblastoma, surgery succeeds, but the recovery is more gradual than with adrenal and pituitary lesions. Œstrin therapy is not so promising as was at first anticipated. Large doses are required to bring about hairfall, and on discontinuing the dosage the hairs return ; [1] moreover, the menstrual rhythm may be disturbed and miscarriage brought on. Courses of strong doses have had success ; [2] lest the pituitary might be affected, I have not ventured to prescribe such. Œstrin therapy may be tried when there is definite evidence of ovarian deficiency, as at the menopause, and in young women with the male type of baldness. On the other hand, when their hirsuties is due to excess of male hormone, œstrin therapy may fail. Some report benefit from rubbing in ointments containing œstrin, and also from intradermal injections ; of these I have little experience. One patient who used an ointment with œstrin reported that the hairs fell off her thighs and legs, but soon returned.

(b) *Local treatment* consists in the removal of the hairs at skin level, or in destruction of the root. There is a choice of many local methods. These may be briefly passed in review : Destruction of the hair papilla with a needle attached to the negative pole of the galvanic current, usually described as " electrolysis," remains the most popular and is probably still the most widely employed method. Diathermy, usually described as electro-coagulation, in skilled hands gives excellent results. Details of these two chief electrical methods are discussed later (see p. 295). Destruction of the hair roots was carried out by means of X-ray even before Sabouraud's introduction of the pastille method of measuring X-ray dosage. The after-results were in many cases disastrous. Soon after the pastille came into use in 1905, Sabouraud and Noiré published a method of hair destruction by X-ray which they believed to be safe. A pastille dose was given once in four weeks, filtered through a half millimetre of aluminium for four or five doses. The hairs were destroyed, and for a varying period of time the skin appeared to be unaffected. But as time passed, in some cases only after an interval of years, fine atrophy and telangiectases developed on the area of skin which had been exposed to the rays. I treated a number of patients with axillary perspiration by this method between 1910 and 1914. The hairs came out and in many cases telangiectases and atrophy developed after intervals of two to ten years. One lady, whose forearm I treated for excessive hairiness in 1916, began to show telangiectases only fifteen years later. From time to time reports are published

[1] A. D. PETERS, *Brit. J. Derm.*, 1934, **46**, 283.
[2] R. LEYTON, *Med. Press and Circular*, 1949, **1**, 44.

of far more serious forms of delayed X-ray reactions. On account of the possibility of late reactions, X-ray and radium cannot be recommended as safe means for bringing about the destruction of hairs. This was the considered opinion of the dermatologists of twenty years ago. Nevertheless, some modern X-ray workers, who do not use gas-filled tubes, are again attempting to find a dose which will epilate and yet have no after-effects upon the skin. With modern tubes pigmentation soon follows an erythema dose ; this did not occur with gas-filled tubes. Until fifteen years and more have passed the results of these doses cannot be known. Andrews has had some success with radon implanted in the follicles. Dr. Hernaman-Johnson [1] advocates one epilation dose of X-ray, followed three weeks later by friction twice a day with smooth pumice stone. The friction should be continued for a few minutes, " against the grain " of the hair, morning and evening, for several months ; then only once a day.

For a time *thallium acetate* offered hope to sufferers. Some years ago mysterious ointments, said to be procurable only from Paris, could be purchased for a guinea a box, and the clients were promised a slow but certain cure if these were conscientiously applied to the affected areas every day for several months. Some electrotherapeutic enthusiasts tried ionization with thallium acetate, and in a small percentage of cases success was claimed. Cases have been recorded in whom, after such treatment, the hairs on the scalp fell out instead of those on the area of ionization. Therefore I tested this method with excessive caution, in several patients, without success. However, Sabouraud claimed some good results. After twenty years of trial, he found that success could be obtained in certain cases, provided that his rules were strictly adhered to. He advised : acétate acide de thallium, 0.30–0.60 ctgm. ; oxyde de zinc, 0.2 gm. ; vaseline blanche, 30 gm. Every evening a little of this ointment, not larger than a pea, was gently rubbed in. Owing to the fact that the drug is dangerous, he emphasized the fact that it was of the utmost importance not to use more than this amount. For three months no result was visible, but if the patient persevered the hairs diminished in size, colour and thickness. After eighteen months the patient noticed improvement in the appearance of the region which had been treated. Patients must be seriously warned of the dangers of thallium ; if more than the prescribed minute quantity of this ointment is used, paralysis may develop as well as a total loss of hair. Experiments have been suggested with thallium by mouth and short X-ray exposures.

The use of a stiff *wax* is successful in some cases, especially with downy

[1] *Brit. Med. J.*, 1933, 1, 121.

hairs. The composition consists of white wax and resin, usually in the proportion of 1 in 4 or 5 ; the two are melted together in turpentine, then allowed to harden into a plaster or a stick. When using them, the plaster or the blunt end of the stick is softened with heat ; then when cooled sufficiently to cause no painful sensation, it is drawn along in the direction of the hairs, and pressed on to the affected region. When cool and hardened, it is rapidly torn off, against the direction of the hair, bringing away the hairs by the roots. When fine hairs have their roots situated very superficially, it is possible that the hair bulbs and papillæ are brought away adhering to the wax composition. Many of the hairs of average size undoubtedly return in a month ; they have fine pointed tips instead of the coarse bristly regrowth after shaving or a depilatory. Yet some observant women have expressed to me their conviction that the regular use of the wax brought about a decrease in the number of fine hairs of the moustache. I was able to follow the result of regular wax epilation in a young woman in the late twenties. After careful experiment she became expert in applying it ; the rate of hair growth on the upper lip certainly diminished. She found she could postpone using the wax for gradually lengthening intervals of time ; eventually she had only to use it every six weeks. Her upper lip had a normal smooth skin. Madame Lilian Grant sent me these notes from Paris concerning her experience with wax. A woman of 43 had so thick a beard that she was obliged to shave twice a day. Madame Grant had to pull the wax with force three times before she could remove all the hairs ; blood oozed from many of the follicles. Six weeks later the hairs had not returned. Some months passed before the hairs began to reappear, at first thin and downy. Another remarkable case was that of a man ; after a forcible treatment with wax the hairs did not show signs of recurrence for a month ; then about 20 per cent. were still absent, apparently those from the follicles which had oozed blood after the treatment.

Other popular methods of dealing with superfluous hairs are : the *pumice stone* and the *depilatory*. Both remove the hair shaft at the skin-level ; the roots remain, the hairs grow again in a few days, and with harsh free ends. With the pumice stone method, the hairs are first cut level with the skin. Then the part is well lathered with soap and water, and a fine pumice stone is gently rubbed over the area every day. After the first cutting of the hair, the daily use of the pumice stone prevents them appearing above the skin. But they may coarsen, and in brunettes, after a few years, a shadow is seen, as in a dark shaven man.

The depilatory is supplied either in the form of fluid or powder. Depilatories form the basis of all the glowing advertisements which are cut out and posted to the physician by anxious patients. So ingenious is the wording of these notices that the public are easily deluded into crediting their seductive tales. A favourite myth is that of the dying Indian who, in gratitude for some benefit received, confided to the advertiser the secret drug employed by women of the East for the removal of their hairs. This romance has been embroidered with variations as long as I can remember; permanent removal is always promised. The credulous patients, who always believe that their doctor is prejudiced, often seek the personal advice of the unscrupulous inventor of the tale. They return completely convinced of his or her sincerity and unselfish interest in their case, and proceed to try the miracle-working drug. However, after trial of the expensive bottle, they soon learn their error, for after a few weeks the removed hairs blossom again. Depilatories vary slightly in composition. All contain barium sulphide with zinc oxide or other inactive ingredient. The usual proportion is barium sulphide, 2 to 4 drachms, and zinc oxide and starch to the ounce. This powder must be kept in a tightly corked bottle. The powder is mixed with water till it has the consistence of a thick cream. The unpleasant odour of rotten eggs is given off with the formation of sulphide of hydrogen. With a wooden spatula the paste is spread thickly over the part and left on for two to four minutes, just until the skin begins to burn or tingle. Then the paste is rapidly scraped off, and the hairs come away with it. If the paste is left on too long, the skin becomes red and irritated. The part is then thoroughly bathed, in order to remove all traces of depilatory, and a soothing ointment or lotion is applied. On an average, the process has to be repeated once a fortnight.

When the hairs are very fine and dark, *bleaching* with hydrogen peroxide can be used. At least 20 vol. strength is necessary, and the bottle should be tightly corked and kept in a dark place. Not only does this agent make dark hairs turn to a pale gold, but it also discourages the growth. If ammonia is applied first, it renders the hair shafts brittle, so that many fall off.[1] The peroxide, or peroxide with ammonia, should be applied with a wad of wool once or twice a week. One must avoid irritating the skin by letting the fluid fall and remain on it. Some object that a pale gold moustache on a brunette skin is even more noticeable in bright sunlight than the normal dark hair.

The *safety razor* is often advised for wide-spread cases; girls have

[1] The following method has been recommended. Pour a little of 10 or 20 vol. hydrogen peroxide into a saucer, together with a piece of litmus paper, which will turn red. Add liq. ammon. fort. drop by drop, until the litmus paper turns blue. This can be applied to the hair at first daily, then at gradually increasing intervals until sufficiently bleached.

to be carefully taught how to use it. *Plucking out* strong hairs should never be advised. In some cases shaving and plucking cause local irritation and may lead to hypertrophy of the hair bulb. Certainly, after years of daily plucking out, inflamed papules, even pustules are often seen. Should the patient decide at some future date to have electrical treatment, the operation is rendered much more lengthy and difficult if the hairs have been previously pulled out. In such cases, the papilla seems to alter from its natural position, and the roots of the pulled hairs are frequently seen to be bent or twisted (Fig. 59).

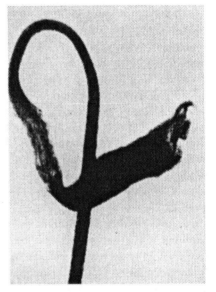

Pulled hairs often return several times before being finally killed by the galvanic or the diathermy current, because the bent or twisted root makes it impossible for the operator to judge the position of the papilla from the angle of the hair. An elderly intelligent woman stated that when hair appeared after the menopause she pulled the hairs out daily, and about her sixtieth year found that new hairs ceased to appear. This effect *does not occur in young people.*

*Surgical Methods.* In severe cases æsthetic surgery has been successful. Flaps of skin are dissected back, and the hair roots pulled out from underneath. The

Fig. 59.—This hair had returned after one removal by electrolysis and came out in this curled position. It had been plucked out frequently before patient was first seen. Microphotograph Mag. × 52.

strips of skin are restored to their position ; the remaining scar is negligible.[1]

*Electrical Methods in the Treatment of Hypertrichosis.* No physician should consider that the work of epilation in cases of hypertrichosis is beneath the dignity of the medical profession. In simple cases few cures bring more happiness to the patient ; in severe cases the physician has the satisfaction of knowing that the patient has been saved from the disastrous future of a mental breakdown.

[1] MOURE, Un moyen chirurgical d'épilation, *Bulletin de la Soc. de Derm. et Syph.*, Nov. 10, 1927.

The work must be carried out in a good light. When sunlight is poor, a strong lamp should be arranged to shine on the area which is receiving treatment. The operator must work in a comfortable position ; without adequate support the arm cannot be kept steady enough for such delicate work. The patient should recline on a couch or low chair with a head rest and adjustable back. The pain caused by the electrical method of hair destruction varies with the individual. Some people are extraordinarily sensitive to electricity ; they demand a local anæsthetic, and describe their sensations as " agonizing." Certainly in some patients the facial contortions and the writhings of the limbs make all treatment impossible without a local anæsthetic. However, I have known only two patients who gave up treatment on account of the pain caused by the removal of hairs. By far the majority of women suffer so little that the eyes and the endurance of the physician are exhausted long before the patient desires the end of the treatment. Indeed, so little do many women object to the current that they carry on interesting discussions during the sittings ; then time flies for both patient and operator. For those who are hyper-sensitive, I order a cocaine solution to be dabbed on frequently during the half-hour preceding treatment. One per cent. phenol or menthol may be added with advantage. For those who suffer severely, Bonain's solution (p. 252) can be applied. There are objections to its use. It makes the area sticky and so glistening that the follicle openings are hidden. Again, as its reaction continues the part becomes blanched,[1] and does not react with the normal degree of erythema round each hair as it is removed ; hence one is tempted to treat many hairs close together, and too many at one sitting. For very sensitive patients the part can be anæsthetized by driving in novocaine, or other anæsthetic, with the positive pole of the galvanic current. This takes time, and few people will pay the extra fee for the extra time required. Because of the swelling and disfigurement entailed by their use, hypodermic injections cannot be recommended. Patients who come for epilation often tell the physician that they have some social engagement soon after the sitting, and cannot allow any disfigurement more than absolutely necessary. In any case, a hypodermic injection affects only a limited area ; when removing hairs, a good operator aims at the destruction of hairs far apart, and extends the treatment over as wide an area as possible. On the Continent and in America some have destroyed 10, 20 or even more hairs at once. Twenty-four needles attached to one pole are placed in the follicles, and a

---

[1] I am now convinced that if work is continued after the part is blanched with adrenalin, healing is delayed and the mark is long in departing.

current of two to ten milliamperes is run for three to five minutes or longer.[1]

It is important to choose a suitable needle for performing epilation. It must have a fine shaft, otherwise the skin would be marked at the surface opening of the follicle. This type of needle is difficult to obtain. Many years ago several preparations were vaunted which were used to insulate the metal above the point. The objection to the use of such insulation was its bulkiness. When the insulating material is fine enough for the purpose it usually requires constant renewal. This prolongs the time of the treatment and renders it wearisome, as well as expensive. However, Bordier recommended a needle with permanent insulation down to near the point, and until Austria was annexed such needles could be obtained from Vienna.

So far as the composition of the needle is concerned, some praise iridium and platinum, but steel is excellent, inexpensive, and firm. A straight needle answers most purposes, but for use in certain positions, such as under the chin, it is easier to work with a needle which is bent at an angle. As the hair root is larger than the follicle, the point of the needle should be larger than the shaft. MacIntosh, of Chicago, makes a needle with a bulb-shaped point which is suitable for this work. For the average case, however, No. 12 ordinary steel sewing needle is fine enough not to mark the skin, and its point can be made blunt by rubbing it over emery paper. The rounded or blunted needle end has another advantage. A needle with a blunt end glides along the follicle and reaches the root more readily because a degree of resistance is felt if the blunt end is pushed against the side of the follicle. When passing the needle with a sharp point down by the side of the hair, the operator often pierces the wall of the follicle, and is quite unaware that this has occurred. This fact probably accounts for many of the failures to destroy a hair root which has been attacked with quite an adequate current.

Several forms of needle holders can be used. Those with an interrupter button are not in favour with expert workers. The usual holder has an insulated handle : at one end is the screw for the wire attaching it to the battery or other source of current ; at the other end is the metal attachment for clasping the needle. The important fact often forgotten by the novice is that the steel needle must be connected only to the negative pole. At the negative pole the body fluids are so acted upon by the passage of the current that there is dilatation of the blood-vessels, softening of the tissues and exudation round the needle. The reaction near the needle is alkaline, because hydrogen and soda are attracted to

[1] M. A. Morton, *Arch. Phys. Therapy*, 1940, **21**, 678.

the region of the negative pole. The steel of the needle is not affected by the chemical reaction of this pole. If by mischance the steel needle is attached to the positive pole, when the current flows, iron is driven off from the needle into the tissues ; a deposit of iron forms, and thus an indelible black stain is left in the track of the needle. When a faulty attachment of the needle to the positive pole has been made, the operator's attention is first struck by the fact that there is an absence of swelling and exudation or " frothing " at the surface of the follicle. Then to his horror he notices the black stain of the iron deposit and finds the needle adhering so strongly to the tissues that its withdrawal is difficult. When an operator frequently makes this mistake of forgetting to make certain that his needle is attached to the negative pole, he should use platinum instead of steel needles ; or, better still, give up doing such work.

Some operators use the galvanic current from a switchboard, or other apparatus connected with the main. It is safer to use a simple galvanic battery with dry Léclanché cells. The number of cells required for the production of sufficient current depends upon their age. With new cells and a large indifferent pad well moistened in slightly salted water, one, two, or four cells may be sufficient for good work. The patient should not be already connected to the positive pole when the operator inserts the needle into the follicle. If the patient is attached to the positive pole, and the cells are already in circuit, so much pain is felt when the needle is inserted that the operator has no freedom to move the needle about whilst endeavouring to find the angle of the follicle. It is better for the operator to begin the delicate process of tracing the path of the follicle and the position of the hair root, and only when this is successfully gauged should the current be put into action by connecting the patient to the positive pole. By this method the operator has adequate time to judge the depth of the follicle by feeling that the needle encounters resistance to its further passage. This indicates that the needle point has reached the hair root or papilla. When this is accomplished, the patient places her hands on a pad or into a bowl of water attached to the positive pole. The current can then be slowly turned on by an assistant, or, as is equally convenient, by the left hand of the operator. However, it is easier to turn on the current first, then tell the patient to place her hand with very gentle pressure on the pad ; the milliamperage gradually increases when the patient makes firmer pressure on the positive pad with one, then both hands. Many unqualified workers bind the patient securely to the indifferent (positive) pole. It is preferable to give the patient the power to make or break the contact at the positive pole. The positive pole can be an electrode held by the insulated handle ; when the operator indicates to the patient that the needle is in position, she starts the flow of the current by pressing the moist electrode on the opposite palm. By this method the patient can control the amount of current. It gives her confidence to know that she can influence the quantity of the current, increasing it by stronger and decreasing it by gentler pressure on the pad ; and that she can even arrest it entirely by breaking her contact with the indifferent pole. This method has a further advantage : both the make and the break of a current are less painful at the positive than at the negative pole. The galvanic current can be administered practically without pain if the current is turned on and off very slowly. The patient herself can arrange this by modifying the pressure on to, and then off the indifferent pad.

The amount of current advisable depends on the thickness of the hair, also upon the sensations of the patient. Every meter varies ; only experience can tell us what current is best for an individual apparatus. With my battery, a fine hair is usually loosened in five to eight seconds with $\frac{1}{2}$ to $\frac{3}{4}$ milliampere. Fine hairs on the upper lip may be removed with scarcely any redness and no frothing. A thick hair may require the passage of $1\frac{1}{2}$ to 2 milliamperes for twenty seconds or even longer. With the larger current the area around the needle reddens and swells, and a fine froth is visible. L. Brocq advised 1 to $2\frac{1}{2}$ m.a. for 4 to 5 seconds for fine hairs ; in sensitive cases only $\frac{1}{2}$ m.a. could be employed and 1 to 2 minutes might be necessary to loosen the hair. For thick hairs he frequently used 4 to 5 m.a. for 5 to 15 seconds.

Hairs lying close together should not be dealt with at the same sitting. A good rule is to leave between the hairs selected for treatment a space as large as the erythematous swelling which occurs round each needle puncture. After the removal of the needle, if the hair root has been effectively destroyed, the hair comes away on the gentlest traction with the epilation forceps. If the hair is not loosened enough to come away without being pulled, it should be left in position and dealt with at a future sitting. It is unwise to enter a follicle more than once at a sitting, lest excessive reaction and consequent scar tissue follow. A sitting should not be longer than half an hour. The amount of redness and swelling after a sitting varies greatly with the patient, as well as with the amount of current used. After the removal of many thick, strong hairs, there is naturally more reaction than with the same number of fine hairs, because it has been necessary to use a greater current. To reduce swelling I have found it useful to apply the positive pole over the treated area, and pass a small current for a few minutes. The anode (positive) pole has a decongestive action which is useful if not continued too long, in which case it is apt to be followed by undue dryness, even scaling of the skin.[1]

After each sitting the patient should bathe the part with water as hot as can be borne, and this can be carried out several times a day for five or ten minutes. There is little marking visible for a day or two ; then the tiny scabs at the mouth of each follicle become more conspicuous. Subsequent treatment should not be given till these scabs have dropped off. For patients who say that their skin is slow to heal, calcium lactate has often proved useful, in ten-grain doses three times a day for three days. It is advisable that the patient should return in a fortnight or three weeks, so that if any hairs show signs of returning, they can be dealt with whilst still short and fine. Some believe that the galvanic current stimulates the growth of hair in the vicinity. Certainly, in a proportion of cases, the downy hairs in the neighbourhood appear to become stronger, but with the majority of patients this does not occur.

In 1932 Bordier of Lyons introduced diathermy for removing hairs. He used steel needles, 0·2 mm. diameter, and insulated to their point. He described their destruction in a fraction of a second ; he stated that the diathermy spark causes less pain than the galvanic current, and that hairs cannot return. The patient is placed on a condenser couch, which acts as one pole ; the needle is attached to the other pole, and used with a current so fine that it cannot be measured. Dr. Turrell used the indirect method—the patient lay on the couch, which was attached to one pole ; the other pole she held with a double handle. The operator passed a fine metal, such as a primus pricker, down the follicle, turned on the current with a foot switch, and let it act for a second or two. I tried four different machines, with the monopolar and the bipolar method, with the condenser, the coagulation and the sparking (desication or fulguration) methods. In my experience most women find the current quite as painful as the galvanic current, and the remarks made about the return of the hairs after electrolysis are also true of those treated with diathermy. Diathermy is a more rapid method than electrolysis ; over a hundred hairs can be dealt with at a sitting. A proportion of the thick hairs return, even when they have come out without pulling, and with the follicle sheath attached to the shaft. Coarse hairs, which have often been plucked out by the patient, may grow again several times, even after apparently successful destruction. Indeed, in the case of " bad healers," the swelling was so marked that I had to abandon the first

---

[1] Every case differs ; no guide can be given as to the amount of current suitable to hasten healing. After the first treatment one learns which current is best for the individual.

piece of apparatus I had had built for the purpose. Some prefer the long wave spark-gap type to the short wave diathermy. The individual apparatus must be studied in order to obtain the best result. Machines vary ; even the same apparatus conveys different sensations according to the condition of the spark gap, whether the surfaces are rough or smooth, closer or farther apart. About 1937 Madame le Docteur Noel of Paris evolved a portable apparatus constructed on the short wave spark-gap current lines, which destroyed the hairs with less pain, less reaction and less time than any other with which I was then acquainted. Many machines have since been put on the market. The treatment is based upon what was called in Europe diathermy coagulation, and in America electrocoagulation. The needles I preferred were made of fine tungsten, insulated to near the tip ; I had them sent regularly from Vienna till war stopped that source of supply. The only disadvantage was the recurring necessity to replace the insulation. With use it wore off ; then it was difficult to prevent the coagulation of the spark continuing from the base of the follicle to the skin surface.

Several articles describing in detail the methods employed by dermatologists in America may be consulted by those who are interested in this subject.[1]

I prefer to work comparatively slowly, giving one to four seconds to each hair. With a foot switch it is easy to give pauses during the time the current is passing ; this method of brief periods of pain renders the treatment more endurable to sensitive patients. There is no frothing, less swelling and a smaller scab formation than with electrolysis. The novice tends to give too long an application of the spark, so that the surface of the follicle shows a white mark of coagulated skin. As over 100 hairs can be treated at a sitting one is tempted to remove too many ; this leads to slower healing than after electrolysis, and may cause anxiety as to the possibility of permanent marking. This, however, except in the case of the upper lip, is more rare than the appearance of the reaction would lead one to expect. If a smaller number of hairs are removed at one time, and these are adequately spaced out, no mark is left. I have seen a few cases develop pigmentation when the depressions have taken long to disappear. This pigmentation appeared in the summer months and eventually vanished with the dark days of winter.

One is continually being asked questions about the return and the complete destruction of the hairs. If a hair offers the slightest resistance

[1] E.g. CHARLES LERNER, New York State Journ. Med., 1942, 42, 879. He advises a current of 60–75 m.a. applied intermittently for three seconds at a time.

to traction after diathermy or electrolysis, and comes out with a jerk, a fresh hair will be seen growing from the follicle in about a fortnight. In many books the statement is made that at least one out of every ten hairs extracted will grow in again. This is somewhat inexact. In my experience, after careful epilation, there are found three types of hairs which return rapidly, even after apparently successful destruction. Hairs which have been plucked out often, and have therefore developed a twisted root, usually show signs of returning in ten to fifteen days, according to the depth of their follicles. Hair with thick roots, and the strong hairs which grow in soft moles, often return as rapidly. Sometimes the hairs will not return for six months. If one gives a strong enough current one can be certain of destroying the root at the first treatment, but one takes the risk of leaving a scar on the skin at the follicle mouth. In the long run it is safer for the patient that the operator should work more slowly. Coarse hairs may return three or four times, but they are finer at every regrowth, and eventually the papilla is so effectively destroyed that the hair cannot grow again.

Once I had the opportunity of treating two sisters with a similar growth of hair on the chin, on the same days, and by the same method. A year later both were examined : one had less than a dozen hairs which had returned, the other had three times as many, and in addition, many downy hairs in the vicinity had grown longer. This development of downy hairs occurs in some cases, but not in others. I noticed it more frequently after electrolysis than after diathermy. It is a curious fact that the few hairs remaining after a course of treatment often grow very long and sometimes curly. Many of these have an unusually superficial and small root ; this fact suggests that the previous treatment had destroyed the more deeply set original papilla.

# FORMULÆ

Soft soap ⎫ equal parts of each.
Industrial spirit ⎭

Sapo mollis ⎫
Oleum cadinum ⎬ equal parts.
Alcohol ⎭

Lavender or other scent may be added.

Liquor potassae, 1 in 6. Rub in carefully with a pledget of cotton-wool and wash off.

Oil of cade, 5% in sweet almond oil ; leave on for 24 hours.

Formulæ with a basis of vaseline and lanolin are retained, but more pleasant preparations are the emulsifying bases. These are more readily washed off the scalp, and enable deeper penetration of remedial agents. In the future, no doubt, many of the drugs applied to the scalp will be incorporated in creams made up with cetyl alcohol, lanette wax, and other similar bases.

Two emulsifying bases are given in the B.P. 1948 :

### UNG. EMULSIFICANS.

| | | |
|---|---|---|
| Emuls. Wax | . . . . | 300 gr. |
| White soft paraffin | . . . | 500 gr. |
| Liquid paraffin | . . . . | 200 gr. |

### UNG. EMULSIFICANS AQUOSUM.

| | | |
|---|---|---|
| Emulsifying ointment | . . . | 300 gr. |
| Chlorocresol . | . . . . | 1 gr. |
| Distilled Water | . . . . | 699 gr. |

The latter is comparable with that of Valogel or H.E.B. simple.

### OINTMENTS FOR USE IN CHRONIC SCALY CONDITIONS

(i) Liq. picis carbonis . . . . . . . m. 30
Hydrarg. ammon. . . . . . . . gr. 5
Paraff. moll. alb. . . . . . . ad 1 oz.
        Salicylic acid gr. 5–15 may be added.

(ii) Liq. picis carbonis . . . . . . . m. 120
Adipis . . . . . . . . . 1 oz.

(iii) Ungt. acid. salicyl.
Ungt. sulph. equal parts.
        (i.e. approximately 10% of each active ingredient).

(iv) Acid. salicyl. . . . . . . . . gr. 15
Liq. picis carb. . . . . . . . m. 15
Ungt. sulph. . . . . . . . ad 1 oz.

### LOTIONS FOR USE WITH PITYRIASIS

(i) Hyd. perchlor. . . . . . . . gr. ½–1½
Liq. carb. deterg. . . . . . . . m. 20–35
Ol. amygd. dulc. . . . . . . . m. 2–30
Industrial spirit . . . . . . . . ½ oz.
Aq. dest. . . . . . . . ad 1 oz.

Modify the proportions of oil and spirit according to the individual hair. Where expense is not considered, use Rectified spirit or alcohol.

(ii) Oil of cedar

Oil of cade (deodorized) . . . . .   āā 2½ drachms

Acetone . . . . . . . . . 1 oz.

Alcohol (95%) . . . . . . ad 4 oz.

(iii) Acid. salicyl. . . . . . . . . gr. 10–20

Ol. ricini . . . . . . . . . m. 2–12

Spt. rosmarini . . . . . . . . m. 60

Industrial spt. . . . . . . . m. 30 to 180

Aq. dest. . . . . . . . ad 1 oz.

### FOR PSORIASIS (Sabouraud)

| | | |
|---|---|---|
| Huile de cade désodorisée . . 10 gm. | Deodorised oil of cade . . | 100 parts |
| Lanoline . . . . . . . 10 gm. | Lanoline . . . . . . | 100 parts |
| Vaseline . . . . . . . 10 gm. | Vaseline . . . . . . | 100 parts |
| Acide pyrogallique . . . . 1 gm. | Acid pyrogallic . . . . | 10 parts |
| Turpeth minéral . . . . 1 gm. | Mercury oxysulphate . . | 10 parts |

and

| | | |
|---|---|---|
| Goudron de houille lavé neutre . 6 gm. | Prepared coal tar (B.P. 1932) | 120 parts |
| Lanoline . . . . . . . 6 gm. | Lanoline . . . . . . | 120 parts |
| Vaseline . . . . . . . 20 gm. | Vaseline . . . . . . | 400 parts |
| Précipité blanc . . . . . 1 gm. | Ammoniated mercury . . | 20 parts |
| Résorcine . . . . . . 1 gm. | Resorcin . . . . . . | 20 parts |

Clear off in the morning with

Alcohol à 90%.

Acetone.

Aq. dest. . . . . . . . . . of each equal parts

*For use on the scalp alone.*

Hydrarg. ammon. . . . . . . . gr. 20–30

Acid. salicyl. . . . . . . . . gr. 20 to 40

Cremor frigid., vaselin. or other base . . ad 1 oz.

The stronger ointments used for pityriasis, especially those with a high percentage of tar and sulphur, are also useful for psoriasis.

### SABOURAUD'S DIRECTIONS FOR THE USE OF CARBON BISULPHIDE WITH SEBORRHŒA OLEOSA

Carbon bisulphide, first introduced for this purpose by Sabouraud, has certain disadvantages. The bottle must be kept well corked, because the vapour is poisonous and it has a foul odour which penetrates far. The fluid is highly inflammable, therefore cannot be employed when there is an open flame in the room. The windows should be kept open when it is being used, and the application should be made close to the open window. The fluid produces a very stinging sensation on the scalp, but this quickly passes. Sabouraud gave the following directions. Every night a few drops are shaken on to a swab of cotton-wool and the scalp is vigorously rubbed for thirty seconds. The eyes should be kept closed all the time ; a long breath should be taken before, and held during the time of application. In the morning the scalp is washed and vigorous friction is given with a brush. With women, the hair must be divided into partings. A piece of cotton-wool is well moistened with the solutions given below. To each parting is given two seconds' friction. A fine deposit of sulphur is removed by the daily washing, an essential part of the course of treatment. When there is little hair, the cotton-wool swab should be well soaked with a lotion consisting of two parts of carbon disulphide with one part of carbon tetrachloride, and applied rapidly over the scalp. Thus the spirit penetrates into the mouths of the follicles ; as the fluid evaporates rapidly from the surface of the scalp this method causes no inconvenience.  Later, tonic lotions with nitrate of potassium or pilocarpine are ordered.

| | | | | | | |
|---|---|---|---|---|---|---|
| Sulfure de carbone | . . . | 120 ctc. | Carbon disulphide | . . . | 180 parts |
| Soufre octaédrique | . . . | 10 gr. | Precipitated sulphur | . . | 15 parts |
| Tétrachlor. de carbone | . . | 180 ctc. | Carbon tetrachloride | . . | 270 parts |
| Verveine et bergamotte āā 1 gm. | | | Oil of verbena | . . . . | 1·5 parts |
| | | (Sabouraud.) | Oil of bergamot. | . . . | 1·5 parts |

### For Greasy Hair

Acid. tannic. . . . . . . . gr. 40
Spirit of lavender . . . . . . . 3 oz.
Spirit of rosemary . . . . . . . 3 oz.

Talc ⎫
Zinci oxidi. ⎪
P. lycopod. ⎬equal parts.
P. iris ⎪
Sulph. praecip. ⎭

Mix with care (Sabouraud).

### Stimulant Lotions for Alopecia Areata

(i) Liq. ammon. fort. . . . . . . ⎫
Tincture of cantharidin . . . . . ⎬āā 1 drachm
Glycerine . . . . . . . ⎭
Distilled water . . . . . . ad 1 oz.
(Erasmus Wilson.)

(ii) Tincture of cantharidin
Dilute acetic acid . . . . . . āā 1½ drachms
Glycerine . . . . . . . . 1 drachm
Indust. spirit . . . . . . . . 2 drachms
Distilled water . . . . . . ad 1 oz.

(iii) Tincture of cantharidin and glycerine, equal parts.

(iv) Oil of cade, oil of turpentine, olive oil, equal parts.     (Stelwagon.)

(v) Pure phenol or phenol diluted 1 in 3 parts spirit.

(vi) Tincture of cantharidin, tincture of capsicum, oil of turpentine, equal parts. The effect of this mixture requires to be watched and it should be diluted with almond or olive oil as indicated.     (Stelwagon.)

(vii) Phenol . . . . . . . . . 4 parts
Tincture of cantharidin . . . . . . 16 parts
Pure castor oil. . . . . . . . 16 parts
Rectified spirit to 128 parts.     (Hyde and Montgomery.)

(viii) Fluid extract of jaborandi boiled down to half its volume and added to 4 parts of lard.     (Jackson.)

### Hair Stimulant Lotions

(i) Potass. nitrat. . . . . . . . 2 parts
Aq. dest. . . . . . . . . 60 parts
Alcohol (90%) . . . . . . . . 500 parts

(ii) Phenol . . . . . . . . . m. 8
Tinct. cantharidin . . . . . . . m. 30
Indust. spirit . . . . . . . . ½ oz.
Bay rum . . . . . . . . 2 drachms
Aq. dest. . . . . . . . . ad 1 oz.

(iii) Tinct. jaborandi . . . . . . . ½ drachm
Tinct. cantharidin . . . . . . . 1 drachm
Acid. salicyl. . . . . . . . . gr. 10
Glycerine . . . . . . . . ½ drachm
Industrial spirit . . . . . . ad 1 oz.

Sir Norman Walker recommended

(iv) Acidi lactici . . . . . . . . 1·5
Ol. ricini. . . . . . . . . 2·5
Spt. myrciae (Bay rum) . . . . . ad 100

Apply twice a day, at first cautiously, then with more and more vigour as the scalp gets used to it.

### SOOTHING, FOR ITCHING

(i) Menthol . . . . . . . . . gr. 4
Industrial spirit . . . . . . . 2 drachms
Ac. acetici. dil. . . . . . . . ½ oz.
Aq. dest. . . . . . . . ad 1 oz.

(ii) Menthol . . . . . . . . . ½% in Ol. ricini.

(iii) Liq. plumb. subacet. dil. . . . . . . 1 drachm
Liq. carb. deterg. . . . . . . . m. 25
Aq. dest. . . . . . . . ad 1 oz.

(iv) Liq. carb. deterg. . . . . . . . 1 in 10

(v) Phenol . . . . . . . . . 1 in 40

Printed in the United Kingdom
by Lightning Source UK Ltd.
119499UK00001BA/3

9 781406 799200